AF675571

# Advancements in Heart Failure Research

# Advancements in Heart Failure Research

Guest Editors

**Tzu-Hurng Cheng**
**Ju-Chi Liu**

MDPI

Basel • Beijing • Wuhan • Barcelona • Belgrade • Novi Sad • Cluj • Manchester

*Guest Editors*

Tzu-Hurng Cheng
Department of Biochemistry
China Medical University
Taichung City
Taiwan

Ju-Chi Liu
Department of Internal Medicine
Taipei Medical University
Taipei
Taiwan

*Editorial Office*
MDPI AG
Grosspeteranlage 5
4052 Basel, Switzerland

This is a reprint of the Special Issue, published open access by the journal *Life* (ISSN 2075-1729), freely accessible at: https://www.mdpi.com/journal/life/special_issues/V2ODCQFXF0.

For citation purposes, cite each article independently as indicated on the article page online and as indicated below:

Lastname, A.A.; Lastname, B.B. Article Title. *Journal Name* **Year**, *Volume Number*, Page Range.

**ISBN 978-3-7258-6488-1 (Hbk)**
**ISBN 978-3-7258-6489-8 (PDF)**
**https://doi.org/10.3390/books978-3-7258-6489-8**

© 2026 by the authors. Articles in this book are Open Access and distributed under the Creative Commons Attribution (CC BY) license. The book as a whole is distributed by MDPI under the terms and conditions of the Creative Commons Attribution-NonCommercial-NoDerivs (CC BY-NC-ND) license (https://creativecommons.org/licenses/by-nc-nd/4.0/).

# Contents

# About the Editors

**Tzu-Hurng Cheng**

Tzu-Hurng Cheng is a professor at China Medical University, affiliated with the Department of Biochemistry. His research focuses on cardiovascular pharmacology, molecular mechanisms of heart failure, and translational therapeutics. He has served as a mentor and editorial advisor for numerous biomedical publications and is actively engaged in promoting ethical publishing and global scientific communication.

**Ju-Chi Liu**

Ju-Chi Liu is a professor in the Department of Internal Medicine at Taipei Medical University and serves as Superintendent of Taipei Medical University Shuang Ho Hospital. His research interests include atherosclerosis, hypertension, and molecular biology of the cardiovascular system. He has led numerous projects in translational cardiovascular medicine and has received multiple awards from the Taiwan Society of Cardiology and international congresses. He is actively engaged in advancing precision medicine approaches for cardiovascular disease and mentoring the next generation of clinicians and researchers.

# Preface

Heart failure remains a leading cause of morbidity and mortality worldwide, necessitating continued exploration of its complex pathophysiology and treatment. This Reprint gathers cutting-edge studies that address emerging molecular targets, novel biomarkers, and therapeutic approaches, including pharmacological and non-pharmacological interventions. The contributions reflect the collaborative efforts of international researchers dedicated to advancing cardiovascular health. This volume is intended for clinicians, researchers, and students seeking to deepen their understanding of heart failure and its evolving management.

**Tzu-Hurng Cheng and Ju-Chi Liu**
*Guest Editors*

*life*

MDPI

*Editorial*

# Bridging Gaps in Heart Failure Science: Toward a More Integrated Future

**Ju-Chi Liu [1,2] and Tzu-Hurng Cheng [3,*]**

1 Division of Cardiology, Department of Internal Medicine, Shuang Ho Hospital, Ministry of Health and Welfare, Taipei Medical University, New Taipei City 23561, Taiwan; liumdcv@tmu.edu.tw
2 Division of Cardiology, Department of Internal Medicine, School of Medicine, College of Medicine, Taipei Medical University, Taipei City 11002, Taiwan
3 Department of Biochemistry, School of Medicine, College of Medicine, China Medical University, Taichung City 404328, Taiwan
* Correspondence: thcheng@mail.cmu.edu.tw

Heart failure remains a significant global health concern, profoundly impacting the lives of millions and placing considerable strain on healthcare systems worldwide. Although diagnostic and therapeutic advancements have led to measurable improvements in patient care, substantial challenges persist—underscoring the need for ongoing research and innovation. Emerging strategies such as remote monitoring, telemedicine, and biomarker-based risk stratification have contributed to better clinical outcomes. Yet, critical gaps remain in our understanding of disease progression, treatment responsiveness, and the development of individualized care pathways. This Special Issue brings together a series of contemporary investigations that address key dimensions of heart failure management. Remote monitoring and telemedicine are reshaping the delivery of care [1]. For instance, the ECOST-CRT study demonstrated that remote monitoring in patients undergoing cardiac resynchronization therapy significantly reduced hospitalizations and enhanced device performance [2]. Broader implementation of digital health programs has further highlighted their potential to reduce acute care utilization and improve access to timely interventions [3]. Biomarker-guided approaches are increasingly informing prognosis and therapeutic decisions. Immune markers—such as the neutrophil-to-lymphocyte ratio and the lymphocyte-to-white blood cell count ratio—have emerged as valuable predictors of adverse outcomes [4,5]. Investigations into innate immunity have also shed light on the inflammatory mechanisms that contribute to heart failure pathophysiology [6]. Pharmacological innovations continue to expand treatment options, particularly for patients with preserved ejection fraction and metabolic comorbidities. The FINEARTS-HF trial demonstrated the efficacy of finerenone in slowing disease progression among heart failure patients with obesity [7]. Similarly, findings from the SUMMIT trial underscored tirzepatide's potential to alleviate circulatory overload and mitigate end-organ damage in obese individuals [8,9]. Lifestyle interventions remain foundational to heart failure management [10]. Dietary modifications have shown promise in lowering lipoprotein(a) levels and reducing overall cardiometabolic risk [11,12]. Remote cardiac rehabilitation programs have emerged as viable alternatives, especially in resource-limited settings, offering improvements in functional capacity and patient adherence [13]. These findings reinforce the importance of integrating behavioral strategies into comprehensive care models. Taken together, the studies featured in this Special Issue advocate for a multidimensional approach to heart failure management—one that combines technological innovation, biomarker refinement, pharmacological advancement, and lifestyle optimization. Nonetheless, several challenges remain, including the need for personalized treatment strategies, enhanced adherence to care protocols, and deeper insights into the immunometabolic underpinnings of heart failure. By synthesizing current evidence and highlighting emerging methodologies, this Special Issue calls for sustained interdisciplinary collaboration and innovation. Bridging existing knowledge gaps and embracing novel approaches will be essential in developing more effective, patient-centered solutions for this pervasive and complex condition.

Recent advances in heart failure management have been driven by technological innovation, refined risk assessment tools, and evolving dietary strategies. These developments have not only enhanced clinical outcomes but also underscored the importance of a cohesive, multidisciplinary approach to this complex condition. Telemedicine and remote monitoring have markedly transformed patient care, enabling earlier detection of physiological changes and facilitating timely clinical interventions. Evidence supports the effectiveness of remote monitoring in improving outcomes by allowing prompt responses to shifts in patient status [1]. Telemedicine, in particular, has broadened access to care for underserved populations, reinforcing the value of sustained investment in digital health infrastructure. Progress in risk stratification has paved the way for more individualized treatment strategies. Biomarkers such as the lymphocyte-to-white blood cell count ratio have emerged as reliable prognostic indicators in heart failure, aiding clinicians in identifying patients at elevated risk [5]. Integrating these markers into routine practice enhances clinical decision-making and supports more targeted therapeutic interventions. Dietary patterns have also gained recognition as key contributors to heart failure prevention and management. The cardioprotective effects of the Mediterranean and DASH diets are well established, particularly in their capacity to reduce heart failure risk [14]. Additionally, dietary modifications that influence lipoprotein(a) levels offer valuable insights into the role of nutrition in cardiovascular care [12]. These findings highlight the critical interplay between diet and heart health, warranting further investigation into nutrition-based strategies as essential components of comprehensive heart failure management.

This Special Issue explores recent advances in heart failure research, emphasizing innovations in diagnostic methodologies, therapeutic strategies, and emerging treatment modalities. Among the promising developments are novel metrics such as the Lipid Accumulation Product (LAP) and Cardiometabolic Index (CMI), which have demonstrated utility in identifying metabolic syndrome risk—even in populations traditionally considered low-risk, such as athletes. These tools offer a pathway toward more personalized and preventive diagnostic frameworks [10]. Nutritional interventions continue to gain prominence in heart failure management. Findings from the OmniHeart trial and related studies underscore the critical link between dietary patterns and metabolic health. In particular, the modulation of lipoprotein(a) levels through tailored nutrition strategies highlights the importance of individualized, lifestyle-based assessments in cardiovascular risk reduction [11,15]. Cardioprotective agents such as grape seed extract (GSE) and L-carnitine have shown encouraging results in mitigating doxorubicin-induced cardiotoxicity. These compounds have been associated with improved histopathological outcomes and preserved cardiac function [16]. GSE's antioxidant properties appear especially beneficial when combined with exercise, offering synergistic protection against oxidative stress [17,18]. Likewise, L-carnitine has demonstrated potential in pediatric oncology settings, where it may serve as a supportive adjunct during high-dose anthracycline therapy [19]. These findings merit further clinical validation through well-designed trials. Antidiabetic therapies—including sodium–glucose cotransporter-2 (SGLT2) inhibitors and glucagon-like peptide-1 receptor agonists (GLP-1 RAs)—are increasingly recognized for their perioperative benefits in cardiac surgery [20]. Liraglutide, a GLP-1 RA, has shown promise in preclinical models by restoring cardiac function following isoprenaline-induced myocardial injury and preventing heart failure progression [21]. Agents such as empagliflozin and semaglutide have also demonstrated efficacy in enhancing myocardial autophagy and reducing inflammation [22,23]. SGLT2 inhibitors contribute to left ventricular remodeling and reduce perioperative complications [24,25], while semaglutide has been shown to improve cardiac function in patients with heart failure and preserved ejection fraction [25]. Electrocardiographic (ECG) parameters are gaining traction as predictive tools in cardiac resynchronization therapy (CRT). Tanasescu's work illustrates how specific ECG features correlate with Kansas City Cardiomyopathy Questionnaire (KCCQ) scores, offering a refined approach to CRT optimization [26]. Advances in pacing techniques, including left bundle branch and biventricular pacing, continue to enhance cardiac performance and underscore the value of integrating ECG insights into individualized care planning [27]. Despite these strides, translating research into routine clinical practice remains a challenge. While the Mediterranean and DASH diets have been associated with reduced heart failure risk, long-term, population-based studies evaluating their sustained impact are still limited [14]. The role of diet in influencing cardiovascular mortality and metabolic health among older adults also warrants further investigation across diverse cohorts [28]. Similarly, the safety and efficacy of cardioprotective agents such as GSE and L-carnitine require confirmation through large-scale clinical trials [16–19]. Implementation barriers—including disparities in healthcare resources, variability in clinical practice, and infrastructural limitations—continue to impede the adoption of evidence-based strategies. Although telemedicine and remote monitoring have expanded access to care in underserved regions, issues such as patient adherence and data reliability remain unresolved [1,29]. Nevertheless, large-scale remote monitoring initiatives have successfully reduced hospitalization rates, reinforcing the need for robust integration and operational frameworks [3]. Looking ahead, interdisciplinary collaboration among cardiologists, nutritionists, pharmacologists, and data scientists will be essential to bridge existing knowledge gaps, harmonize care standards, and accelerate global progress in heart failure research.

Heart failure research continues to evolve, propelled by technological innovation and methodological refinement. This Special Issue highlights emerging trends that are poised to shape the future of heart failure management, with particular emphasis on artificial intelligence (AI), nutritional strategies, biomarker development, and personalized care. AI is rapidly transforming cardiovascular medicine by enhancing predictive modeling and supporting data-driven clinical decisions. AI-enabled platforms have shown efficacy in detecting early complications and stratifying risk through the analysis of large-scale datasets, particularly in remote monitoring contexts [1]. Telemedicine and AI-integrated patient monitoring systems are improving adherence and reducing hospitalizations by capturing symptom-specific biometric data [3,28]. In parallel, AI applications in cardiac rehabilitation and chronic disease management are expanding access to care and optimizing resource utilization [13]. When embedded into clinical workflows, these technologies facilitate timely and informed decision-making, marking a paradigm shift in heart failure care delivery. Despite these advances, several areas warrant further investigation. Long-term adherence to heart-healthy dietary patterns—such as the Mediterranean and DASH diets—and their cumulative effects on heart failure prevention and progression remain underexplored [14]. Given the influence of nutrition on cardiometabolic risk factors, including lipoprotein(a), developing strategies to improve dietary compliance may contribute meaningfully to risk reduction [11,12]. Tailored interventions for older adults and individuals with multiple comorbidities are also essential, as population-specific studies can inform more nuanced clinical approaches [27]. Progress in biomarker research offers promising avenues for refining patient stratification and monitoring. Ratios such as lymphocyte-to-white blood cell count and neutrophil-to-lymphocyte have emerged as potential prognostic indicators [4,5].

Further exploration of immune-related mechanisms—particularly those involving innate and adaptive immunity—may reveal novel therapeutic targets and deepen our understanding of heart failure pathophysiology [6,29]. Addressing the complexities of heart failure with preserved ejection fraction remains a critical priority [30]. This subset of patients presents unique diagnostic and therapeutic challenges, underscoring the need for continued research and innovation.

This Special Issue brings together a diverse collection of studies that advance the field of heart failure research, highlighting the value of a multidisciplinary approach to diagnosis, treatment, and prevention. Through the exploration of emerging innovations—including telemedicine, biomarker refinement, and dietary interventions—these contributions address critical gaps in current knowledge and lay the groundwork for future inquiry. The findings presented offer meaningful insights with the potential to reshape heart failure management and improve patient outcomes. Collectively, they reflect the transformative capacity of collaborative research to drive progress and inform clinical practice. As the burden of heart failure continues to grow, sustained engagement among researchers, clinicians, and policymakers will be essential to overcoming persistent challenges. By building on these advancements, the global scientific community moves closer to a more comprehensive understanding of heart failure and its multifaceted treatment landscape. This Special Issue serves not only as a reflection of current progress but also as a call to action—urging continued innovation and unified efforts in addressing one of the most pervasive conditions in cardiovascular medicine.

**Author Contributions:** J.-C.L. and T.-H.C. contributed to the conceptualization and drafting of the manuscript. J.-C.L. provided critical revisions and insights on heart failure management strategies. T.-H.C. supervised the study, ensured the accuracy of the content, and provided final approval. All authors have read and agreed to the published version of the manuscript.

**Conflicts of Interest:** The authors declare no conflicts of interest.

## Abbreviations

The following abbreviations are used in this manuscript:

| | |
|---|---|
| HF | Heart Failure |
| CRT | Cardiac Resynchronization Therapy |
| ECG | Electrocardiogram |
| KCCQ | Kansas City Cardiomyopathy Questionnaire |
| AI | Artificial Intelligence |
| SGLT2 | Sodium–Glucose Cotransporter-2 |
| GLP-1 RA | Glucagon-Like Peptide-1 Receptor Agonist |
| GSE | Grape Seed Extract |
| LAP | Lipid Accumulation Product |
| CMI | Cardiometabolic Index |
| DASH | Dietary Approaches to Stop Hypertension |
| LVEF | Left Ventricular Ejection Fraction |
| OmniHeart | Optimal Macronutrient Intake Trial for Heart Health |

## References

1. Liu, J.C.; Cheng, C.Y.; Cheng, T.H.; Liu, C.N.; Chen, J.J.; Hao, W.R. Unveiling the Potential: Remote Monitoring and Telemedicine in Shaping the Future of Heart Failure Management. *Life* **2024**, *14*, 936. [CrossRef]
2. Klein, C.; Kouakam, C.; Lazarus, A.; de Groote, P.; Bauters, C.; Marijon, E.; Mouquet, F.; Degand, B.; Guyomar, Y.; Mansourati, J.; et al. Comprehensive vs. standard remote monitoring of cardiac resynchronization devices in heart failure patients: Results of the ECOST-CRT study. *EP Eur.* **2024**, *26*, euae233. [CrossRef]

3. Margosian, S.; Crossley, H.; Riggs, M.; Henkemeyer, T.; Fisher, M.; Patel, A.; Ellimoottil, C.; Jenq, G.; Toma, G. Impact of a Large-Scale Remote Patient Monitoring Program on Hospitalization Reduction. *Telemed. J. E-Health* **2025**, *31*, 914–918. [CrossRef] [PubMed]
4. Huang, Y.; Huang, L.H.; Su, H.B.; Li, Y.X.; Chen, H.; Li, J.H.; Yang, L.H.; Su, Q.; Gui, C. Prognostic potential of neutrophil-to-lymphocyte ratio for adverse outcomes in dilated cardiomyopathy: A retrospective cohort study. *Sci. Rep.* **2025**, *15*, 10339. [CrossRef]
5. Charach, L.; Spitzer, A.; Zusmanovitch, L.; Charach, G. Lymphocyte to White Blood Cell Count Ratio an Independent Risk Factor for Heart Failure. *Life* **2024**, *14*, 1266. [CrossRef]
6. Wang, J.; Zhang, Z.; Sun, Y.; Yu, B.; Wang, Y.; Lu, Y.; Yu, J.; Wang, N.; Xia, F. Association of innate versus specific immunity with heart failure incidence: A prospective study. *Heart* **2024**, *111*, 76–82. [CrossRef]
7. Butt, J.H.; Henderson, A.D.; Jhund, P.S.; Claggett, B.L.; Desai, A.S.; Lay-Flurrie, J.; Viswanathan, P.; Lage, A.; Scheerer, M.F.; Lam, C.S.P.; et al. Finerenone, Obesity, and Heart Failure with Mildly Reduced/Preserved Ejection Fraction: Prespecified Analysis of FINEARTS-HEART FAILURE. *J. Am. Coll. Cardiol.* **2025**, *85*, 140–155. [CrossRef] [PubMed]
8. Packer, M.; Zile, M.R.; Kramer, C.M.; Baum, S.J.; Litwin, S.E.; Menon, V.; Ge, J.; Weerakkody, G.J.; Ou, Y.; Bunck, M.C.; et al. Tirzepatide for Heart Failure with Preserved Ejection Fraction and Obesity. *N. Engl. J. Med.* **2025**, *392*, 427–437. [CrossRef]
9. Borlaug, B.A.; Zile, M.R.; Kramer, C.M.; Baum, S.J.; Hurt, K.; Litwin, S.E.; Murakami, M.; Ou, Y.; Upadhyay, N.; Packer, M. Effects of tirzepatide on circulatory overload and end-organ damage in heart failure with preserved ejection fraction and obesity: A secondary analysis of the SUMMIT trial. *Nat. Med.* **2025**, *31*, 544–551. [CrossRef] [PubMed]
10. Di Gioia, G.; Ferrera, A.; Celeski, M.; Mistrulli, R.; Lemme, E.; Mango, F.; Squeo, M.R.; Pelliccia, A. Lipid Accumulation Product and Cardiometabolic Index as Effective Tools for the Identification of Athletes at Risk for Metabolic Syndrome. *Life* **2024**, *14*, 1452. [CrossRef]
11. Haring, B.; von Ballmoos, M.C.; Appel, L.J.; Sacks, F.M. Healthy dietary interventions and lipoprotein (a) plasma levels: Results from the Omni Heart Trial. *PLoS ONE* **2014**, *9*, e114859. [CrossRef] [PubMed]
12. Stojko, M.; Spychał, A.; Nikel, K.; Kołodziej, R.; Zalejska-Fiolka, J. The Impact of Diet on Lipoprotein(a) Levels. *Life* **2024**, *14*, 1403. [CrossRef]
13. Itoh, H.; Amiya, E.; Jimba, T.; Shimbo, M.; Narita, K.; Taya, M.; Kadokami, T.; Yasu, T.; Oka, H.; Sogawa, M.; et al. Efficacy and safety of remote cardiac rehabilitation in the recovery phase of cardiovascular diseases (RecRCR study): A multicenter, nonrandomized, and interventional trial in Japan. *Int. J. Cardiol. Heart Vasc.* **2024**, *52*, 101421. [CrossRef] [PubMed]
14. Arayici, M.E.; Kilic, M.E.; Yilmaz, M.B. High and Low Adherence to Mediterranean and DASH Diet Patterns and the Risk of Heart Failure: A Meta-Analysis of Observational Studies. *Life* **2025**, *15*, 63. [CrossRef] [PubMed]
15. Law, H.G.; Stanhope, K.L.; Zhang, W.; Myagmarsuren, M.; Jamshed, Z.M.; Khan, M.A.; Bang, H.; Havel, P.J.; Berglund, L.; Enkhmaa, B. Lipoprotein(a) and diet: Consuming sugar-sweetened beverages lowers lipoprotein(a) levels in obese and overweight adults. *J. Lipid Res.* **2024**, *65*, 100588. [CrossRef]
16. Aldayel, T.S.; Kilany, O.E.; El-Hak, H.N.G.; Abdelrazek, H.M.A.; Abdallah, O.; Omar, D.E. Clinicopathological Studies on the Impact of Grape Seed Extract and L-Carnitine as Cardioprotective Agents Against Doxorubicin-Induced Toxicity in Rats. *Life* **2024**, *14*, 1656. [CrossRef]
17. Sergazy, S.; Shulgau, Z.; Fedotovskikh, G.; Chulenbayeva, L.; Nurgozhina, A.; Nurgaziyev, M.; Krivyh, E.; Kamyshanskiy, Y.; Kushugulova, A.; Gulyayev, A.; et al. Cardioprotective effect of grape polyphenol extract against doxorubicin induced cardiotoxicity. *Sci. Rep.* **2020**, *10*, 14720. [CrossRef]
18. Belhadjali, F.; Ghrir, S.; Ksia, F.; Limam, F.; Aouani, E.; Mokni, M. Protective effect of grape seed extract and exercise training on tissues toxicities in doxorubicin-treated healthy rat. *Biomarkers* **2023**, *28*, 544–554. [CrossRef]
19. Lin, C.; Narayan, H.K.; Trovillion, E.; Armenian, S.; Alejandro, L.; Kuo, D.J. Serum Carnitine Concentrations and Cardiac Function in Pediatric, Adolescent and Young Adult Oncology Patients Receiving High-Dose Anthracyclines. *J. Pediatr. Pharmacol. Ther.* **2024**, *29*, 475–481. [CrossRef]
20. Wang, A.; Bitzas, S.; Perez, D.; Schwartz, J.; Zaidi, S.; Oster, J.; Bergese, S.D. Perioperative Considerations of Novel Antidiabetic Agents in Heart Failure Patients Undergoing Cardiac Surgery. *Life* **2025**, *15*, 427. [CrossRef]
21. Bajic, Z.; Sobot, T.; Smitran, A.; Uletilovic, S.; Mandić-Kovačević, N.; Cvjetkovic, T.; Malicevic, U.; Stanetic, B.; Đukanović, Đ.; Maticic, M.; et al. Liraglutide Treatment Restores Cardiac Function After Isoprenaline-Induced Myocardial Injury and Prevents Heart Failure in Rats. *Life* **2025**, *15*, 443. [CrossRef]
22. Endo, S.; Kanamori, H.; Yoshida, A.; Naruse, G.; Komura, S.; Minatoguchi, S.; Watanabe, T.; Kawaguchi, T.; Yamada, Y.; Mikami, A.; et al. Sodium-glucose cotransporter 2 inhibitor empagliflozin enhances autophagy and reverses remodeling in hearts with large, old myocardial infarctions. *Eur. J. Pharmacol.* **2025**, *992*, 177355. [CrossRef]
23. Lin, K.; Wang, A.; Zhai, C.; Zhao, Y.; Hu, H.; Huang, D.; Zhai, Q.; Yan, Y.; Ge, J. Semaglutide protects against diabetes-associated cardiac inflammation via Sirt3-dependent RKIP pathway. *Br. J. Pharmacol.* **2025**, *182*, 1561–1581. [CrossRef]

24. Brekke, H.K.; Holmaas, G.; Astor, M.C.; Steien, E.; Haaverstad, R.; Ghavidel, F.Z.; Farstad, M. Metabolic acidosis in patients with diabetes 2 undergoing cardiac surgery: The impact of SGLT2 inhibitor use: A retrospective cohort study. *Eur. J. Anaesthesiol.* **2025**, *42*, 152–161. [CrossRef]
25. Rosu, A.M.; Tomescu, L.F.; Badea, T.G.; Radu, E.S.; Rosu, A.L.; Brezeanu, L.N.; Tanasescu, M.D.; Isac, S.; Isac, T.; Popa, O.A.; et al. The Relationship Between the Kansas City Cardiomyopathy Questionnaire and Electrocardiographic Parameters in Predicting Outcomes After Cardiac Resynchronization Therapy. *Life* **2024**, *14*, 564. [CrossRef] [PubMed]
26. Diaz, J.C.; Tedrow, U.B.; Duque, M.; Aristizabal, J.; Braunstein, E.D.; Marin, J.; Niño, C.; Bastidas, O.; Lopez Cabanillas, N.; Koplan, B.A.; et al. Left Bundle Branch Pacing vs. Left Ventricular Septal Pacing vs. Biventricular Pacing for Cardiac Resynchronization Therapy. *JACC Clin. Electrophysiol.* **2024**, *10*, 295–305. [CrossRef] [PubMed]
27. Li, S.Y.; Lu, Z.H.; Leung, J.; Su, Y.; Yu, B.; Kwok, T. Dietary patterns modify the association between body mass index and mortality in older adults. *Clin. Nutr.* **2025**, *46*, 20–29. [CrossRef] [PubMed]
28. Mohapatra, S.; Issa, M.; Ivezic, V.; Doherty, R.; Marks, S.; Lan, E.; Chen, S.; Rozett, K.; Cullen, L.; Reynolds, W.; et al. Increasing adherence and collecting symptom-specific biometric signals in remote monitoring of heart failure patients: A randomized controlled trial. *J. Am. Med. Inform. Assoc.* **2025**, *32*, 181–192. [CrossRef]
29. Maeda, D.; Matsue, Y.; Kagiyama, N.; Fujimoto, Y.; Sunayama, T.; Dotare, T.; Nakade, T.; Jujo, K.; Saito, K.; Kamiya, K.; et al. Lymphocyte-to-C-reactive protein ratio and score in patients with heart failure: Nutritional status, physical function, and prognosis. *ESC Heart Fail.* **2024**, *11*, 3723–3731. [CrossRef]
30. Man, D.E.; Motofelea, A.C.; Buda, V.; Velimirovici, D.E.; Bodea, O.; Duda-Seiman, D.M.; Luca, C.T.; Dragan, S.R. Left Atrial Strain in Patients with Chronic Heart Failure with Preserved Ejection Fraction: A Narrative Review. *Life* **2025**, *15*, 313. [CrossRef]


**Disclaimer/Publisher's Note:** The statements, opinions and data contained in all publications are solely those of the individual author(s) and contributor(s) and not of MDPI and/or the editor(s). MDPI and/or the editor(s) disclaim responsibility for any injury to people or property resulting from any ideas, methods, instructions or products referred to in the content.

*life*

MDPI

*Article*

# A Prospective Clinical Study of Ferric Citrate Hydrate for Chronic Heart Failure with Iron Deficiency Anemia

**Akira Sezai [1,*], Hisakuni Sekino [2], Makoto Taoka [1], Kazuaki Obata [2], Sakie Kanno [2] and Masashi Tanaka [1]**

[1] Department of Cardiovascular Surgery, Nihon University School of Medicine, Tokyo 173-8610, Japan; taoka.makoto@nihon-u.ac.jp (M.T.); tanaka.masashi@nihon-u.ac.jp (M.T.)
[2] Sekino Hospital, Tokyo 171-0014, Japan; sekinoh@sekino-hospital.com (H.S.); obatak@sekino-hospital.com (K.O.); s.kanno.mt@gmail.com (S.K.)
* Correspondence: asezai.med@gmail.com; Tel.: +81-3-3972-8111

**Abstract:** Background: The efficacy of intravenous iron preparations for chronic heart failure with iron deficiency has been reported, but the efficacy of oral iron preparations has not been demonstrated. In this study, we conducted a prospective clinical study using ferric citrate hydrate tablets in patients with chronic heart failure complicated by iron deficiency anemia. Methods and Results: A prospective study was conducted using ferric citrate hydrate in patients with chronic heart failure complicated by iron deficiency anemia. The registered patients were divided into two groups: those administered ferric citrate hydrate and those switched from iron sulfate sustained-release to ferric citrate hydrate. The primary endpoint was hemoglobin level. The secondary endpoints included hematocrit, serum iron, saturation, ferritin, and cardiac-, renal-, and hepatic-related biomarkers. A total of 141 patients were enrolled in this study, including 95 patients who were newly administered ferric citrate hydrate and 46 patients who were switched from iron sulfate sustained-release to ferric citrate hydrate. Conclusions: Ferric citrate hydrate significantly increased hemoglobin, serum iron, transferrin saturation (TSAT), and ferritin levels, and decreased atrial natriuretic peptide (ANP), brain natriuretic peptide (BNP), and N-terminal pro-brain natriuretic peptide (NT-proBNP) levels. Ferric citrate hydrate could be continued without side effects such as gastrointestinal symptoms. Improvement in iron metabolism and anemia due to iron supplementation with ferric citrate hydrate led to improvement in heart failure biomarkers.

**Keywords:** iron-deficiency anemia; anemia; heart failure; ferric citrate hydrate; chronic heart failure

## 1. Introduction

The combination of heart failure and anemia is common, with anemia (hemoglobin (Hb) < or = 12.0 g/dL) present in 12% of the 912 patients with chronic heart failure enrolled in the RENAISSANCE trial. For every 1 g/dL higher baseline Hb, a 15.8% reduction in risk of mortality and a 14.2% reduction in risk of death or hospitalization for heart failure were reported. In addition, more severe chronic heart failure was associated with significantly lower Hb levels and was a significant and independent predictor of death or heart failure hospitalization [1]. Reports from Japan indicate that anemia was present in 60% of patients with acute decompensated heart failure [2,3] and in 35% of patients with chronic heart failure (C). In these reports, anemia is also considered an independent prognostic factor for heart failure patients [2,4].

 https://doi.org/10.3390/life15040598

The causes of anemia in heart failure include (1) hemofiltration due to fluid retention, (2) decreased erythropoietin production due to chronic kidney disease, (3) decreased bone marrow hematopoietic function due to inflammatory cytokine activity stimulation, (4) iron deficiency, etc. [5], but there is no established evidence on how to treat anemia. Furthermore, it has also been reported that heart failure patients often have iron deficiency [6,7]. The cause is a disturbance in iron utilization due to hepcidin, which is thought to play an important role in anemia and iron metabolism in heart failure [8,9]. Hepcidin is mainly produced by hepatocytes, and excess hepcidin causes iron deficiency and anemia by inhibiting iron absorption from the intestine and inhibiting the release of iron from macrophage stores [10]. Inflammation is also involved, and it induces hepcidin expression via interleukin-6 [11].

Clinical studies of iron administration for heart failure with iron deficiency are being conducted regardless of whether or not the patient has anemia. There was reported that iron deficiency was found in 62% of 7160 patients diagnosed with chronic heart failure, while anemia, according to WHO criteria, was found in 35% of these patients [12]. Intravenous iron preparations for patients with chronic heart failure have been reported to improve symptoms, increase the distance walked in six minutes, and reduce the number of hospitalizations due to worsening heart failure, regardless of whether the patient has anemia or not [13,14], and intravenous iron preparations are recommended for heart failure with iron deficiency in the European Society of Cardiology guidelines [15]. However, no results have been shown to indicate the effectiveness of oral iron supplements. In the IRONOUT HF study, which was a trial of oral iron preparations, an iron polysaccharide formulation was used, and it was hoped that it would be possible to ingest the most elemental iron of any commercially available oral supplement and that its tolerability profile would help with medication compliance and minimize the risk of subjects being unblinded, but it was not possible to demonstrate efficacy [16]. In addition, most of the clinical research has been on chronic heart failure with iron deficiency, and there has been little clinical research on chronic heart failure with iron deficiency anemia.

In Japan, there are currently five types of oral iron deficiency anemia medication: Ssodium ferrous citrate tablets, ferric fumarate capsules, iron sulfate sustained-release tablets, soluble ferric pyrophosphate syrup, and ferric citrate hydrate tablets. In this study, a prospective clinical study was conducted using ferric citrate hydrate tablets in patients with chronic heart failure complicated by iron deficiency anemia, and the enrolled patients were divided into two groups: those who were newly administered ferric citrate hydrate tablets and those who were switched from iron sulfate sustained-release tablets (Fero-Gradumet Tablets) to ferric citrate hydrate tablets.

## 2. Materials and Methods

### 2.1. Study Protocol

The subjects of this study were patients with chronic heart failure and iron deficiency anemia. The definition of chronic heart failure in this study was cases with a history of heart failure hospitalization and taking two or more standard heart failure medications (angiotensin II receptor blockers (ARBs), angiotensin-converting enzyme (ACE) inhibitors, angiotensin receptor neprilysin inhibitors (ARNIs), mineralocorticoid receptor antagonists (MRAs), beta blockers, diuretics, or inotropic agents). Furthermore, the subjects were limited to patients whose prescriptions, including those for heart failure medications, had remained unchanged for at least 6 months. In this study, we did not specify the left ventricular ejection fraction.

The definition of iron deficiency anemia was an Hb level of less than 11 g/dL for men and less than 10.5 g/dL for women, and a ferritin level of less than 100 ng/mL or a ferritin level of 100 to 299 ng/mL with a TSAT of less than 20%. In addition, patients were defined as having a negative occult blood test and having other types of anemia ruled out by measuring vitamin B12, lactate dehydrogenase (LDH), and haptoglobin. Although this is an open label study, assessors were blinded.

The age range of eligible patients was ≥20 years to <100 years. The exclusion criteria were (1) patients who did not meet the definition of chronic heart failure and iron deficiency anemia specified in the inclusion criteria, (2) patients who were judged by the investigator to be unable to take oral medications properly due to dementia or other reasons, (3) patients with unstable heart failure, (4) pregnant women, and (5) women who were breastfeeding. Finally, patients who were judged by the investigator to be unsuitable for this study were excluded.

Patients were assigned to oral treatment with ferric citrate hydrate (Riona®, 500 mg/once/day after dinner, Torii Pharmaceutical Co., Ltd., Tokyo, Japan). Ferric citrate hydrate is a drug covered by insurance since 2021 to treat iron deficiency anemia. When the Hb level was 13 g/dL or higher after administration of ferric citrate hydrate, the dose was reduced to 250 mg; if the level was still 13 g/dL or higher after that, the drug was discontinued. The extraction and statistical processing of the test data was carried out by a third party not involved in this study. Blood samples were taken in the morning. The iron content of the ferric citrate hydrate tablets used in this study was 124 mg per 500 mg, and that of the iron sulfate sustained-release tablets (Fero-Gradumet®, 105 mg/one time/day, Viatris Inc., Tokyo, Japan) was 105 mg.

The study details were explained to each patient, and informed consent was obtained. The study was approved by the hospital's institutional review board (protocol no. 20210401 and approval on 1 June 2021), and the study was registered with the Hospital Medical Information Network (study ID: UMIN000050436).

The primary endpoint was the Hb level. The secondary endpoints were as follows: New York Heart Association (NYHA) classification; hematocrit (Ht); serum iron; TSAT = (Fe/total iron binding capacity (TIBC)) × 100; ferritin; cardiac-related biomarkers (ANP, BNP, NT-proBNP); renal-related biomarkers (blood urea nitrogen (BUN), creatinine (Cr), estimated glomerular filtration rate (eGFR)); hepatic-related biomarkers (aspartate aminotransferase (AST), alanine aminotransferase (ALT)); oxidized low-density lipoprotein (Ox-LDL); and high-sensitivity C-reactive protein (hs-CRP).

The definition of MACCE in this study included death, ischemic heart disease, cerebrovascular disease, heart failure, and arrhythmia requiring hospitalization for treatment.

All blood samples were measured before administration. ANP, BNP, NT-proBNP, and Ox-LDL were measured at 3 and 6 months after administration, while the other parameters were measured at 1, 3, and 6 months after administration.

Adverse reactions were classified as renal dysfunction (increased Cr by 50%), hepatic dysfunction (increased AST/ALT by ≥50%), and allergic reactions. The attending physician decided the management of the reactions.

### 2.2. Statistical Analysis

Measured values were expressed as the mean standard deviation (SD). A $p$ value of less than 0.05 was considered statistically significant. Each dataset was analyzed using repeated measures ANOVA, and Bonferroni's method was used to adjust for multiple comparisons. NYHA classification data were analyzed using Student's $t$-test. All analyses were performed with SPSS software (SPSS Inc., Chicago, IL, USA, version number: 28.0.0.0, copyright holder: IBM SPSS Statistics). Data aggregation was performed by Sekino Laboratory staff who were not involved in this study, and statistical analysis was supported by Data Seed Inc. (Tokyo, Japan). Data Seed Inc. was not involved in conducting the study.

## 3. Results

A total of 141 patients were enrolled in this study, with 95 patients receiving ferric citrate hydrate for the first time and 46 patients switching from iron sulfate sustained-release tablets to ferric citrate hydrate. Among the newly administered cases, there were seven where the patient had taken iron supplements in the past and was unable to continue taking them due to digestive symptoms.

The baseline characteristics are shown in Table 1. Regarding classifications of heart failure in this study, in the new administration cases, 25% had heart failure with reduced ejection fraction (HFrEF), 21% had heart failure with mildly reduced ejection fraction (HFmrEF), and 54% had heart failure with preserved ejection fraction (HFpEF). In the switching cases, 35% had HFrEF, 19% had HFmrEF, and 46% had HFpEF, so about half of the cases were HFpEF. In terms of age, there were 33 (35%) and 71 (74%) cases of new administration in patients aged 80 and over, and 25 (54%) and 38 (83%) cases of switching in patients aged 80 and over. Regarding CKD, there were 48 cases (51%) of new administration cases with CKD stage G3a or below, 40 cases (42%) with stage G3b or below, and 12 cases (13%) with stage G4 or below. For the switching group, there were 26 cases (57%) with CKD stage G3a or below, 24 cases (52%) with stage G3b or below, and eight cases (17%) with stage G4 or below. There were 77 (81%) in the new treatment group and 11 (24%) in the switching group. Regarding ferritin levels of less than 100 ng/mL, there were 90 (95%) in the new treatment group and 24 (52%) in the switching group.

**Table 1.** Patient characteristics.

| | **Newly Administered Cases** | **Switching Cases** |
|---|---|---|
| Number | 95 | 46 |
| Age (years) | 74.7 ± 1.2 (43–97) | 77.4 ± 1.6 (47–92) |
| Gender (male:female) | 64:31 | 29:17 |
| Duration of Heart Failure (months) | 11.6 ± 3.6 | 14.9 ± 5.7 |
| NYHA classification | 1.87 ± 0.65 | |
| I | 11 | 13 |
| II | 62 | 26 |
| III | 22 | 7 |
| Average | 2.12 ± 0.58 | 1.87 ± 0.65 |
| Classifications of heart failure | | |
| HFrEF | 24 (25%) | 16 (35%) |
| HFmrEF | 20 (21%) | 9 (19%) |
| HFpEF | 51 (54%) | 21 (46%) |
| Causes of heart failure | | |
| Ischemic heart disease | 25 (26%) | 14 (30%) |
| Valve disease | 49 (52%) | 19 (41%) |
| Cardiomyopathy | 4 (4%) | 7 (15%) |
| Arrhythmia | 4 (4%) | 1 (2%) |
| Hypertension | 12 (13%) | 5 (11%) |
| Amyloidosis | 1 (1%) | 0 (0%) |
| Complication | | |
| Hypertension | 58 (61%) | 25 (54%) |
| Diabetes mellitus | 30 (32%) | 20 (43%) |
| Dyslipidemia | 68 (72%) | 35 (76%) |
| Hyperuricemia | 34 (36%) | 21 (46%) |
| CKD (stage G3a>) | 48 (51%) | 26 (57%) |
| CKD (stage G3b>) | 40 (42%) | 24 (52%) |
| CKD (stage G4>) | 12 (13%) | 8 (17%) |

**Table 1.** *Cont.*

| | Newly Administered Cases | Switching Cases |
|---|---|---|
| Obesity | 21 (22%) | 7 (15%) |
| Cerebral infarct | 3 (3%) | 2 (4%) |
| Peripheral atrial disease | 5 (5%) | 4 (9%) |
| Treatment for heart failure | | |
| ACE-I or ARB | 31 (33%) | 11 (24%) |
| ARNI | 39 (41%) | 23 (50%) |
| MRA | 64 (67%) | 30 (65%) |
| Beta-blockers | 77 (81%) | 39 (85%) |
| SGLT2 inhibitor | 33 (35%) | 17 (37%) |
| Ivabradine | 2 (2%) | 2 (4%) |
| Loop diuretics | 40 (42%) | 24 (52%) |
| Tolvaptan | 11 (12%) | 4 (9%) |
| Calcium channel blocker | 31 (33%) | 14 (30%) |
| Digoxin | 3 (3%) | 1 (2%) |
| Pimobendan | 2 (2%) | 2 (4%) |
| HIF-PH inhibitor use | 24 (25%) | 16 (35%) |

NYHA, New York Heart Association; HFrEF, Heart Failure with Reduced Ejection Fraction; HFmrEF, Heart Failure with mildly reduced Ejection Fraction; HFpEF, Heart Failure with preserved Ejection Fraction; CKD, chronic kidney disease; ACE-I, Angiotensin-Converting Enzyme Inhibitor; ARB, Angiotensin II Receptor Blocker; ARNI, Angiotensin Receptor Neprilysin Inhibitor; MRA, Mineralocorticoid Receptor Antagonist; SGLT2, Sodium-Glucose Cotransporter 2 Inhibitor; HIF-PH, hypoxia-inducible factor prolyl-hydroxylase.

*Adverse Events*

There were no readmissions due to heart failure or cardiovascular events during the 6-month period of this study. In the new administration group, there were no patients who were unable to continue taking ferric citrate hydrate due to gastrointestinal symptoms, but in the switching group, there was one case of nausea and one case of diarrhea. The patient who experienced diarrhea discontinued the drug after 2 months of administration. The patient who discontinued treatment was excluded from the primary analysis.

- <Newly administered cases:>
- Primary endpoint:

Hb (Figure 1): Before the administration of ferric citrate hydrate, the hemoglobin level was 10.3 $\pm$ 1.0 g/dL. After 1 month of treatment, it increased to 12.0 $\pm$ 1.3 g/dL; after 3 months, it was 12.9 $\pm$ 1.5 g/dL; and after 6 months, it remained at 12.9 $\pm$ 1.5 g/dL. These values show a statistically significant increase compared to baseline (all; $p < 0.001$). Furthermore, hemoglobin levels at 3 and 6 months were significantly higher than those at 1 month ($p < 0.001$ for both comparisons).

- Secondary endpoints:

NYHA classification (Table 2): No patients experienced worsening of NYHA classification following ferric citrate hydrate treatment. Compared to baseline, NYHA classification improved significantly after treatment ($p < 0.001$).

**Table 2.** Changes in New York Heart Association classification and each biomarker in the newly administered cases.

| Newly Administered Cases | Pre | 1 Month | 3 Months | 6 Months |
|---|---|---|---|---|
| NYHA classification | 2.12 ± 0.58 | - | - | 1.74 ± 0.53 |
| *p* value | - | - | - | <0.001 |
| Hematocrit (%) | 32.8 ± 0.3 | 37.8 ± 0.4 | 39.9 ± 0.5 | 39.6 ± 0.5 |
| *p* value | - | <0.001 | <0.001 | <0.001 |
| Serum iron (µg/dL) | 47.5 ± 2.9 | 95.5 ± 6.2 | 84.6 ± 3.8 | 94.6 ± 3.7 |
| *p* value | - | <0.001 | <0.001 | <0.001 |
| TSAT (%) | 15.1 ± 1.1 | 33.0 ± 2.3 | 29.8 ± 1.5 | 32.9 ± 1.4 |
| *p* value | - | <0.001 | <0.001 | <0.001 |
| Ferritin (ng/mL) | 39.5 ± 6.4 | 66.3 ± 12.0 | 80.4 ± 11.5 | 114.9 ± 16.2 |
| *p* value | - | <0.001 | <0.001 | <0.001 |
| BUN (mg/dL) | 20.5 ± 0.8 | 20.3 ± 0.7 | 20.0 ± 0.8 | 20.6 ± 0.8 |
| *p* value | - | 0.638 | 0.381 | 0.895 |
| Serum creatine (mg/dL) | 1.14 ± 0.05 | 1.13 ± 0.05 | 1.12 ± 0.05 | 1.11 ± 0.05 |
| *p* value | - | 0.377 | 0.226 | 0.023 |
| eGFR (mL/dL/1.73 m$^2$) | 51.2 ± 1.8 | 50.8 ± 1.7 | 51.0 ± 1.8 | 51.6 ± 1.7 |
| *p* value | - | 0.403 | 0.787 | 0.518 |
| AST (U/L) | 24.2 ± 1.1 | 24.6 ± 0.9 | 24.9 ± 1.1 | 25.8 ± 1.1 |
| *p* value | - | 0.545 | 0.480 | 0.156 |
| ALT (U/L) | 16.3 ± 0.9 | 17.1 ± 0.8 | 17.5 ± 1.0 | 17.6 ± 0.9 |
| *p* value | - | 0.244 | 0.253 | 0.108 |
| hs-CRP (mg/dL) | 0.50 ± 0.11 | 0.38 ± 0.10 | 0.50 ± 0.10 | 0.33 ± 0.07 |
| *p* value | - | 0.088 | 0.959 | 0.092 |
| Oxidized LDL (U/L) | 57.6 ± 2.0 | - | 53.5 ± 2.0 | 51.3 ± 1.9 |
| *p* value | - | - | 0.025 | 0.001 |

NYHA, New York Heart Association; TSAT, transferrin saturation index; BUN, urea nitrogen; eGFR, estimated glomerular filtration rate; AST, aspartate aminotransferase; ALT, alanine aminotransferase; hs-CRP, high-sensitivity C-reactive protein; oxidized LDL, Oxidized low-density lipoprotein.

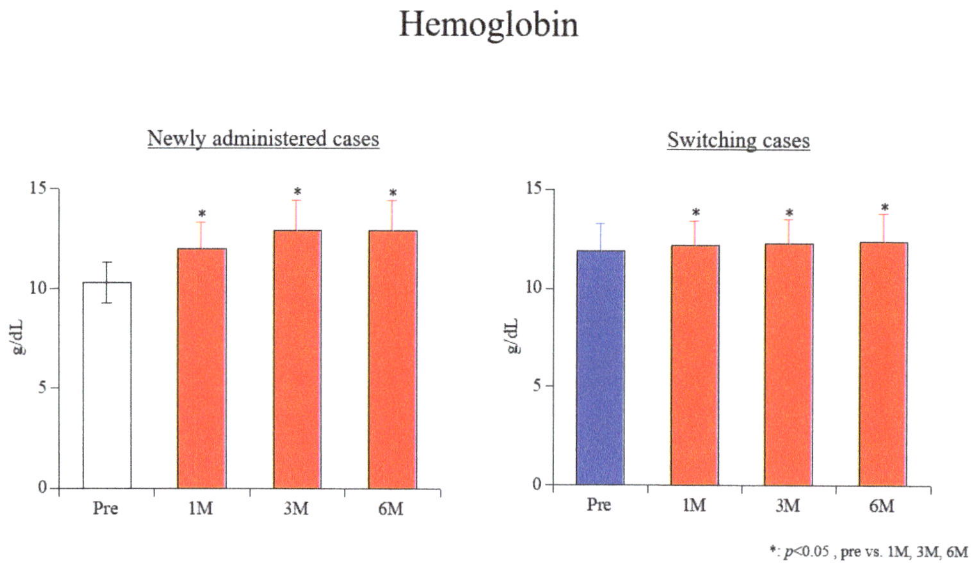


**Figure 1.** Changes in hemoglobin levels.

Ht, Fe, TSAT, and ferritin (Table 2): Ht, serum iron, TSAT, and ferritin levels all increased significantly after ferric citrate hydrate administration compared to baseline (all $p < 0.001$). Ht increased significantly at 3 and 6 months compared to 1 month (both $p < 0.001$). Serum iron levels were significantly higher at 6 months than at 3 months ($p = 0.014$). TSAT did not differ significantly across the treatment periods (1 vs. 3 months: $p = 0.109$; 1 vs. 6 months: $p = 0.964$; 3 vs. 6 months: $p = 0.056$). Ferritin levels increased significantly at 3 and 6 months compared to 1 month (1 vs. 3 months: $p = 0.002$; 1 vs. 6 months: $p < 0.001$), and levels at 6 months were also significantly higher than at 3 months ($p < 0.001$).

Cardiac-related biomarkers (ANP, BNP, NT-proBNP) (Figure 2): ANP levels were 154.8 ± 25.8 pg/mL at baseline, 140.8 ± 25.3 pg/mL at 3 months, and 121.3 ± 16.9 pg/mL at 6 months. A significant decrease was observed at 6 months compared to baseline ($p = 0.018$), but there was no significant difference between 3 and 6 months ($p = 0.137$). BNP levels were 148.7 ± 19.2 pg/mL at baseline, 133.4 ± 23.1 pg/mL at 3 months, and 124.4 ± 18.8 pg/mL at 6 months. A statistically significant decrease was observed at 6 months compared to baseline ($p = 0.022$), with no significant difference between 3 and 6 months ($p = 0.491$). NT-proBNP levels were 777.4 ± 109.8 pg/mL at baseline, 645.3 ± 85.1 pg/mL at 3 months, and 658.2 ± 82.8 pg/mL at 6 months. Statistically significant decreases were observed at both 3 months ($p = 0.025$) and 6 months ($p = 0.046$) compared to baseline, but no significant difference was found between 3 and 6 months ($p = 0.475$).

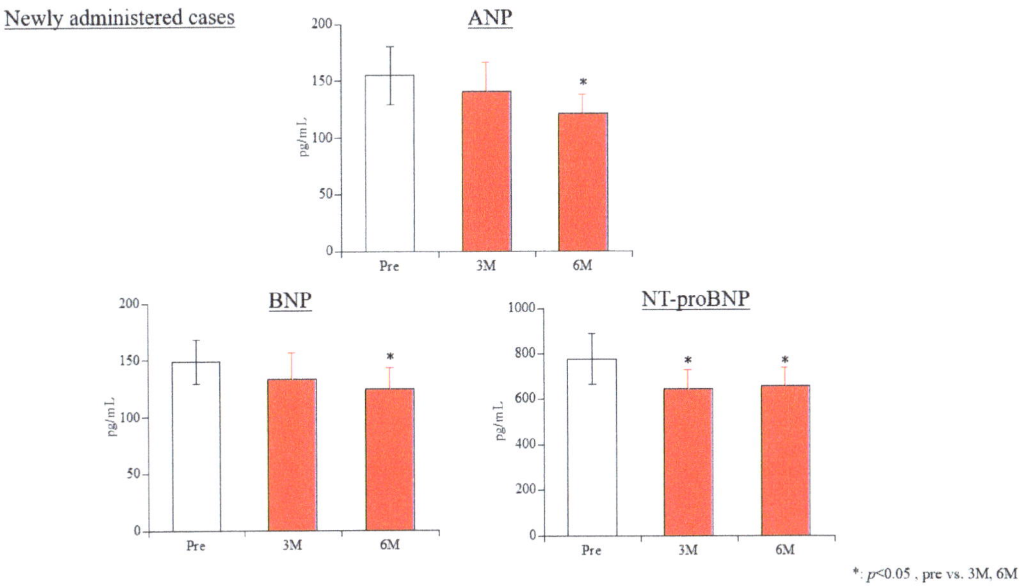


**Figure 2.** Changes in cardiac hormones in newly administered cases. ANP, atrial natriuretic peptide; BNP, brain natriuretic peptide; NT-proBNP, N-terminal pro-brain natriuretic peptide.

Renal-related biomarkers (BUN, Cr, eGFR) (Table 2): There was no significant change in BUN before and after treatment, nor across treatment time points. Serum creatinine (Cr) significantly decreased at 6 months compared to baseline ($p = 0.023$), although there were no significant differences between treatment periods. eGFR showed no significant change before and after treatment, or across time points.

Hepatic-related biomarkers (AST, ALT) (Table 2): No statistically significant changes were observed in AST or ALT levels before and after ferric citrate hydrate administration, or between treatment periods.

Other biomarkers (hs-CRP, Ox-LDL) (Table 2): There were no significant changes in hs-CRP levels before and after treatment, nor between treatment periods. Oxidized LDL (Ox-LDL) levels were significantly reduced at 3 and 6 months compared to baseline (3 months: $p = 0.025$; 6 months: $p = 0.001$), with no significant difference between 3 and 6 months ($p = 0.164$).

- <Switching cases>
- Primary endpoint:

Hb (Figure 1): In patients who switched from iron sulfate sustained-release tablets to ferric citrate hydrate, the hemoglobin level was 11.9 ± 1.4 g/dL before switching. After switching, the hemoglobin level increased significantly to 12.2 ± 1.2 g/dL at 1 month, 12.3 ± 1.2 g/dL at 3 months, and 12.4 ± 1.4 g/dL at 6 months (1 month: $p < 0.001$; 3 months: $p = 0.009$; 6 months: $p = 0.004$). There were no significant differences between post-switch time points (1 vs. 3 months: $p = 0.503$; 1 vs. 6 months: $p = 0.156$; 3 vs. 6 months: $p = 0.214$).

- Secondary endpoints:

NYHA classification (Table 3): No patients experienced worsening of NYHA classification after switching to ferric citrate hydrate. Compared to baseline, NYHA classification improved significantly ($p = 0.044$).

**Table 3.** Changes in New York Heart Association classification and each biomarker in the switching cases.

| Switching Cases | Pre | 1 Month | 3 Months | 6 Months |
|---|---|---|---|---|
| NYHA classification | 1.87 ± 0.65 | - | - | 1.78 ± 0.59 |
| *p* value | - | - | - | 0.044 |
| Hematocrit (%) | 36.7 ± 0.7 | 37.8 ± 0.6 | 38.2 ± 0.6 | 38.7 ± 0.6 |
| *p* value | - | 0.003 | 0.012 | 0.02 |
| Serum iron (μg/dL) | 82.0 ± 4.8 | 95.2 ± 6.8 | 83.8 ± 4.1 | 89.8 ± 6.6 |
| *p* value | - | 0.117 | 0.753 | 0.327 |
| TSAT (%) | 28.9 ± 1.8 | 48.8 ± 4.1 | 42.6 ± 2.9 | 32.8 ± 1.9 |
| *p* value | - | <0.001 | <0.001 | 0.125 |
| Ferritin (ng/mL) | 192.4 ± 33.8 | 208.7 ± 36.2 | 197.8 ± 30.7 | 206.5 ± 30.5 |
| *p* value | - | 0.002 | 0.673 | 0.273 |
| BUN (mg/dL) | 25.4 ± 1.5 | 25.1 ± 1.2 | 24.5 ± 1.2 | 24.7 ± 1.5 |
| *p* value | - | 0.748 | 0.199 | 0.440 |
| Serum creatine (mg/dL) | 1.26 ± 0.10 | 1.25 ± 0.08 | 1.22 ± 0.08 | 1.23 ± 0.08 |
| *p* value | - | 0.753 | 0.289 | 0.498 |
| eGFR (mL/dL/1.73 $m^2$) | 47.3 ± 2.9 | 46.0 ± 2.8 | 47.2 ± 2.8 | 46.5 ± 2.7 |
| *p* value | - | 0.090 | 0.905 | 0.471 |
| AST (U/L) | 25.7 ± 2.0 | 26.3 ± 1.8 | 24.8 ± 1.7 | 27.3 ± 2.9 |
| *p* value | - | 0.493 | 0.299 | 0.374 |
| ALT (U/L) | 18.5 ± 2.2 | 18.6 ± 1.8 | 17.5 ± 1.7 | 20.3 ± 2.8 |
| *p* value | - | 0.906 | 0.240 | 0.223 |
| hs-CRP (mg/dL) | 0.33 ± 0.06 | 0.25 ± 0.05 | 0.34 ± 0.06 | 0.43 ± 0.15 |
| *p* value | - | 0.113 | 0.842 | 0.388 |
| Oxidized LDL (U/L) | 56.2 ± 2.9 | - | 51.3 ± 2.5 | 53.9 ± 2.5 |
| *p* value | - | - | 0.050 | 0.425 |

NYHA, New York Heart Association; TSAT, transferrin saturation index; BUN, urea nitrogen; eGFR, estimated glomerular filtration rate; AST, aspartate aminotransferase; ALT, alanine aminotransferase; hs-CRP, high-sensitivity C-reactive protein; Oxidized LDL, oxidized low-density lipoprotein.

Ht, Fe, TSAT, and ferritin (Table 3): After switching, hematocrit values increased significantly compared to pre-switch levels (1 month: $p = 0.003$; 3 months: $p = 0.012$; 6 months: $p = 0.020$). However, there were no significant differences between the post-switch time points (1 vs. 3 months: $p = 0.366$; 1 vs. 6 months: $p = 0.052$; 3 vs. 6 months:

$p = 0.108$). Serum iron levels did not differ significantly before and after switching, nor among the post-switch time points. Ferritin levels increased significantly from pre-switch to 1 month post-switch ($p = 0.002$), but no significant changes were observed between 3 and 6 months or among time points thereafter. TSAT levels increased significantly at 1 and 3 months post-switch (both $p < 0.001$). Additionally, TSAT continued to rise significantly at 3 and 6 months compared to 1 month (1 vs. 3 months: $p = 0.009$; 1 vs. 6 months: $p < 0.001$), and at 6 months compared to 3 months ($p = 0.003$).

Cardiac-related biomarkers (ANP, BNP, NT-proBNP) (Figure 3): ANP levels were 258.4 ± 60.2 pg/mL before switching, 267.1 ± 69.2 pg/mL at 3 months post-switch, and 261.2 ± 66.1 pg/mL at 6 months. There were no statistically significant changes before and after switching, nor among the post-switch time points. BNP levels were 225.4 ± 58.2 pg/mL before switching, 218.2 ± 62.9 pg/mL at 3 months, and 212.2 ± 58.7 pg/mL at 6 months. No statistically significant differences were found. NT-proBNP levels were 1727.9 ± 553.0 pg/mL before switching, 1408.2 ± 384.0 pg/mL at 3 months, and 1459.2 ± 421.5 pg/mL at 6 months. There were no statistically significant changes observed before and after switching or between post-switch time points.

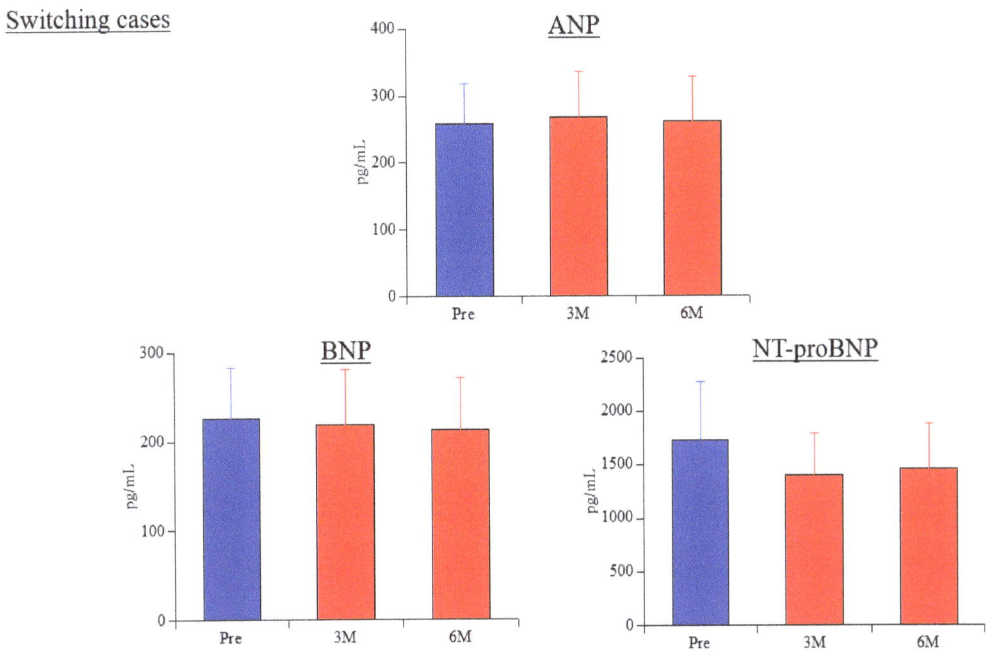


**Figure 3.** Changes in cardiac hormones in switching cases. ANP, atrial natriuretic peptide; BNP, brain natriuretic peptide; NT-proBNP, N-terminal pro-brain natriuretic peptide.

Renal-related biomarkers (BUN, Cr, eGFR) (Table 3): There were no statistically significant changes in BUN, serum creatinine (Cr), or estimated glomerular filtration rate (eGFR) before and after switching to ferric citrate hydrate, nor between post-switch time points.

Hepatic-related biomarkers (AST, ALT) (Table 3): No significant differences were observed in AST or ALT levels before and after treatment, or across post-switch time points.

Other biomarkers (hs-CRP, Ox-LDL) (Table 3): No significant changes were observed in hs-CRP levels before and after switching, or between the 3- and 6-month post-switch periods. Similarly, no statistically significant differences were observed in Ox-LDL levels before and after switching, or between the post-switch time points.

## 4. Discussion

Ferric citrate hydrate, the formulation used in this study, was approved in 2014 as a drug for treating hyperphosphatemia in chronic kidney disease and in 2021 as a drug for iron deficiency anemia. It is a drug that suppresses phosphorus absorption by combining with phosphate ions derived from food in the digestive tract to form a poorly soluble precipitate. Although there have been clinical study reports on ferric citrate hydrate in relation to hyperphosphatemia or iron deficiency anemia [17–19], there have been no reports of studies on heart failure with iron deficiency anemia. The results of this study showed that ferric citrate hydrate not only improves anemia but also improves iron metabolism and the heart failure biomarkers ANP, BNP, and NT-proBNP in patients with chronic heart failure complicated by iron deficiency anemia. Furthermore, improvement in NYHA classification was observed. In addition, there was no worsening of heart failure during treatment with ferric citrate hydrate, and it was thought to be a safe drug that could be used. In a switching study from iron sulfate sustained-release tablets, an increase in Hb was observed after switching to ferric citrate hydrate. There was no difference in serum iron levels before and after switching, but ferritin levels increased significantly after switching, and TSAT increased significantly after 1 month and 3 months of switching. Although there were no differences in ANP, BNP, or NT-proBNP, biomarkers for heart failure, before and after switching, NYHA classification was improved. These results suggest the following: (1) in patients with heart failure complicated by anemia, shortness of breath may have been due in part to anemia, and improvement in anemia led to relief of symptoms; (2) improvement in anemia may have contributed to symptom relief in heart failure, which could have subsequently led to improvements in ANP, BNP, or NT-proBNP levels.

According to WHO criteria, anemia is defined as a hemoglobin level of less than 13 g/dL for men and less than 12 g/dL for women, and in most previous clinical studies, WHO criteria have been used. In the present study, the authors examined lowering these hemoglobin levels and considered that the hemoglobin levels that should be treated clinically for anemia were less than 11 g/dL for men and less than 10.5 g/dL for women. They believe that this may have resulted in the improvement of each dataset.

Many clinical studies have been conducted on administering iron supplements to patients with chronic heart failure. In a report on oral iron supplements, the IRONOUT HF study, which targeted 225 HFrEF patients with iron deficiency, found no significant difference between the oral iron supplement group and the placebo group in terms of peak VO2 ($p = 0.46$), 6-min walk distance ($p = 0.19$), NT-proBNP levels ($p = 0.48$), or KCCQ clinical scores ($p = 0.57$) [16]. The reasons why no difference was seen were: (1) the mean Hb level before iron administration in the target patients was high at 12.6 (11.8–13.3) g/dL, (2) the mean NT-proBNP level before iron administration in the target patients was low at 1111 (453–2412) pg/mL compared to our study, (3) the TSAT level only increased by 2 (−3 to 7) % after iron treatment, (4) ferritin levels did not increase significantly after treatment with iron supplements, (5) the observation period was short (16 weeks), (6) adverse events were reported in 35% of cases, serious adverse events in 109% of cases, and permanent discontinuation of treatment in 14% of cases, and (7) it was stated that 113 out of 114 subjects received at least one dose of the study drug, so it was thought that the doses may not have been administered in sufficient quantities every day. Our research results have demonstrated that, in patients with heart failure, it is important to improve anemia as well as to supplement iron, and although there are many clinical studies on iron deficiency regardless of the presence or absence of anemia, there are few studies on iron deficiency anemia, so we believe that the results of this study are significant.

On the other hand, there are reports of the effectiveness of intravenous iron preparations, and the ESC guidelines also recommend intravenous iron supplementation for

HFrEF and HFmrEF [15]. In the CONFIRM-HF study (observation period: 52 weeks), which included 304 patients with chronic heart failure and iron deficiency, patients in the intravenous iron group were given one or two vials (500 mg or 1000 mg of iron) at Day 0 and Weeks 6, 12, 24, and 36, depending on the patient's weight and hemoglobin level. The results showed that the iron supplementation group had significantly better results than the placebo group in terms of the Patient Global Assessment, NYHA functional classification, 6-min walk test, fatigue score, and quality of life (KCCQ, EQ-5D). In addition, there was a 61% reduction in hospitalizations due to worsening heart failure compared to the placebo group ($p = 0.009$) [14]. In the FAIR-HF study (observation period: 24 months), which targeted 459 patients with chronic heart failure (NYHA II, III, HFrEF) with Hb 9.5 to 13.5 g/dL + iron deficiency, the iron supplementation group had significantly better results than the placebo group in terms of Patient Global Assessment ($p < 0.001$), NYHA classification ($p < 0.001$), and 6-min walking distance ($p < 0.001$) [13]. In the AFFIRM-AHF study (observation period: 52 weeks), which targeted 1110 patients with acute heart failure and iron deficiency (EF < 50%), the primary endpoint events (heart failure hospitalization, cardiovascular death) were reduced in the intravenous iron group ($p = 0.059$), and heart failure hospitalization was significantly reduced in the intravenous iron group ($p = 0.013$). In patients with heart failure, regardless of whether they have anemia or not, intravenous iron supplementation is effective [20]. In the IRONMAN trial (mean observation period: 2.5 years) of 1137 patients with chronic heart failure with EF < 45% who had iron deficiency, the impact of the COVID-19 pandemic meant that the trial was unable to show a significant difference in the primary endpoint (recurrent hospitalization for heart failure and cardiovascular death) ($p = 0.07$), but numerically, hospitalization and cardiovascular death decreased, and the quality of life of the participants in the intervention group improved significantly after 4 months [21]. The high iron content of the intravenous iron and the fact that it could be administered appropriately in the hospital meant that it was possible to provide sufficient iron supplementation, which may have contributed to the positive results. The author also believes that one of the reasons why large-scale studies have not shown the effectiveness of oral iron preparations is that oral iron preparations often cause gastrointestinal symptoms as side effects, which can make it difficult to continue taking them.

In our study, none of the patients who were newly introduced to ferric citrate hydrate had to discontinue taking it due to gastrointestinal symptoms. In our study, none of the patients who were newly introduced to Ferric Citrate Hydrate discontinued treatment due to gastrointestinal symptoms. Among the patients who switched to Ferric Citrate Hydrate, two experienced issues, but only one ultimately discontinued treatment. Furthermore, in the new cases, seven patients had previously taken iron sulfate sustained-release tablets and had been unable to continue taking them due to gastrointestinal symptoms. All seven of these patients were able to continue taking ferric citrate hydrate, indicating that its impact on gastrointestinal symptoms was minimal. Iron supplementation and anemia treatment could be carried out appropriately and continuously. The problem with conventional oral iron preparations is that they cannot be continued due to side effects such as gastrointestinal symptoms [22–24]. Ferric citrate hydrate, which was examined in this study, has been reported to cause fewer gastrointestinal complications than conventional iron preparations. A clinical study was conducted on 739 Japanese patients with iron deficiency anemia and no heart failure, and a comparison study was conducted on ferric citrate hydrate and the oral drug sodium ferrous citrate. In this study, ferric citrate hydrate was divided into high-dose (1000 mg/day) and low-dose (500 mg/day) and compared with sodium ferrous citrate (100 mg/day). Most of the adverse events that led to early discontinuation of the study treatment were related to gastrointestinal symptoms, and there was no difference in the incidence of diarrhea among the three groups. However, the incidence of nausea was 15.5% in the low-dose group, 10.5% in the high-dose group, and 32.7% in the sodium ferrous citrate group, and the incidence of vomiting was 5.2% in the low-dose group, 1.2% in the high-dose group, and 15.2% in the sodium ferrous citrate group. The incidence of these events was significantly lower in the ferric citrate hydrate group than in the sodium ferrous citrate group [25]. In terms of economic evaluation, it has been reported that switching to ferric citrate hydrate is more cost-effective when gastrointestinal side effects are observed with sodium ferrous citrate [26].

The signal pathways that induce nausea and vomiting remain unclear, but it has been suggested that serotonin and free radicals are involved in nausea and vomiting [27,28]. Machida et al. hypothesized that, since ferrous iron is more likely to produce free radicals and cause gastrointestinal disorders than ferric iron, the difference in the incidence of vomiting between sodium ferrous citrate and ferric citrate hydrate is due to the effect of iron supplements on small intestinal EC cell counts. They conducted a rat study to investigate effects of sodium ferrous citrate and ferric citrate hydrate. The sodium ferrous citrate group resulted in a significant increase in the number of EC cells in the duodenum and jejunum and the associated expression of substance, whereas the ferric citrate hydrate group did not demonstrate such effects. In addition, the sodium ferrous citrate group showed a significant decrease in food intake that continued from 48 h after the start of administration, while the ferric citrate hydrate group did not show such an effect [29]. With conventional oral iron preparations, there are many cases where patients are unable to continue taking the medication due to gastrointestinal symptoms, and this is one of the reasons why they do not produce the same results as intravenous iron preparations. The author believes that if the medication can be taken continuously and appropriately, it is possible to achieve the same results as intravenous medication, and based on our research results, ferric citrate hydrate produced very few gastrointestinal symptoms. In addition, the fact that all patients were able to continue taking the medication throughout the study period is also thought to be a reason for the good results.

In this study, 25% of newly administered cases and 35% of switching cases were taking HIF-PH inhibitors, which are drugs used to treat renal anemia, prior to the study. As many of the patients in this study were elderly, it was thought that renal anemia and iron deficiency anemia were relatively common in this group. Furthermore, it is said that HIF-PH inhibitors lower hepcidin and increase iron metabolism (iron utilization), and it is possible that the administration of HIF-PH inhibitors caused the decrease in ferritin and TSAT levels. Decreases in hepcidin, ferritin, and TSAT levels have been reported with HIF-PH inhibitors [30,31], and in some cases, the administration of iron supplements is necessary. It has also been reported that there are differences depending on the type of HIF-PH inhibitor [32,33]. In the results of our clinical study, in which we switched from ESA to four types of HIF-PH inhibitors, there was variation in the TSAT and ferritin data, and no difference in iron metabolism was observed between the types of HIF-PH inhibitors [34].

There is no fixed view on this. This point should be studied in the future, and the necessity of iron supplements should be clarified. The subjects in this study were patients with stable iron metabolism whose doses of HIF-PH inhibitors had remained unchanged for at least six months. As the next step, we plan to conduct a sub-analysis comparing patients with and without HIF-PH inhibitor treatment. Furthermore, we consider it necessary to investigate the potential effects of HIF-PH inhibitors on iron metabolism and heart failure.

## 5. Conclusions

This study found that ferric citrate hydrate significantly increased Hb, serum iron, TSAT, and ferritin levels in patients with chronic heart failure complicated by iron deficiency anemia, and decreased ANP, BNP, and NT-proBNP levels. Ferric citrate hydrate could be continued without side effects such as gastrointestinal symptoms. In a study comparing ferric citrate hydrate with iron sulfate sustained-release tablets, ferric citrate hydrate had better results for ferritin and TSAT, but there was no difference in Hb or serum iron levels. There was also no difference in ANP, BNP, or NT-proBNP.

We believe that improvement in iron metabolism and anemia due to iron supplementation led to improvements in heart failure biomarkers.

## 6. Limitations

There are several limitations to this study. First, this was a single-center, observational study evaluating the effects of ferric citrate hydrate, and not a randomized controlled trial with a placebo or alternative iron preparations. Although ferric citrate hydrate did not lead to worsening heart failure or re-hospitalization, the primary limitation is that the study endpoints were limited to biomarkers, without detailed assessments of quality of life (QOL) or exercise capacity. Including these parameters in future studies would allow for a more comprehensive evaluation of the efficacy of oral iron supplementation.

Second, increasing the sample size in future studies would help to better demonstrate the effectiveness of oral iron preparations in patients with chronic heart failure complicated by iron deficiency anemia. A comparative study including a control group would also be warranted.

Third, although the observation period in this study was 6 months, a longer-term follow-up would provide more clinically relevant data. Finally, for the treatment of heart failure, medications such as ARNIs and SGLT2 inhibitors may influence long-term outcomes. While the current study only included patients whose pharmacologic treatment had remained unchanged for at least 6 months, the specific effects of each drug should be investigated in future studies.

**Author Contributions:** Conceptualization, A.S., H.S., M.T. (Makoto Taoka) and M.T. (Masashi Tanaka); methodology, A.S., H.S., M.T. (Makoto Taoka) and M.T. (Masashi Tanaka); software, A.S.; validation, A.S., H.S., M.T. (Makoto Taoka), K.O., S.K. and M.T. (Masashi Tanaka); formal analysis, A.S.; investigation, A.S.; resources, A.S., K.O. and S.K.; data curation, A.S.; writing—original draft preparation, A.S.; writing—review and editing, A.S.; visualization, A.S.; supervision, A.S.; project administration, A.S.; funding acquisition, H.S. All authors have read and agreed to the published version of the manuscript.

**Funding:** This research received no external funding.

**Institutional Review Board Statement:** The study was conducted in accordance with the Declaration of Helsinki and approved by the Institutional Review Board of Sekino Hospital (protocol no. 20210401 and approval on 1 June 2021) and the study was registered with our Hospital Medical Information Network (study ID: UMIN000050436).

**Informed Consent Statement:** Informed consent was obtained from all subjects involved in the study.

**Data Availability Statement:** The data that support the findings of this study are available on request from the corresponding author, [A.S]. The data are not publicly available due to restrictions e.g., their containing information that could compromise the privacy of research participants.

**Acknowledgments:** We would like to express our sincere appreciation to Yoshitarou Shimizu, Medical Technologists at Sekino Hospital, for their constructive cooperation.

**Conflicts of Interest:** The authors declare no conflicts of interest.

## References


1. Anand, I.; McMurray, J.J.; Whitmore, J.; Warren, M.; Pham, A.; McCamish, M.A.; Burton, P.B. Anemia and its relationship to clinical outcome in heart failure. *Circulation* **2004**, *110*, 149–154. [PubMed]
2. Kajimoto, K.; Sato, N.; Takano, T.; Investigators of the Acute Decompensated Heart Failure Syndromes (ATTEND) Registry. Association between anemia, clinical features, and outcome in patients hospitalized for acute heart failure syndromes. *Eur. Heart J. Acute Cardiovasc. Care* **2015**, *4*, 568–576. [PubMed]
3. Hamaguchi, S.; Tsuchihashi-Makaya, M.; Kinugawa, S.; Yokota, T.; Takeshita, A.; Yokoshiki, H.; Tsutsui, H.; JCARE-CARD Investigators. Anemia is an independent predictor of long-term adverse outcomes in patients hospitalized with heart failure in Japan. A report from the Japanese Cardiac Registry of Heart Failure in Cardiology (JCARE-CARD). *Circ. J.* **2009**, *73*, 1901–1908.
4. Yamauchi, T.; Sakata, Y.; Takada, T.; Nochioka, K.; Miura, M.; Tadaki, S.; Ushigome, R.; Sato, K.; Onose, T.; Tsuji, K.; et al. Prognostic impact of anemia in patients with chronic heart failure—With special reference to clinical background: Report from the CHART-2 study. *Circ. J.* **2015**, *79*, 1984–1993. [CrossRef]
5. Inder, S.; Anand, I.S. Anemia and iron deficiency in heart failure: Current concepts and emerging therapies. *Circulation* **2018**, *138*, 80–98.
6. Jankowska, E.A.; Rozentryt, P.; Witkowska, A.; Nowak, J.; Hartmann, O.; Ponikowska, B.; Borodulin-Nadzieja, L.; Banasiak, W.; Polonski, L.; Filippatos, G.; et al. Iron deficiency: An ominous sign in patients with systolic chronic heart failure. *Eur. Heart J.* **2010**, *31*, 1872–1880.
7. Cohen-Solal, A.; Damy, T.; Terbah, M.; Kerebel, S.; Baguet, J.P.; Hanon, O.; Zannad, F.; Laperche, T.; Leclercq, C.; Concas, V.; et al. High prevalence of iron deficiency in patients with acute decompensated heart failure. *Eur. J. Heart Fail.* **2014**, *16*, 984–991.
8. Matsumoto, M.; Tsujino, T.; Lee-Kawabata, M.; Naito, Y.; Akahori, H.; Sakoda, T.; Ohyanagi, M.; Tomosugi, N.; Masuyama, T. Iron regulatory hormone hepcidin decreases in chronic heart failure patients with anemia. *Circ. J.* **2010**, *74*, 301–306.
9. Jankowska, E.A.; Malyszko, J.; Ardehali, H.; Koc-Zorawska, E.; Banasiak, W.; von Haehling, S.; Macdougall, I.C.; Weiss, G.; McMurray, J.J.; Anker, S.D.; et al. Iron status in patients with chronic heart failure. *Eur. Heart J.* **2013**, *34*, 827–834.
10. Ganz, T. Hepcidin, a key regulator of iron metabolism and mediator of anemia of inflammation. *Blood* **2003**, *102*, 783–788. [CrossRef]
11. Nemeth, E.; Valore, E.V.; Territo, M.; Schiller, G.; Lichtenstein, A.; Ganz, T. Hepcidin, a putative mediator of anemia of inflammation, is a type II acute-phase protein. *Blood* **2003**, *101*, 2461–2463. [PubMed]
12. Masini, G.; Graham, F.J.; Pellicori, P.; Cleland, J.G.F.; Cuthbert, J.J.; Kazmi, S.; Inciardi, R.M.; Clark, A.L. Criteria for iron deficiency in patients with heart failure. *J. Am. Coll. Cardiol.* **2022**, *79*, 341–351. [PubMed]
13. Anker, S.D.; Comin Colet, J.; Filippatos, G.; Willenheimer, R.; Dickstein, K.; Drexler, H.; Lüscher, T.F.; Bart, B.; Banasiak, W.; Niegowska, J.; et al. Ferric carboxymaltose in patients with heart failure and iron deficiency. *N. Engl. J. Med.* **2009**, *361*, 2436–2448. [PubMed]
14. Ponikowski, P.; van Veldhuisen, D.J.; Comin-Colet, J.; Ertl, G.; Komajda, M.; Mareev, V.; McDonagh, T.; Parkhomenko, A.; Tavazzi, L.; Levesque, V.; et al. Beneficial effects of long-term intravenous iron therapy with ferric carboxymaltose in patients with symptomatic heart failure and iron deficiency. *Eur. Heart J.* **2015**, *36*, 657–668.
15. McDonagh, T.A.; Metra, M.; Adamo, M.; Gardner, R.S.; Baumbach, A.; Böhm, M.; Burri, H.; Butler, J.; Čelutkienė, J.; Chioncel, O.; et al. 2023 Focused Update of the 2021 ESC Guidelines for the diagnosis and treatment of acute and chronic heart failure. *Eur. Heart J.* **2023**, *44*, 3627–3639.
16. Lewis, G.D.; Malhotra, R.; Hernandez, A.F.; McNulty, S.E.; Smith, A.; Felker, G.M.; Tang, W.H.W.; LaRue, S.J.; Redfield, M.M.; Semigran, M.J.; et al. Effect of oral iron repletion on exercise capacity in patients with heart failure with reduced ejection fraction and iron deficiency: The IRONOUT HF randomized clinical trial. *JAMA* **2017**, *317*, 1958–1966.
17. Yokoyama, K.; Hashimoto, T.; Okuda, Y.; Matsumoto, Y.; Ito, K.; Yamada, R.; Susai, H.; Nishino, N. Safety and effectiveness of ferric citrate hydrate in serum phosphorus management of patients with chronic kidney disease: A long-term, real-world, observational, post-marketing surveillance study. *Clin. Exp. Nephrol.* **2022**, *26*, 688–699.
18. Yokoyama, K.; Fukagawa, M.; Akiba, T.; Nakayama, M.; Ito, K.; Hanaki, K.; Wolf, M.; Hirakata, H. Randomised clinical trial of ferric citrate hydrate on anaemia management in haemodialysis patients with hyperphosphataemia: ASTRIO study. *Sci. Rep.* **2019**, *9*, 8877.
19. Tomosugi, N.; Koshino, Y.; Ogawa, C.; Maeda, K.; Shimada, N.; Tomita, K.; Daimon, S.; Shikano, T.; Ryu, K.; Takatani, T.; et al. Oral iron absorption of ferric citrate hydrate and hepcidin-25 in hemodialysis patients: A prospective, multicenter, observational trial. *Int. J. Mol. Sci.* **2023**, *24*, 13799.
20. Ponikowski, P.; Kirwan, B.A.; Anker, S.D.; McDonagh, T.; Dorobantu, M.; Drozdz, J.; Fabien, V.; Filippatos, G.; Göhring, U.M.; Keren, A.; et al. Ferric carboxymaltose for iron deficiency at discharge after acute heart failure: A multicentre, double-blind, randomised, controlled trial. *Lancet* **2020**, *396*, 1895–1904.

21. Kalra, P.R.; Cleland, J.G.F.; Petrie, M.C.; Thomson, E.A.; Kalra, P.A.; Squire, I.B.; Ahmed, F.Z.; Al-Mohammad, A.; Cowburn, P.J.; Foley, P.W.X.; et al. Intravenous ferric derisomaltose in patients with heart failure and iron deficiency in the UK (IRONMAN): An investigator-initiated, prospective, randomised, open-label, blinded-endpoint trial. *Lancet* **2022**, *400*, 2199–2209. [PubMed]
22. Clark, S.F. Iron deficiency anemia: Diagnosis and management. *Curr. Opin. Gastroenterol.* **2009**, *25*, 122–128. [PubMed]
23. Gereklioglu, C.; Asma, S.; Korur, A.; Erdogan, F.; Kut, A. Medication adherence to oral iron therapy in patients with iron deficiency anemia. *Pak. J. Med. Sci.* **2016**, *32*, 604–607. [PubMed]
24. Galloway, R.; McGuire, J. Determinants of compliance with iron supplementation: Supplies, side effects, or psychology? *Soc. Sci. Med.* **1994**, *39*, 381–390.
25. Komatsu, N.; Arita, K.; Mitsui, H.; Nemoto, T.; Hanaki, K. Efficacy and safety of ferric citrate hydrate compared with sodium ferrous citrate in Japanese patients with iron deficiency anemia: A randomized, double-blind, phase 3 non-inferiority study. *Int. J. Hematol.* **2021**, *114*, 8–17.
26. Momoeda, M.; Ito, K.; Inoue, S.; Shibahara, H.; Mitobe, Y.; Komatsu, N. Cost-effectiveness of ferric citrate hydrate in patients with iron deficiency anemia. *Int. J. Hematol.* **2024**, *121*, 467–475. [CrossRef]
27. Andrews, P.L.; Rapeport, W.G.; Sanger, G.J. Neuropharmacology of emesis induced by anti-cancer therapy. *Trends Pharmacol. Sci.* **1988**, *9*, 334–341.
28. Torii, Y.; Mutoh, M.; Saito, H.; Matsuki, N. Involvement of free radicals in cisplatin-induced emesis in *Suncus murinus*. *Eur. J. Pharmacol.* **1993**, *248*, 131–135.
29. Machida, T.; Hiraide, S.; Yamamoto, T.; Shiga, S.; Hasebe, S.; Fujibayashi, A.; Iizuka, K. Ferric citrate hydrate has little impact on hyperplasia of enterochromaffin cells in the rat small intestine compared to sodium ferrous citrate. *Pharmacology* **2022**, *107*, 574–583.
30. Fishbane, S.; Pollock, C.A.; El-Shahawy, M.; Escudero, E.T.; Rastogi, A.; Van, B.P.; Frison, L.; Houser, M.; Maksym, P.; Dustin, J.L.; et al. Roxadustat versus epoetin alfa for treating anemia in patients with chronic kidney disease on dialysis: Results from the randomized phase 3 ROCKIES Study. *J. Am. Soc. Nephrol.* **2022**, *33*, 850–866.
31. Akizawa, T.; Nangaku, M.; Yamaguchi, T.; Koretomo, R.; Maeda, K.; Miyazawa, Y.; Hirakata, H. A phase 3 study of enarodustat in anemic patients with CKD not requiring dialysis: The SYMPHONY ND study. *Kidney Int. Rep.* **2021**, *6*, 1840–1849. [CrossRef] [PubMed]
32. Yang, J.; Xing, J.; Zhu, X.; Xie, X.; Wang, L.; Zhang, X. Effects of hypoxia-inducible factor-prolyl hydroxylase inhibitors vs. erythropoiesis-stimulating agents on iron metabolism in non-dialysis-dependent anemic patients with CKD: A network meta-analysis. *Front. Endocrinol.* **2023**, *14*, 1131516. [CrossRef] [PubMed]
33. Takkavatakarn, K.; Thammathiwat, T.; Phannajit, J.; Katavetin, P.; Praditpornsilpa, K.; Eiam-Ong, S.; Susantitaphong, P. The impacts of hypoxia-inducible factor stabilizers on laboratory parameters and clinical outcomes in chronic kidney disease patients with renal anemia: A systematic review and meta-analysis. *Clin. Kidney J.* **2023**, *16*, 845–858. [CrossRef]
34. Sezai, A.; Abe, M.; Maruyama, T.; Taoka, M.; Sekino, H.; Tanaka, M. A prospective randomized controlled clinical study to investigate the efficacy and safety of hypoxia-inducible factor-prolyl hydroxylase inhibitors in non-dialysis patients with chronic heart failure and renal anemia switched from continuous erythropoietin receptor activator treatment. *J. Clin. Med.* **2024**, *13*, 2764. [CrossRef]

**Disclaimer/Publisher's Note:** The statements, opinions and data contained in all publications are solely those of the individual author(s) and contributor(s) and not of MDPI and/or the editor(s). MDPI and/or the editor(s) disclaim responsibility for any injury to people or property resulting from any ideas, methods, instructions or products referred to in the content.

*life* MDPI

*Article*

# Liraglutide Treatment Restores Cardiac Function After Isoprenaline-Induced Myocardial Injury and Prevents Heart Failure in Rats

**Zorislava Bajic [1,2,*], Tanja Sobot [1,2], Aleksandra Smitran [3], Snezana Uletilovic [2,4], Nebojša Mandić-Kovačević [2,5], Tanja Cvjetkovic [2,4], Ugljesa Malicevic [2,6], Bojan Stanetic [7], Đorđe Đukanović [2,8], Milka Maticic [2], Sanja Jovicic [2,9], Dragan M. Djuric [10], Milos P. Stojiljkovic [2,11] and Ranko Skrbic [2,11,12,13]**

1 Department of Physiology, Faculty of Medicine, University of Banja Luka, 78000 Banja Luka, The Republic of Srpska, Bosnia and Herzegovina; tanja.sobot@med.unibl.org
2 Centre for Biomedical Research, Faculty of Medicine, University of Banja Luka, 78000 Banja Luka, The Republic of Srpska, Bosnia and Herzegovina; snezana.uletilovic@med.unibl.org (S.U.); nebojsa.mandic-kovacevic@med.unibl.org (N.M.-K.); tanja.cvjetkovic@med.unibl.org (T.C.); ugljesa.malicevic@med.unibl.org (U.M.); djordje.djukanovic@med.unibl.org (Đ.Đ.); milka.maticic@med.unibl.org (M.M.); sanja.jovicic@med.unibl.org (S.J.); milos.stojiljkovic@med.unibl.org (M.P.S.); ranko.skrbic@med.unibl.org (R.S.)
3 Department of Microbiology and Immunology, Faculty of Medicine, University of Banja Luka, 78000 Banja Luka, The Republic of Srpska, Bosnia and Herzegovina; aleksandra.smitran@med.unibl.org
4 Department of Medical Biochemistry and Chemistry, Faculty of Medicine, University of Banja Luka, 78000 Banja Luka, The Republic of Srpska, Bosnia and Herzegovina
5 Department of Pharmacy, Faculty of Medicine, University of Banja Luka, 78000 Banja Luka, The Republic of Srpska, Bosnia and Herzegovina
6 Department of Pathophysiology, Faculty of Medicine, University of Banja Luka, 78000 Banja Luka, The Republic of Srpska, Bosnia and Herzegovina
7 Department of Cardiology, University Clinical Centre of the Republic of Srpska, 78000 Banja Luka, The Republic of Srpska, Bosnia and Herzegovina; bojan.stanetic@kc-bl.com
8 Department of Pharmaceutical Chemistry, Faculty of Medicine, University of Banja Luka, 78000 Banja Luka, The Republic of Srpska, Bosnia and Herzegovina
9 Department of Histology and Embryology, Faculty of Medicine, University of Banja Luka, 78000 Banja Luka, The Republic of Srpska, Bosnia and Herzegovina
10 Faculty of Medicine, Institute of Medical Physiology "Richard Burian", University of Belgrade, 11000 Belgrade, Serbia; dr_djuric@yahoo.com
11 Department of Pharmacology, Toxicology and Clinical Pharmacology, Faculty of Medicine, University of Banja Luka, 78000 Banja Luka, The Republic of Srpska, Bosnia and Herzegovina
12 Academy of Science and Arts of the Republic of Srpska, 78000 Banja Luka, The Republic of Srpska, Bosnia and Herzegovina
13 Department of Pathologic Physiology, I.M. Sechenov First Moscow State Medical University, 119435 Moscow, Russia
* Correspondence: zorislava.bajic@med.unibl.org

**Abstract:** Background: Myocardial injury (MI) is characterized by an increased level of at least one cardiac troponin. Experimental MI can be induced by isoprenaline, a β-adrenergic agonist, and it can lead to heart failure (HF). Liraglutide is glucagon-like 1 peptide receptor agonist used in diabetes management, but it has anti-inflammatory and antioxidative effects, which can be beneficial in treatment of HF. The aim of this study was to investigate the effects of liraglutide on isoprenaline-induced MI and prevention of HF. Methods: Male Wistar albino rats were divided into four groups: Con—received saline the first 2 days + saline the next 7 days; Iso—isoprenaline the first 2 days + saline the next 7 days; Lir—saline the first 2 days + liraglutide the next 7 days; Iso + Lir—isoprenaline the first 2 days + liraglutide the next 7 days. On day 10, blood samples were taken for biochemical analysis and oxidative stress marker evaluation, and hearts were isolated for pathohistological analysis. Cardiac function was assessed by electrocardiography (ECG) and echocardiography (ECHO). Results: Liraglutide treatment significantly attenuated oxidative stress, repaired ECG and ECHO parameters, and mitigated myocardial morphological changes induced by isoprenaline. Conclusions: Liraglutide restores cardiac function in isoprenaline-induced HF.

**Keywords:** isoprenaline-induced heart failure; liraglutide; oxidative stress; electrocardiography; echocardiography

## 1. Introduction

Myocardial injury (MI) is characterized by at least one of the cardiac troponin levels exceeding the 99th percentile of the upper reference limit [1]. Generally, a relative increase of 20% in troponin concentration is considered to be significant enough for diagnosing MI [2,3]. The term myocardial injury encompasses a wide range of conditions. The key difference between myocardial injury and myocardial infarction is determined by the source of elevated troponin. MI refers to the death of myocardial cells from nonischemic causes, whereas myocardial infarction is linked to ischemic factors, including plaque disruption and compromised oxygen supply to the myocardium [4]. The release of cardiac troponin into the bloodstream is associated with cardiomyocyte necrosis and apoptosis, an increase in membrane permeability, and mechanical stretching from pressure or volume overload without myocardial ischemia [5]. It is acknowledged that numerous conditions can lead to MI, such as tachyarrhythmia, myocarditis, Takotsubo syndrome, and valvular heart disease [2].

MI is marked by oxidative stress and the activation of the inflammatory cytokine response [6]. Accumulation of reactive oxygen species (ROS) in the mitochondria can result in a harmful cycle that causes damage to mitochondrial DNA and a reduction in mitochondrial functionality, subsequently leading to the production of more ROS. These ROS can promote cardiomyocyte hypertrophy, cardiomyocyte apoptosis, and interstitial fibrosis through the activation of matrix metalloproteinases (MMPs), thus perpetuating a detrimental cycle of adverse ventricular remodeling and the progression to heart failure (HF) [7,8]. MI initiates an inflammatory response designed to eliminate necrotic cellular debris and commence the process of anti-inflammatory repair. The occurrence of cellular necrosis and apoptosis is crucial for the activation of the inflammatory immune system. This activation has a dual purpose: while the chronic inflammatory state can lead to maladaptive remodeling, the infiltration of inflammatory cells has the capacity to recruit leukocytes, clear tissue debris, and initiate the healing response, ultimately facilitating the formation of scar tissue [8]. There is a reciprocal relationship between oxidative stress and inflammatory cytokines: oxidative stress promotes inflammation, which in turn increases oxidative stress. This interplay exacerbates changes in the heart after an MI, affecting cardiac function and prognosis [6]. All of these processes can lead to HF [9]. Notably, this progression to HF can occur even while the patient is still receiving treatment and care in a hospital setting. It is noteworthy that 75% of individuals affected by MI die within five years following the event [5]. This highlights the urgent need for effective prevention and early intervention for individuals at risk of or recovering from MI.

In the context of translational medicine, there is an ongoing pursuit of suitable experimental models that accurately replicate human diseases. As a result, isoprenaline is commonly used in studies of MI [10]. The myocardial injury caused by isoprenaline is distinguished by the presence of oxidative stress and an inflammatory response [11,12].

Many drugs and procedures have been used in order to prevent the development of HF following MI. Liraglutide is an established GLP-1 receptor agonist (GLP-1 RA) that is commonly used in the treatment of diabetes. The use of GLP-1 RAs is supported by their beneficial effects on glucose metabolism and the functioning of the pancreas. These agents not only enhance the survival of pancreatic cells but also decrease glycemic levels. Given the serious complications that can arise from diabetes and its various comorbidities, the therapeutic effects of GLP-1 RAs are being studied in a wide range of diseases and conditions associated with diabetes. There is evidence that GLP-1 RAs can also improve neurological impairments, including cognitive decline and Alzheimer's disease [13], dermatological conditions such as psoriasis [14], and renal diseases [15]. Recent studies have revealed that liraglutide exhibits beneficial effects, including its role in reducing inflammation [16] and oxidative stress [17].

We have recently established that pretreatment with liraglutide has significant cardioprotective effects in acute MI [18]. Based on the previous study, we aimed to evaluate the potential role of liraglutide in the treatment of MI and in the prevention of HF. For this purpose, the rats were treated with two consecutive doses of isoprenaline followed by liraglutide treatment for the next seven days.

## 2. Materials and Methods

### 2.1. Experimental Animals

In this study, male Wistar albino rats were used. The animals were kept under specific laboratory conditions, with a room temperature of 21 ± 2 °C, humidity level of 55 ± 5%, and a light and dark cycle of 12 h each, commencing at 08:00 a.m. This research, along with all procedures, protocols, and experimental animals, was approved by the Ethics Committee for the Protection of Welfare of Experimental Animals at the Faculty of Medicine, University of Banja Luka (approval number 18/1.190-13/22, dated 1 June 2022). The housing of the animals adhered to the guidelines established by the National Institute of Health (NIH) for the care and use of laboratory animals.

### 2.2. Experimental Grouping

The animals were categorized into four distinct groups. Over a period of 7 days, they received either 0.9% of NaCl (saline) or liraglutide treatment after isoprenaline-induced MI. The control group (Con, n = 6) was administered 1 mL/kg of 0.9% NaCl subcutaneously (s.c.) on the first 2 days, followed by 1 mL/kg of 0.9% NaCl s.c. for the subsequent 7 days. The isoprenaline group (Iso, n = 8) was given isoprenaline at a dosage of 85 mg/kg dissolved in 1 mL/kg of saline, administered s.c. on the first 2 days, and then received 1 mL/kg of 0.9% NaCl s.c. for the next 7 days. The liraglutide group (Lir, n = 6) was treated with 0.9% NaCl s.c. on the first 2 days, followed by liraglutide at a dosage of 1.8 mg/kg s.c. for 7 days. Lastly, the liraglutide + isoprenaline group (Iso + Lir, n = 8) received isoprenaline at 85 mg/kg s.c. on the first 2 days, followed by liraglutide at 1.8 mg/kg subcutaneously for the remaining 7 days (Figure 1).

### 2.3. Obtaining Blood and Tissue Samples

At the end of the experiment, all rats were anesthetized, and blood samples were drawn from the aorta into Vacutainer tubes intended for serum and plasma citrate. To obtain serum, the blood samples were left at room temperature for 20 min to allow clotting, followed by centrifugation at 3000 rpm for 5 min. Plasma samples underwent centrifugation at 3000 rpm for 10 min. After separating the plasma, red blood cells were washed three times with three volumes of cold 0.9% NaCl. All samples were preserved at −80 °C until further analysis. The hearts were removed and placed in small plastic containers filled with 10% formalin for histological examination.

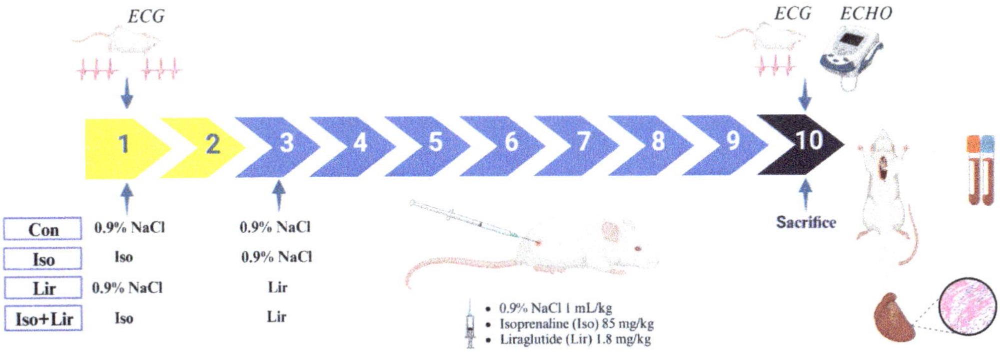


**Figure 1.** Study design: animal grouping and study protocol. Con—0.9% NaCl s.c. on the first 2 days + 0.9% NaCl s.c. for the next 7 days; Iso—isoprenaline 85 mg/kg s.c. on the first 2 days + 0.9% NaCl s.c. for the next 7 days; Lir—0.9% NaCl s.c. on the first 2 days + liraglutide 1.8 g/kg for the next 7 days; Iso + Lir—isoprenaline 85 mg/kg s.c. on the first 2 days + liraglutide 1.8 g/kg for the next 7 days.

### *2.4. Biomarkers of Myocardial Injury and Other Biochemical Parameters*

The concentration of serum high sensitive troponin I (hs TnI) was assessed on the Abbot Alinity ci-series platform utilizing chemiluminescent microparticle immunoassay (CMIA). Measurements of serum glucose, level of lipids (total cholesterol—TC, high-density lipoprotein—HDL, low-density lipoprotein—LDL, triglycerides—TG), and the activities of aspartate aminotransferase (AST), alanine aminotransferase (ALT), and lactate dehydrogenase (LDH) were conducted using the same Abbot Alinity ci-series through chemiluminescence immunoassay (CLIA). N-terminal pro-brain natriuretic peptide (NT-proBNP) was measured by enzyme-linked immunosorbent assay (ELISA) with the FineTest Rat NT-proBNP (N-Terminal Pro-Brain Natriuretic Peptide) ELISA Kit, Wuhan Fine Biotech Co., Ltd., Wuhan, China.

### *2.5. Prooxidative and Antioxidative Markers*

Prooxidative markers, including thiobarbituric acid reactive substances (TBARS), superoxide anion radical ($O_2^-$), and hydrogen peroxide ($H_2O_2$), and nitrite ($NO_2^-$), were assessed in plasma. The TBARS level, indicative of lipid peroxidation, was quantified using 1% TBA and 0.05 M sodium hydroxide (NaOH), measured at wavelength of 530 nm. The plasma concentration of $O_2^-$ was evaluated by using nitro blue tetrazolium (NTB) in conjunction with the TRIS buffer, with a measurement also of 530 nm. The concentration of plasma $H_2O_2$ was determined using the Pick and Keisari method, which relies on the oxidation of phenol red by $H_2O_2$, with measurements taken at a wavelength of 610 nm. For the determination of nitrite levels, the Green method was employed, utilizing 30% sulfosalicylic acid and Griess reagent [19]. The antioxidative markers catalase (CAT) and superoxide dismutase (SOD), along with reduced glutathione (GSH) levels, were analyzed in red blood cell lysates according to Beutler methods, with results obtained through spectrophotometric measurement [19].

### *2.6. ECG Recording*

ECG recordings were conducted on three separate occasions. The initial two recordings took place on the first day of the experiment, specifically before and 10 min following the administration of the first dose of isoprenaline. The third recording was executed at the end of the experiment, before the sacrifice of the animals, on day 10. Prior to the recordings, the rats were anesthetized using a combination of ketamine (30 mg/kg) and xylazine (5 mg/kg) [20]. The ECGs were captured with a sensitivity setting of 2 cm per 1 mV and a speed of paper of 25 mm/s. Lead II was used to analyze the heart rate (beats per minute, bpm), QT interval (seconds, s), and QRS peak-to-peak voltage amplitude (millivolts, mV) [21] in each tracing.

### 2.7. ECHO

On the tenth day of the experiment, all rats were subjected to anesthesia via intraperitoneal administration of 30 mg/kg ketamine and 5 mg/kg xylazine An ECHO was conducted following the ECG. Transthoracic two-dimensional (2D) echocardiography was performed using a Logio 400 CL ultrasound device with an 11 MHz phased array transducer to assess cardiac structure and function. M-mode echocardiographic images were captured in parasternal long-axis and short-axis views at the papillary muscle tips. Measurements included systolic and diastolic septal (IVSs and IVSd) and posterior wall thickness (PDWs, PDWd) and left ventricular internal diameters (LVIDs and LVIDd). Left ventricular ejection fraction (EF), fractional shortening (FS), and end-systolic (ESV) and end-diastolic volume (EDV) were calculated [22]. All measurements were conducted by the same observer following the American Society of Echocardiography guidelines [23,24].

### 2.8. Pathohistological Findings

Isolated hearts were initially preserved in 10% formalin, followed by the formation of tissue blocks using paraffin wax. Each block was subsequently sectioned into 4 μm slices using a microtome and stained with hematoxylin and eosin (H&E). Myocardial injuries were assessed and assigned a score ranging from 1 to 4. A score of 1 indicates no pathological changes in the myocardium; a score of 2 reflects mild damage characterized by multifocal degeneration and slight inflammatory infiltration or localized damage of cardiomyocytes; a score of 3 denotes moderate damage, featuring significant degeneration of cardiomyocytes and/or widespread inflammation; and a score of 4 signifies severe damage, including necrosis accompanied by diffuse inflammation [18,25]. The heart slices were evaluated, and the average score for each group was computed. The assessment of myocardial fibrosis is done by Masson's trichrome stain, which distinctly marks the deposition of collagen within the myocardial tissue [26].

### 2.9. Statistical Analysis

Statistical analysis was conducted utilizing IBM-SPSS Statistics version 29.0 software (SPSS, Inc., Chicago, IL, USA). The ANOVA test was employed to assess the means of parametric variables. For nonparametric variables, the Kruskal–Wallis and Mann–Whitney U tests were used to compare differences among groups. Post hoc analysis was carried out using Tukey, Bonferroni, and LSD tests. The results are expressed as mean ± standard error, with a $p$-value of less than 0.05 deemed statistically significant.

## 3. Results

### 3.1. Effects of Liraglutide Treatment on Body Weight (BW), Heart Weight (HW), and Heart-to-Body Weight (H/BW) Ratio in Rats with Isoprenaline-Induced HF

Liraglutide significantly reduced body weight ($p < 0.05$ versus Con), and the combination of isoprenaline and liraglutide further enhanced this body weight-loss effect. Ten days after the first dose of isoprenaline, heart weight and size increased (Table 1, Figure 2). The H/BW ratio is often used as a more accurate measure of heart size and of heart hypertrophy, and it was increased in isoprenaline-treated rats. However, liraglutide was able to alleviate this alteration.

**Table 1.** Effects of liraglutide treatment on BW, HW, and H/BW in rats with isoprenaline-induced HF.

| Parameters | Groups (Mean ± SE) | | | |
|---|---|---|---|---|
| | Con | Iso | Lir | Iso + Lir |
| BW (g) | 261.33 ± 10.78 | 228.33 ± 6.31 | 216.33 ± 8.16 * | 199.56 ± 8.86 ** † |
| HW (g) | 0.80 ± 0.02 | 0.82 ± 0.02 | 0.71 ± 0.03 † | 0.68 ± 0.03 * † |
| H/BW ratio | 3.05 ± 0.07 | 3.62 ± 0.09 * | 3.22 ± 0.06 † | 3.40 ± 0.09 * |

BW—body weight; HW—heart weight; H/BW—heart-to-body weight ratio; Con—0.9% NaCl s.c. on the first 2 days + 0.9% NaCl s.c. for the next 7 days; Iso—isoprenaline 85 mg/kg s.c. on the first 2 days + 0.9% NaCl s.c. for the next 7 days; Lir—0.9% NaCl s.c. on the first 2 days + liraglutide 1.8 g/kg for the next 7 days; Iso + Lir—isoprenaline 85 mg/kg s.c. on the first 2 days + liraglutide 1.8 g/kg for the next 7 days; * $p < 0.05$ versus Con, ** $p < 0.001$ versus Con, † $p < 0.05$ versus Iso.

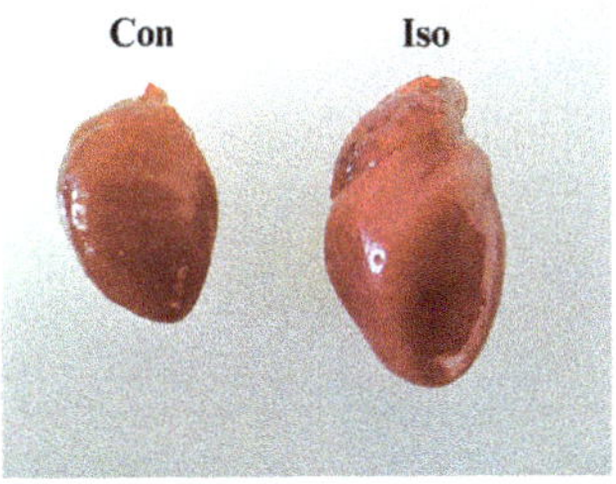


**Figure 2.** Isoprenaline-induced cardiac hypertrophy: comparison of normal (Con group) and isoprenaline-treated heart (Iso group).

### 3.2. Effects of Liraglutide Treatment on Biomarkers of MI and Other Biochemical Parameters in Rats with Isoprenaline-Induced HF

An elevation in cardiac troponin levels is indicative of MI, and elevation in NT-proBNP of HF. A notable rise in the levels of these markers was observed ten days after the initial dose of isoprenaline, and the administration of liraglutide effectively mitigated that increase (Figure 3a,b).

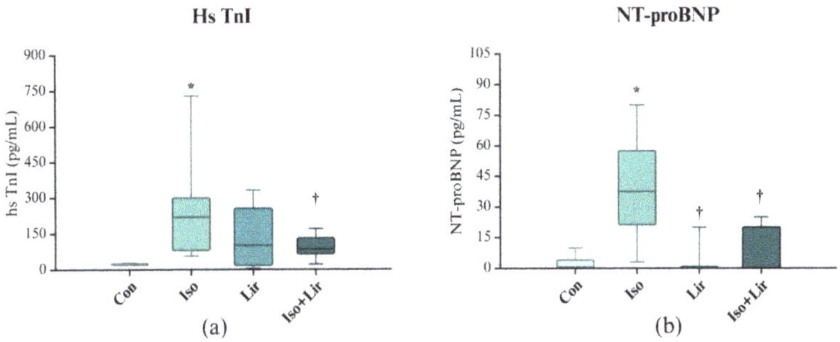


**Figure 3.** Markers of myocardial damage: (**a**) high sensitive troponin I (hs TnI) and (**b**) N-terminal pro-brain natriuretic peptide (NT-proBNP). Con—0.9% NaCl s.c. on the first 2 days + 0.9% NaCl s.c. for the next 7 days; Iso—isoprenaline 85 mg/kg s.c. on the first 2 days + 0.9% NaCl s.c. for the next 7 days; Lir—0.9% NaCl s.c. on the first 2 days + liraglutide 1.8 g/kg for the next 7 days; Iso + Lir—isoprenaline 85 mg/kg s.c. on the first 2 days + liraglutide 1.8 g/kg for the next 7 days; * $p < 0.05$ versus Con, † $p < 0.05$ versus Iso.

Enzymes related to MI, including AST and LDH, were also assessed. Ten days after the first dose of isoprenaline, activities of these enzymes were elevated. Furthermore, ALT activity was measured and revealed a significant rise ($p < 0.05$ Iso versus Con). Moreover, treatment with liraglutide effectively reduced the activities of these enzymes (Table 2).

**Table 2.** Effect of liraglutide treatment on serum biochemical parameters in rats with isoprenaline-induced HF.

| Parameters | Groups (Mean ± SE) | | | |
|---|---|---|---|---|
| | Con | Iso | Lir | Iso + Lir |
| AST (U/L) | 250.58 ± 39.95 | 363.78 ± 41.80 | 284.50 ± 36.84 | 350.67 ± 49.68 |
| ALT (U/L) | 108.67 ± 32.53 | 130.11 ± 7.94 * | 80.17 ± 12.46 † | 123.83 ± 18.64 |
| LDH (U/L) | 1202.67 ± 355.89 | 1968.67 ± 299.43 | 1491.00 ± 264.07 | 1916.67 ± 399.24 |
| Glucose (mmol/L) | 24.58 ± 3.02 | 17.07 ± 2.47 * | 22.38 ± 1.62 | 21.30 ± 1.01 |

AST—aspartate aminotransferase; ALT—alanine aminotransferase; LDH—lactate dehydrogenase; Con—0.9% NaCl s.c. on the first 2 days + 0.9% NaCl s.c. for the next 7 days; Iso—isoprenaline 85 mg/kg s.c. on the first 2 days + 0.9% NaCl s.c. for the next 7 days; Lir—0.9% NaCl s.c. on the first 2 days + liraglutide 1.8 g/kg for the next 7 days; Iso + Lir—isoprenaline 85 mg/kg s.c. on the first 2 days + liraglutide 1.8 g/kg for the next 7 days; * $p < 0.05$ versus Con, † $p < 0.05$ versus Iso.

The administration of isoprenaline, liraglutide, and their combination decreased glucose levels.

The administration of isoprenaline induced a significant change in lipid profile; it increased serum TC, HDL, LDL, and TG (Table 3). The administration of liraglutide significantly restored the levels of TC and HDL ($p < 0.05$ Iso + Lir versus Iso).

**Table 3.** Effect of liraglutide treatment on serum lipid profile in rats with isoprenaline-induced HF.

| Parameters | Groups (Mean ± SE) | | | |
|---|---|---|---|---|
| | Con | Iso | Lir | Iso + Lir |
| TC (mmol/L) | 1.00 ± 0.08 | 1.80 ± 0.23 * | 0.75 ± 0.02 * †† | 1.13 ± 0.17 † ‡ |
| HDL (mmol/L) | 0.37 ± 0.03 | 0.69 ± 0.07 * | 0.28 ± 0.02 †† | 0.46 ± 0.07 † |
| LDL (mmol/L) | 0.16 ± 0.02 | 0.19 ± 0.03 | 0.10 ± 0.00 † | 0.14 ± 0.02 |
| TG (mmol/L) | 0.75 ± 0.15 | 1.03 ± 0.45 | 0.66 ± 0.41 | 0.88 ± 0.16 |

TC—total cholesterol; HDL—high-density lipoprotein; LDL—low-density lipoprotein; TG—triglycerides; Con—0.9% NaCl s.c. on the first 2 days + 0.9% NaCl s.c. for the next 7 days; Iso—isoprenaline 85 mg/kg s.c. on the first 2 days + 0.9% NaCl s.c. for the next 7 days; Lir—0.9% NaCl s.c. on the first 2 days + liraglutide 1.8 g/kg for the next 7 days; Iso + Lir—isoprenaline 85 mg/kg s.c. on the first 2 days + liraglutide 1.8 g/kg for the next 7 days; * $p < 0.05$ versus Con, † $p < 0.05$ versus Iso, †† $p < 0.001$ versus Iso, ‡ $p < 0.05$ versus Lir.

### 3.3. *Effects of Liraglutide Treatment on Prooxidative and Antioxidative Markers in Rats with Isoprenaline-Induced HF*

A significant rise in TBARS, $O_2^-$, and $H_2O_2$ ($p < 0.05$ Con versus Iso) in rats with isoprenaline-induced HF indicates a substantial level of oxidative stress (Figure 4a–d). However, these prooxidative markers were reduced in rats treated with liraglutide. Furthermore, there was a decrease in $NO_2^-$ level, which was alleviated by liraglutide treatment.

Following the first dose of isoprenaline, decreased activities of CAT, SOD, and the level of GSH were recorded ten days later. However, liraglutide managed to restore the reduced levels ($p < 0.05$ Iso + Lir versus Iso) of CAT, SOD, and GSH (Figure 4e–g).

### 3.4. *Effects of Liraglutide Treatment on Electrocardiogram (ECG) in Rats with Isoprenaline-Induced HF*

Isoprenaline administration resulted in a significant increase in heart rate—HR ($p < 0.001$ versus Con)—following the initial injection in both the Iso and Iso + Lir groups, as these groups were identical at that stage (Table 4). Additionally, isoprenaline caused an increase in QRS amplitude following the first dose ($p < 0.05$ Iso versus Con, $p < 0.05$ Iso + Lir versus Con) and a decrease by the end of the experiment ($p < 0.05$ versus Con). After the first dose of isoprenaline, all rats exhibited negative T waves, but ten days later, on the day of sacrifice, the T waves in all animals were positive.

**Table 4.** Effects of liraglutide treatment on ECG parameters in rats with isoprenaline-induced HF.

| Parameters | Groups (Mean ± SE) | | | |
|---|---|---|---|---|
| | Con | Iso | Lir | Iso + Lir |
| HR 1 (bpm) | 243.22 ± 13.09 | 436.51 ± 7.94 ** | 245.67 ± 10.75 †† | 439.28 ± 14.87 ** ‡‡ |
| HR 2 (bpm) | 240.38 ± 4.30 | 220.88 ± 6.28 | 237.64 ± 6.05 | 226.13 ± 11.90 |
| QT 1 (s) | 0.173 ± 0.007 | 0.089 ± 0.005 ** | 0.167 ± 0.004 †† | 0.094 ± 0.004 ** ‡‡ |
| QT 2 (s) | 0.170 ± 0.010 | 0.200 ± 0.017 | 0.173 ± 0.008 | 0.188 ± 0.010 |
| QRS 1 (mV) | 0.280 ± 0.018 | 0.405 ± 0.045 * | 0.268 ± 0.009 † | 0.411 ± 0.042 * ‡ |
| QRS 2 (mV) | 0.302 ± 0.033 | 0.204 ± 0.024 * | 0.290 ± 0.019 † | 0.210 ± 0.027 * ‡ |

HR 1—heart rate after the first dose of isoprenaline; HR 2—heart rate before sacrifice; QT 1—QT interval after the first dose of isoprenaline; QT 2—QT interval before sacrifice; QRS 1—QRS peak-to-peak after the first dose of isoprenaline; QRS 2—QRS peak-to-peak before sacrifice; Con—0.9% NaCl s.c. on the first 2 days + 0.9% NaCl s.c. for the next 7 days; Iso—isoprenaline 85 mg/kg s.c. on the first 2 days + 0.9% NaCl s.c. for the next 7 days; Lir—0.9% NaCl s.c. on the first 2 days + liraglutide 1.8 g/kg for the next 7 days; Iso + Lir—isoprenaline 85 mg/kg s.c. on the first 2 days + liraglutide 1.8 g/kg for the next 7 days; * $p < 0.05$ versus Con, ** $p < 0.001$ versus Con, † $p < 0.05$ versus Iso, †† $p < 0.001$ versus Iso, ‡ $p < 0.05$ versus Lir, ‡‡ $p < 0.001$ versus Lir.

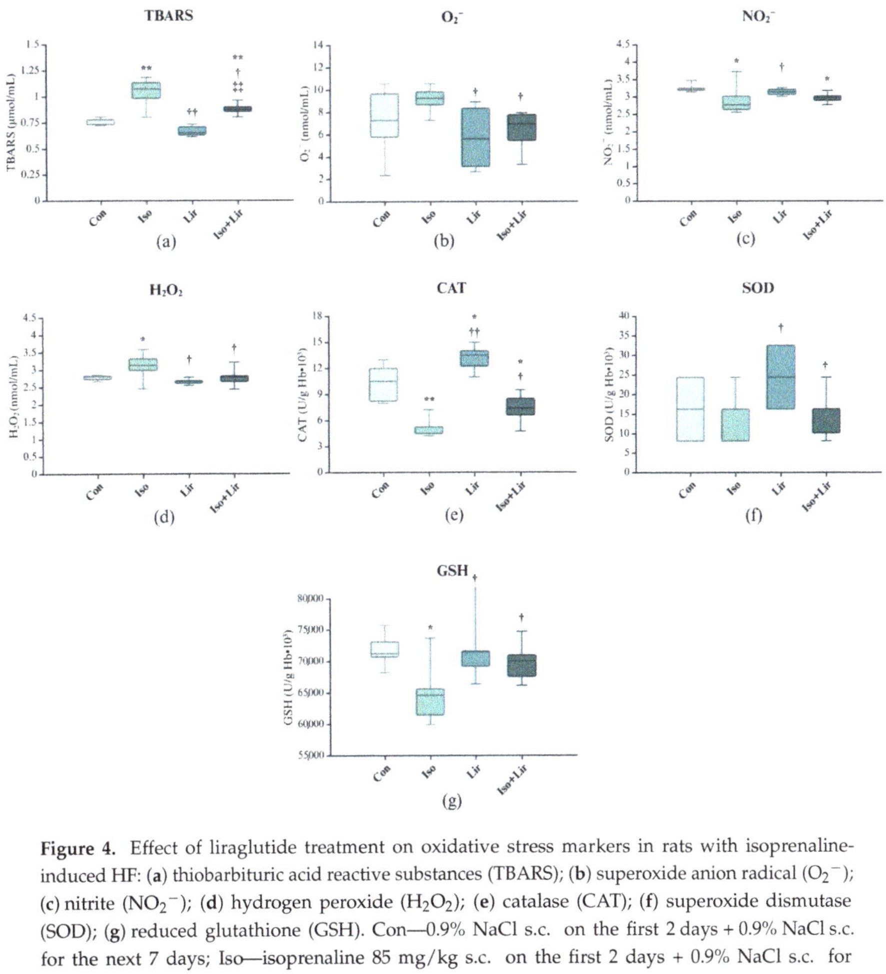


**Figure 4.** Effect of liraglutide treatment on oxidative stress markers in rats with isoprenaline-induced HF: (**a**) thiobarbituric acid reactive substances (TBARS); (**b**) superoxide anion radical ($O_2^-$); (**c**) nitrite ($NO_2^-$); (**d**) hydrogen peroxide ($H_2O_2$); (**e**) catalase (CAT); (**f**) superoxide dismutase (SOD); (**g**) reduced glutathione (GSH). Con—0.9% NaCl s.c. on the first 2 days + 0.9% NaCl s.c. for the next 7 days; Iso—isoprenaline 85 mg/kg s.c. on the first 2 days + 0.9% NaCl s.c. for the next 7 days; Lir—0.9% NaCl s.c. on the first 2 days + liraglutide 1.8 g/kg for the next 7 days; Iso + Lir—isoprenaline 85 mg/kg s.c. on the first 2 days + liraglutide 1.8 g/kg for the next 7 days; * $p < 0.05$ versus Con, ** $p < 0.001$ versus Con, † $p < 0.05$ versus Iso, †† $p < 0.001$ versus Iso, ‡‡ $p < 0.001$ versus Lir.

### 3.5. Effects of Liraglutide Treatment on Echocardiogram (ECHO) in Rats with Isoprenaline-Induced HF

Ten days after the first dose of isoprenaline, the left ventricle internal diameter in systole (LVIDs) was increased (Figure 5). The treatment with liraglutide effectively inhibited the rise of LVIDs ($p < 0.05$ Iso + Lir versus Iso).

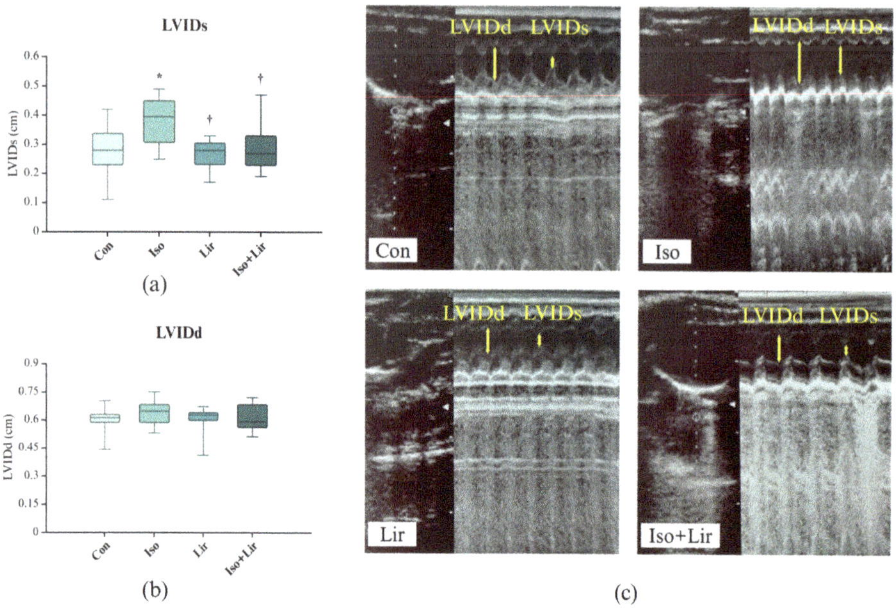


**Figure 5.** Effect of liraglutide treatment on left ventricle internal diameter (LVID) in rats with isoprenaline-induced HF: (**a**) in systole (LVIDs); (**b**) in diastole (LVIDd); (**c**) ECHO image of LVIDs and LVIDd (marked with yellow arrows) in all groups. Con—0.9% NaCl s.c. on the first 2 days + 0.9% NaCl s.c. for the next 7 days; Iso—isoprenaline 85 mg/kg s.c. on the first 2 days + 0.9% NaCl s.c. for the next 7 days; Lir—0.9% NaCl s.c. on the first 2 days + liraglutide 1.8 g/kg for the next 7 days; Iso + Lir—isoprenaline 85 mg/kg s.c. on the first 2 days + liraglutide 1.8 g/kg for the next 7 days; * $p < 0.05$ versus Con, † $p < 0.05$ versus Iso.

The thickness of the interventricular septum showed a reduction ten days after the administration of the first dose of isoprenaline, with a more pronounced effect observed during systole compared to diastole (Figure 6a,b); however, this change did not achieve statistical significance. Treatment with liraglutide appeared to mitigate this change.

The administration of isoprenaline also influenced various echocardiographic parameters related to systolic function, including an increase in ESV)and a decrease in PDWs, EF, and FS ($p < 0.05$ versus Con, Figure 6c,e,g,h). Treatment with liraglutide alleviated these modifications ($p < 0.05$ versus Iso + Lir versus Iso).

The relationship of NT-proBNP with ECHO parameters is shown in Figure 7. A significant negative correlation was found between NT-proBNP and PWDd, as well as between NT-proBNP and PWDs. Furthermore, NT-proBNP exhibited a positive correlation with LVIDs and ESV, while it showed negative correlations with both EF and FS.

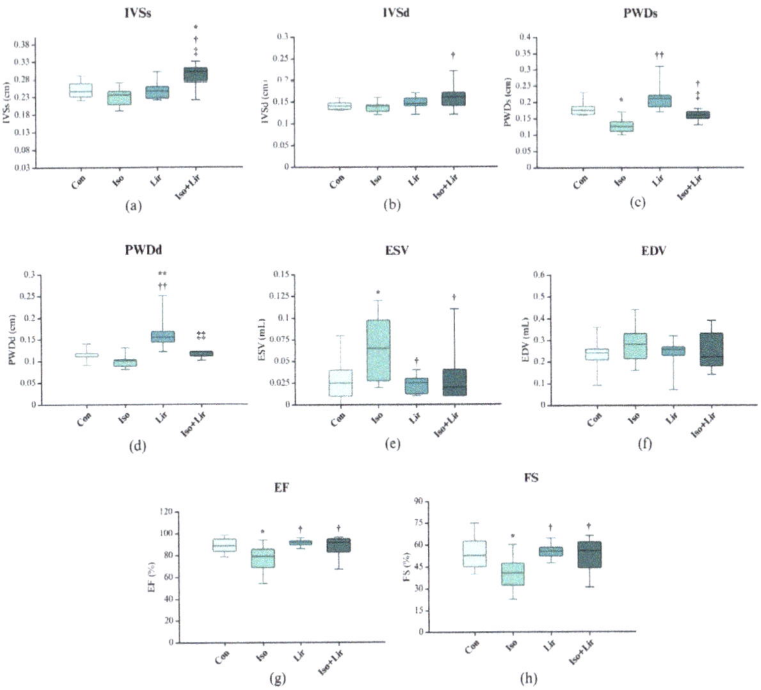


**Figure 6.** Effect of liraglutide treatment on ECHO parameters in rats with isoprenaline-induced HF: (**a**) interventricular septum thickness in systole (IVSs); (**b**) interventricular septum thickness in diastole (IVSd); (**c**) posterior wall diameter in systole (PWDs); (**d**) posterior wall diameter in diastole (PWDd); (**e**) end-systolic volume; (**f**) end-diastolic volume (EDV); (**g**) ejection fraction (EF); (**h**) fractional shortening (FS). Con—0.9% NaCl s.c. on the first 2 days + 0.9% NaCl s.c. for the next 7 days; Iso—isoprenaline 85 mg/kg s.c. on the first 2 days + 0.9% NaCl s.c. for the next 7 days; Lir—0.9% NaCl s.c. on the first 2 days + liraglutide 1.8 g/kg for the next 7 days; Iso + Lir—isoprenaline 85 mg/kg s.c. on the first 2 days + liraglutide 1.8 g/kg for the next 7 days; * $p < 0.05$ versus Con, ** $p < 0.001$ versus Con, † $p < 0.05$ versus Iso, †† $p < 0.001$ versus Iso, ‡ $p < 0.05$ versus Lir, ‡‡ $p < 0.001$ versus Lir.

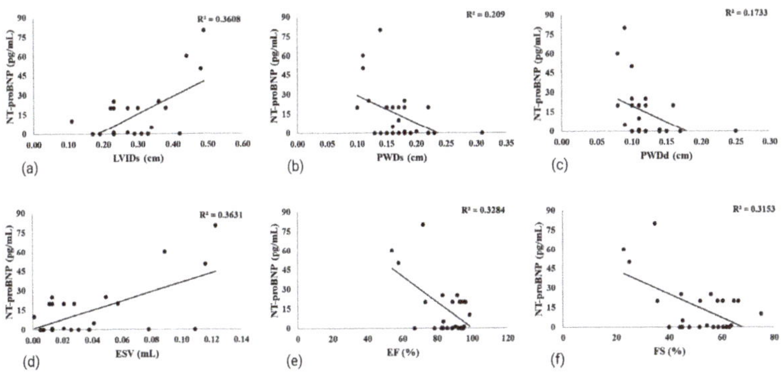


**Figure 7.** The relationship of NT-proBNP with ECHO parameters: (**a**) LVIDs (Pearson correlation R = 0.601, $p < 0.05$); (**b**) PWDs (Pearson correlation R = −0.416, $p < 0.05$); (**c**) PWDs (Pearson correlation R = −0.457, $p < 0.05$) (**d**) ESV (Pearson correlation R = 0.603, $p < 0.05$); (**e**) EF (Pearson correlation R = −0.573, $p < 0.05$); (**f**) FS (Pearson correlation R = −0.562, $p < 0.05$).

### 3.6. Effects of Liraglutide Treatment on Myocardium Morphology in Rats with Isoprenaline-Induced HF

Ten days after the administration of an initial dose of isoprenaline, considerable damage to the myocardium was observed. It was characterized by prominent fragmentation of cardiomyocytes, intercellular edema, infiltration of leukocytes, and hemorrhaging (Figure 8b). A seven-day liraglutide treatment markedly reduced these morphological alterations (Figure 8d,e).

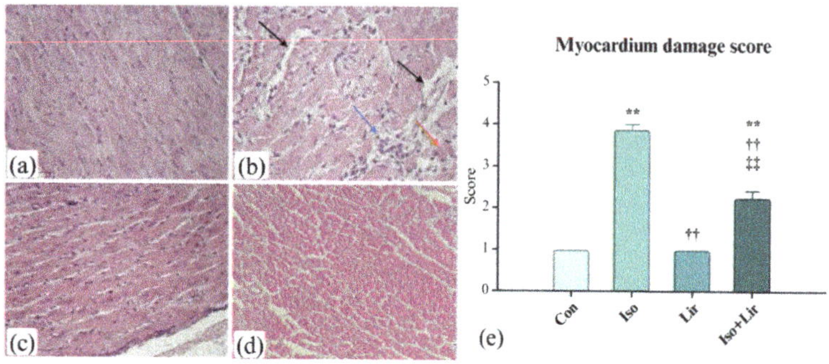


**Figure 8.** Histological characteristics of myocardium after the liraglutide treatment in rats with isoprenaline-induced HF (H&E, magnification ×20): (**a**) Con group—normal histological morphology; (**b**) Iso group—interstitial edema (black arrow), bleeding (red arrow), inflammation (blue arrow); (**c**) Lir group—normal histological morphology; (**d**) Iso + Lir group—reduction of morphological changes caused by isoprenaline; (**e**) myocardium damage score. Con—0.9% NaCl s.c. on the first 2 days + 0.9% NaCl s.c. for the next 7 days; Iso—isoprenaline 85 mg/kg s.c. on the first 2 days + 0.9% NaCl s.c. for the next 7 days; Lir—0.9% NaCl s.c. on the first 2 days + liraglutide 1.8 g/kg for the next 7 days; Iso + Lir—isoprenaline 85 mg/kg s.c. on the first 2 days + liraglutide 1.8 g/kg for the next 7 days; ** $p < 0.001$ versus Con, †† $p < 0.001$ versus Iso, ‡‡ $p < 0.001$ versus Lir.

Figure 9 shows the extent of collagen deposition in myocardium ten days after the first dose of isoprenaline.

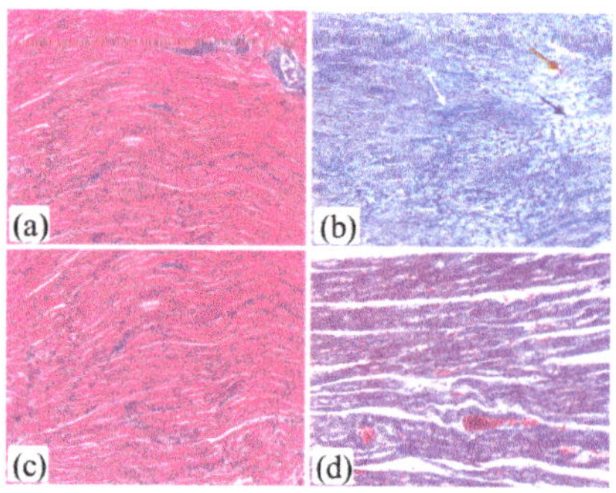


**Figure 9.** The extent of cardiac fibrosis after the liraglutide treatment in rats with isoprenaline-induced HF (Masson trichrome stain, magnification ×20): (**a**) Con group—normal morphology of myocardium; (**b**) Iso group—fibrosis (blue color) with collagen deposits (white arrow), inflammation (purple arrow), bleeding (red arrow), myofibrillar degeneration; (**c**) Lir group—normal morphology of myocardium; (**d**) Iso + Lir group—mild myofibrillar degeneration, dilated blood vessels with extravasation of red blood cells, without inflammation and fibrosis.

## 4. Discussion

Isoprenaline is recognized as a model for MI because it provides adequate mimicry and maintains a low mortality rate, reflecting its considerable reliability in translational medicine [10,27]. The administration of isoprenaline has been associated with heart enlargement [28], represented by the rise in H/BW in this study. Similar observations were made in other studies [29,30].

The findings from this study indicated a reduction in body weight among rats treated with isoprenaline and liraglutide. The observed weight loss in the isoprenaline-treated group may be attributed to the activation of β-adrenoceptors, leading to a decrease in plasma leptin levels, potentially mediated by an increase in cyclic AMP (cAMP) within the adipose tissue. Catecholamines are significant lipolytic hormones, primarily acting through β-adrenoceptors [31]. Liraglutide, a GLP-1 receptor agonist, is used not only for the management of diabetes but also for the treatment of obesity. It demonstrates a considerable impact on body weight reduction [32]. This study noted similar effects of liraglutide on weight loss, and it was particularly pronounced in rats treated with both liraglutide and isoprenaline.

The diagnosis of MI was substantiated by an elevated level of hs TnI. The results of other studies involving the isoprenaline model of MI demonstrated an increase in cardiac troponins [10,33–35]. Natriuretic peptides are recognized as significant biomarkers for diagnosing HF, assessing its severity, and predicting outcomes, as well as potentially aiding in its management. B-type natriuretic peptide (BNP) and NT-proBNP are considered indicators of ventricular stretch, produced in response to the wall stress. As a result, these peptides have become essential components in the evaluation of HF, with their concentration generally increasing in correlation with the deterioration of the condition [36]. An increase in NT-proBNP levels suggests the development of HF. Liraglutide treatment was associated with a significant reduction in hs TnI and NT-proBNP levels, emphasizing the important function of liraglutide in the prevention of HF.

Liraglutide reduces blood glucose by stimulating glucose-dependent insulin secretion and inhibiting glucagon. It effectively lowers glycated hemoglobin and glycemia in adults and may improve pancreatic beta cell function [37]. This study's results demonstrated a lower glucose concentration in animals receiving liraglutide treatment. Additionally, rats treated with isoprenaline also exhibited a decrease in glucose levels, consistent with the observations made by Sobot et al. [10]. Results from the in vitro study of Fiserova et al. [38] demonstrated that acute exposure of cardiomyocytes to isoprenaline led to an elevation in glucose flux at the high dosage of isoprenaline. However, an extended exposure to isoprenaline did not produce a significant impact on glucose flux. The research conducted by Chang et al. [39] indicated that the administration of isoprenaline in obese rats led to an exacerbation of hyperglycemia. It is important to observe that the impact of isoprenaline on glucose metabolism is influenced by both the dosage and the duration of exposure.

The study also revealed an increase in AST, LDH, and ALT enzymes in rats treated with isoprenaline, but significance was noted only for ALT. The findings from multiple studies suggest that the rise in these enzymes is characteristic of the isoprenaline model of MI [11,34,35,40–44]. The activities of LDH, AST, and ALT serve as indicators of changes in the integrity and permeability of cardiomyocyte membranes. An elevation in these cytosolic enzymes in the plasma points to a leakage into the bloodstream, likely resulting from an increased permeability or damaged membranes [35]. Seven-day liraglutide treatment corrected the alterations observed in the activity of these enzymes, but not significantly. The meta-analysis conducted by Malik et al. [45] did not show a statistically significant effect of liraglutide on the reduction of ALT and AST.

This study indicated a rise in TC, LDL, HDL, and TG in rats treated with isoprenaline; however, the rise was significant only in TC and HDL levels. The observed increases in TC, LDL, and TG align with findings from other studies examining isoprenaline-induced MI [46–49]. While Sudha et al. [46] reported an increase in HDL levels, Galal et al. [47] documented a decrease in HDL. Treatment with liraglutide improved the lipid profile in isoprenaline-treated rats, significantly in TC and HDL levels. Similar results were noted in clinical studies [45,50,51].

Increased levels of TBARS, $H_2O_2$, and $O_2^-$ suggest that isoprenaline induced significant oxidative stress. Similar results have been found by other researchers [11,43,49]. In contrast, the level of $NO_2^-$ decreased, which is supported by the study of Rankovic et al. [52], but in a different model of MI, a doxorubicin model. Oxidative stress, along with the generation of oxygen-derived free radicals, is considered a fundamental cause of the various processes that lead to myocardial damage induced by isoprenaline [43]. The presence of highly reactive radicals can lead to lipid peroxidation and initiate cell death through various mechanisms, including apoptosis and autophagy [43,53]. The findings of this study indicated a decline in the activities of SOD and CAT, as well as a reduction in GSH levels, in rats treated with isoprenaline. These findings align with the results of other studies [11,12,35,40,43,49,54]. However, liraglutide demonstrated significant antioxidative properties in both healthy rats and those with isoprenaline-induced HF. The administration of liraglutide resulted in elevated SOD and CAT activities as well as GSH level. Results of the experimental studies showed antioxidative effects [55,56] of the liraglutide treatment similar to ours.

In the current study, an ECG was conducted to assess cardiac function, and to, alongside cardiac troponin levels, confirm the occurrence of MI. Following the administration of isoprenaline, there was a notable increase in heart rate and consequently a decrease in QT interval, which aligns with expectations of isoprenaline as a β-adrenergic agonist. This observation is consistent with findings from other researchers [40]. In addition to the elevated heart rate and the presence of negative T waves, which support the diagnosis of MI [57], alterations in the peak-to-peak amplitude of the QRS complex were observed. The QRS amplitude was elevated in rats treated with isoprenaline, indicating modifications in ventricular depolarization and suggesting ventricular dysfunction. The administration of liraglutide resulted in improvements in electrocardiographic changes.

The ECHO analysis demonstrated that isoprenaline significantly affected cardiac function, with a predominant impact on systolic activity. This influence is characterized by an increase in LVIDs, ESV, and EDV, and a reduction in IVSs, IVSd, PWDs, PWDd, EF, and FS. The alterations in LVIDs, IVs, PDWs, ESV, EF, and FS were significant, suggesting that isoprenaline has a more pronounced effect on systolic function. Similar conclusions were drawn by Li et al. [34]. Decreased EF and FS highlight the substantial impact of isoprenaline on cardiac performance [26,36,58]. Some studies have reported increases in LVIDd, PWDs, and PWDd [36,48]. These differences might result from the distinct experimental protocols and the varying doses of isoprenaline, or the extent of remodeling of the left ventricle. The geometric changes occurring in the ventricle, such as those of shape and size, are the primary driving forces behind the remodeling of the left ventricle. In the early stages of MI, there is an increase in cardiac load as a compensatory response to mechanical and physiological stress. This leads to cardiomyocyte hypertrophy, resulting in myocardial hypertrophy. The decline in cardiac systolic function, along with a subsequent increase in LV volume, can elevate wall stress and oxygen requirements, ultimately contributing to maladaptive tissue remodeling and the onset of HF [8]. The findings of this study indicate that liraglutide has the potential to restore compromised cardiac function and prevent the onset of HF.

Pathohistological assessment showed that administration of isoprenaline resulted in considerable myocardial damage, reflected by a heightened myocardial damage score. The presence of granulocyte infiltration signifies the initiation of myocardial repair after isoprenaline-induced MI. Collagen accumulation indicates the beginning of the heart's remodeling phase [8]. Similar results were presented in other studies [26,27,44,49]. Liraglutide reduced changes in the myocardium induced by isoprenaline, such as inflammation, interstitial edema, myofibrillar degeneration, and fibrosis.

## 5. Conclusions

Liraglutide administration diminishes markers associated with MI and HF, such as hs TnI and NT-proBNP, and facilitates the repair of MI induced by isoprenaline. Furthermore, liraglutide therapy mitigates oxidative stress by lowering levels of TBARS, $H_2O_2$, and $O_2^-$, while simultaneously increasing the activity of CAT and SOD as well as GSH levels. It also restores impaired systolic cardiac function by reducing LVIDs and enhancing EF and FS, effectively preventing HF. Pathohistological examinations reveal that liraglutide effectively reduces inflammation and fibrosis, thereby inhibiting heart remodeling and HF in isoprenaline-treated rats.

**Author Contributions:** Conceptualization, R.S.; methodology, R.S., M.P.S. and D.M.D.; validation, R.S., M.P.S., D.M.D., Z.B. and T.S.; formal analysis, U.M., T.C., S.U., N.M.-K., S.J., Đ.Đ., M.M., A.S. and B.S.; investigation, Z.B. and T.S.; data curation, Z.B. and T.S.; writing—original draft preparation, Z.B.; writing—review and editing, R.S., M.P.S. and D.M.D.; visualization, Z.B.; supervision, R.S. All authors have read and agreed to the published version of the manuscript.

**Funding:** This research received no external funding.

**Institutional Review Board Statement:** The animal study protocol was approved by the Institutional Ethics Committee for the Protection and Welfare of Experimental Animals, Faculty of Medicine, University of Banja Luka, Bosnia and Herzegovina (protocol code 18/1.190-13/22, dated 1 June 2022).

**Informed Consent Statement:** Not applicable.

**Data Availability Statement:** The authors confirm that the data supporting the findings of this study are available within the article.

**Conflicts of Interest:** The authors declare no conflicts of interest.

## References

1. McCarthy, C.; Murphy, S.; Cohen, J.A.; Rehman, S.; Jones-O'Connor, M.; Olshan, D.S.; Singh, A.; Vaduganathan, M.; Januzzi, J.L.; Wasfy, J.H. Misclassification of Myocardial Injury as Myocardial Infarction: Implications for Assessing Outcomes in Value-Based Programs. *JAMA Cardiol.* **2019**, *4*, 460–464. [CrossRef]
2. Taggart, C.; Wereski, R.; Mills, N.L.; Chapman, A.R. Diagnosis, investigation and management of patients with acute and chronic myocardial injury. *J. Clin. Med.* **2021**, *10*, 2331. [CrossRef] [PubMed]
3. Thygesen, K.; Alpert, J.S.; Jaffe, A.S.; Chaitman, B.R.; Bax, J.J.; Morrow, D.A.; White, H.D. Fourth Universal Definition of Myocardial Infarction (2018). *Glob. Heart* **2018**, *13*, 305–338. [CrossRef] [PubMed]
4. Takahashi, J.; Onuma, S.; Hao, K.; Godo, S.; Shiroto, T.; Yasuda, S. Pathophysiology and diagnostic pathway of myocardial infarction with non-obstructive coronary arteries. *J. Cardiol.* **2024**, *83*, 17–24. [CrossRef] [PubMed]
5. Chapman, A.R.; Adamson, P.D.; Mills, N.L. Assessment and classification of patients with myocardial injury and infarction in clinical practice. *Heart* **2017**, *103*, 10–18. [CrossRef]
6. Duan, D.; Li, H.; Chai, S.; Zhang, L.; Fan, T.; Hu, Z.; Feng, Y. The relationship between cardiac oxidative stress, inflammatory cytokine response, cardiac pump function, and prognosis post-myocardial infarction. *Sci. Rep.* **2024**, *14*, 8985. [CrossRef]
7. Bhatt, A.S.; Ambrosy, A.P.; Velazquez, E.J. Adverse Remodeling and Reverse Remodeling After Myocardial Infarction. *Curr. Cardiol. Rep.* **2017**, *19*, 71. [CrossRef]
8. Jiang, H.; Fang, T.; Cheng, Z. Mechanism of heart failure after myocardial infarction. *J. Int. Med. Res.* **2023**, *51*, 03000605231202573. [CrossRef]

9. Jenča, D.; Melenovský, V.; Stehlik, J.; Staněk, V.; Kettner, J.; Kautzner, J.; Adámková, V.; Wohlfahrt, P. Heart failure after myocardial infarction: Incidence and predictors. *ESC Heart Fail.* **2021**, *8*, 222–237. [CrossRef]
10. Sobot, T.; Bajic, Z.; Skrbic, R.; Uletilovic, S.; Mandic-Kovacevic, N.; Cvjetkovic, T.; Malicevic, U.; Djukanovic, D.; Bojic, M.G.; Jovicic, S.; et al. Effect of folic acid on isoprenaline-induced myocardial injury in rats. *Physiol. Int.* **2024**, *111*, 80–96. [CrossRef]
11. Asdaq, S.M.B.; Alamri, A.S.; Alsanie, W.F.; Alhomrani, M. Cardioprotective potential of garlic oil and its active constituent, diallyl disulphide, in presence of carvedilol during chronic isoprenaline injection-mediated myocardial necrosis in rats. *Molecules* **2021**, *26*, 5137. [CrossRef] [PubMed]
12. Mi, X.; Zhang, Z.; Cheng, J.; Xu, Z.; Zhu, K.; Ren, Y. Cardioprotective effects of Schisantherin A against isoproterenol-induced acute myocardial infarction through amelioration of oxidative stress and inflammation via modulation of PI3K-AKT/Nrf2/ARE and TLR4/MAPK/NF-κB pathways in rats. *BMC Complement. Med. Ther.* **2023**, *23*, 277. [CrossRef] [PubMed]
13. Hansen, H.H.; Fabricius, K.; Barkholt, P.; Niehoff, M.L.; Morley, J.E.; Jelsing, J.; Pyke, C.; Knudsen, L.B.; Farr, S.A.; Vrang, N. The GLP-1 Receptor Agonist Liraglutide Improves Memory Function and Increases Hippocampal CA1 Neuronal Numbers in a Senescence-Accelerated Mouse Model of Alzheimer's Disease. *J. Alzheimer's Dis.* **2015**, *46*, 877–888. [CrossRef] [PubMed]
14. Petković-Dabić, J.; Binić, I.; Carić, B.; Umičević-Šipka, S.; Bednarčuk, N.; Dabić, S.; Šitum, M.; Popović-Pejičić, S.; Stojiljković, M.P.; Škrbić, R. Effects of Semaglutide Treatment on Psoriatic Lesions in Obese Patients with Type 2 Diabetes Mellitus: An Open-Label, Randomized Clinical Trial. *Biomolecules* **2025**, *15*, 46. [CrossRef]
15. Shaman, A.M.; Bain, S.C.; Bakris, G.L.; Buse, J.B.; Idorn, T.; Mahaffey, K.W.; Mann, J.F.E.; Nauck, M.A.; Rasmussen, S.; Rossing, P.; et al. Effect of the Glucagon-Like Peptide-1 Receptor Agonists Semaglutide and Liraglutide on Kidney Outcomes in Patients With Type 2 Diabetes: Pooled Analysis of SUSTAIN 6 and LEADER. *Circulation* **2022**, *145*, 575–585. [CrossRef]
16. Savchenko, L.G.; Digtiar, N.I.; Selikhova, L.G.; Kaidasheva, E.I.; Shlykova, O.A.; Vesnina, L.E.; Kaidashev, I.P. Liraglutide exerts an anti-inflammatory action in obese patients with type 2 diabetes. *Rom. J. Intern. Med.* **2019**, *57*, 233–240. [CrossRef]
17. Liu, X.; Huang, J.; Li, J.; Mao, Q.; He, J. Effects of liraglutide combined with insulin on oxidative stress and serum MCP-1 and NF-B levels in type 2 diabetes. *J. Coll. Physicians Surg. Pak.* **2019**, *29*, 218–221. [CrossRef]
18. Bajic, Z.; Sobot, T.; Uletilovic, S.; Mandic-Kovacevic, N.; Cvjetkovic, T.; Malicevic, U.; Djukanovic, D.; Duran, M.; Vesic, N.; Avram, S.; et al. Cardioprotective effects of liraglutide pretreatment on isoprenaline-induced myocardial injury in rats. *Can. J. Physiol. Pharmacol.* **2023**, *101*, 258–267. [CrossRef]
19. Mandić-Kovačević, N.; Kukrić, Z.; Latinović, S.; Cvjetković, T.; Šobot, T.; Bajić, Z.; Maličević, U.; Marinković, S.; Đukanović, Đ.; Uletilović, S.; et al. Antioxidative Potential of Pomegranate Peel Extract: In Vitro and In Vivo Studies. *Scr. Medica* **2023**, *54*, 9–18. [CrossRef]
20. Redfors, B.; Shao, Y.; Omerovic, E. Influence of anesthetic agent, depth of anesthesia and body temperature on cardiovascular functional parameters in the rat. *Lab. Anim.* **2014**, *48*, 6–14. [CrossRef]
21. Taşkıran, E.; Erdoğan, M.A.; Yiğittürk, G.; Erbaş, O. Therapeutic Effects of Liraglutide, Oxytocin and Granulocyte Colony-Stimulating Factor in Doxorubicin-Induced Cardiomyopathy Model: An Experimental Animal Study. *Cardiovasc. Toxicol.* **2019**, *19*, 510–517. [CrossRef] [PubMed]
22. Brown, L.; Fenning, A.; Chan, V.; Loch, D.; Wilson, K.; Anderson, B.; Burstow, D. Echocardiographic Assessment of Cardiac Structure and Function in Rats. *Heart Lung Circ.* **2002**, *11*, 167–173. [CrossRef] [PubMed]
23. Hubesch, G.; Hanthazi, A.; Acheampong, A.; Chomette, L.; Lasolle, H.; Hupkens, E.; Jespers, P.; Vegh, G.; Wembonyama, C.W.M.; Verhoeven, C.; et al. A Preclinical Rat Model of Heart Failure With Preserved Ejection Fraction With Multiple Comorbidities. *Front. Cardiovasc. Med.* **2022**, *8*, 809885. [CrossRef] [PubMed]
24. Dohi, K. Echocardiographic assessment of cardiac structure and function in chronic renal disease. *J. Echocardiogr.* **2019**, *17*, 115–122. [CrossRef]
25. Hamed, A.B.; Mantawy, E.M.; El-Bakly, W.M.; Abdel-Mottaleb, Y.; Azab, S.S. Putative anti-inflammatory, antioxidant, and anti-apoptotic roles of the natural tissue guardian methyl palmitate against isoproterenol-induced myocardial injury in rats. *Futur. J. Pharm. Sci.* **2020**, *6*, 31. [CrossRef]
26. Qi, C.; Shao, Y.; Liu, X.; Wang, D.; Li, X. The cardioprotective effects of icariin on the isoprenaline-induced takotsubo-like rat model: Involvement of reactive oxygen species and the TLR4/NF-κB signaling pathway. *Int. Immunopharmacol.* **2019**, *74*, 105733. [CrossRef]
27. Elshaer, A.; El-Awady, W.S.; Masoud, M.M.; Elmenshawy, M.D.; Wageeh, S.; Shehata, I.E. Comparative Study Among Three Different Models for Induction of Acute Myocardial Infarction in Rats. *Eur. Heart J. Suppl.* **2021**, *23*, D1–D7. [CrossRef]
28. Zhou, D.; Liu, W.; Zhang, J.; Dong, Y.; Wu, J.; Zhang, Y.; Dai, C.; Zhang, T.; Yang, G.; Zhang, Y.; et al. Bellidifolin ameliorates isoprenaline-induced cardiac hypertrophy by the Nox4/ROS signalling pathway through inhibiting BRD4. *Cell Death Discov.* **2023**, *9*, 279. [CrossRef]
29. Li, Y.; He, B.; Zhang, C.; Xia, T.; Zeng, C. Naringenin Attenuates Isoprenaline-Induced Cardiac Hypertrophy by Suppressing Oxidative Stress through the AMPK/NOX2/MAPK Signaling Pathway. *Nutrients* **2023**, *15*, 1340. [CrossRef]

30. Yoon, J.J.; Tai, A.L.; Kim, H.Y.; Han, B.H.; Shin, S.; Lee, H.S.; Kang, D.G. TongGuanWan Alleviates Doxorubicin- and Isoproterenol-Induced Cardiac Hypertrophy and Fibrosis by Modulating Apoptotic and Fibrotic Pathways. *Int. J. Mol. Sci.* **2024**, *25*, 10573. [CrossRef]
31. Baynes, K.C.R.; Nicholas, M.D.; Shojaee-Moradie, F.; Umpleby, A.M.; Giannoulis, M.G. Acute regulation of plasma leptin by isoprenaline in lean and obese fasted subjects. *Diabetes Obes. Metab.* **2006**, *8*, 412–418. [CrossRef] [PubMed]
32. Gasoyan, H.; Pfoh, E.R.; Schulte, R.; Le, P.; Butsch, W.S.; Rothberg, M.B. One-Year Weight Reduction With Semaglutide or Liraglutide in Clinical Practice. *JAMA Netw. Open* **2024**, *7*, e2433326. [CrossRef] [PubMed]
33. Anamalley, R.; Rajassageran, L.; Apparoo, Y.; Jauri, M.H.; Kamisah, Y.; Yunos, N.M.; Zainalabidin, S. Repeated Administration of Low Dose Isoprenaline on the Rat's Cardiovascular System. *Sains Malays.* **2022**, *51*, 2147–2157. [CrossRef]
34. Li, L.; Fang, H.; Yu, Y.H.; Liu, S.X.; Yang, Z.Q. Liquiritigenin attenuates isoprenaline-induced myocardial fibrosis in mice through the tgf-β1/smad2 and akt/erk signaling pathways. *Mol. Med. Rep.* **2021**, *24*, 686. [CrossRef]
35. Pham, V.A.; Tran, H.T.; Mai, T.P.; Nguyen, L.H.; Nguyen, V.H.; Nguyen, T.H.; Bui, S.S.; Van Vu, A.; Do, H.T.; Trinh, Q.V. Myocardial infarction model induced by isoproterenol in rats and potential cardiovascular protective effect of a nattokinase-containing hard capsule. *Phytomed. Plus* **2023**, *3*, 100472. [CrossRef]
36. Keihanian, F.; Moohebati, M.; Saeidinia, A.; Mohajeri, S.A.; Madaeni, S. Therapeutic effects of medicinal plants on isoproterenol-induced heart failure in rats. *Biomed. Pharmacother.* **2021**, *134*, 111101. [CrossRef]
37. Jensen, S.B.K.; Juhl, C.R.; Janus, C.; Lundgren, J.R.; Martinussen, C.; Wiingaard, C.; Knudsen, C.; Frikke-Schmidt, R.; Stallknecht, B.M.; Holst, J.J.; et al. Weight loss maintenance with exercise and liraglutide improves glucose tolerance, glucagon response, and beta cell function. *Obesity* **2023**, *31*, 977–989. [CrossRef]
38. Fiserova, I.; Trinh, M.D.; Elkalaf, M.; Vacek, L.; Heide, M.; Martinkova, S.; Bechynska, K.; Kosek, V.; Hajslova, J.; Fiser, O.; et al. Isoprenaline modified the lipidomic profile and reduced β-oxidation in HL-1 cardiomyocytes: In vitro model of takotsubo syndrome. *Front. Cardiovasc. Med.* **2022**, *9*, 917989. [CrossRef]
39. Chang, G.R.; Chen, W.K.; Hou, P.H.; Mao, F.C. Isoproterenol exacerbates hyperglycemia and modulates chromium distribution in mice fed with a high fat diet. *J. Trace Elem. Med. Biol.* **2017**, *44*, 315–321. [CrossRef]
40. Tawfik, M.K.; Ameen, A.M. Cardioprotective effect of ranolazine in nondiabetic and diabetic male rats subjected to isoprenaline-induced acute myocardial infarction involves modulation of AMPK and inhibition of apoptosis. *Can. J. Physiol. Pharmacol.* **2019**, *97*, 661–674. [CrossRef]
41. Hosseini, A.; Rajabian, A.; Sobhanifar, M.A.; Alavi, M.S.; Taghipour, Z.; Hasanpour, M.; Iranshahi, M.; Boroumand-Noughabi, S.; Banach, M.; Sahebkar, A. Attenuation of isoprenaline-induced myocardial infarction by Rheum turkestanicum. *Biomed. Pharmacother.* **2022**, *148*, 112775. [CrossRef]
42. Marinković, S.T.; Đukanović, Đ.; Duran, M.; Bajic, Z.; Sobot, T.; Uletilović, S.; Mandić-Kovacević, N.; Cvjetković, T.; Maksimović, Ž.M.Ž.M.; Maličević, U.; et al. Pomegranate peel extract attenuates isoprenaline-induced Takotsubo-like myocardial injury in rats. *Pharmaceutics* **2023**, *15*, 1697. [CrossRef]
43. Abdelrahaman, D.; Habotta, O.A.; Taher, E.S.; El-Ashry, E.S.; Ibrahim, I.; Abdeen, A.; Ibrahim, A.M.; Ibrahim, R.M.; Anwer, H.; Mihaela, O.; et al. Suppression of NLRP3 inflammasome orchestrates the protective efficacy of tiron against isoprenaline-induced myocardial injury. *Front. Pharmacol.* **2024**, *15*, 1379908. [CrossRef] [PubMed]
44. Sajid, A.; Ahmad, T.; Ikram, M.; Khan, T.; Shah, A.J.; Mahnashi, M.H.; Alhasaniah, A.H.; Al Awadh, A.A.; Almazni, I.A.; Alshahrani, M.M. Cardioprotective Potential of Aqueous Extract of Fumaria indica on Isoproterenol-Induced Myocardial Infarction in SD Rats. *Oxid. Med. Cell. Longev.* **2022**, *2022*, 2112956. [CrossRef] [PubMed]
45. Malik, A.; Amjad, W.; Inayat, F.; Nadeem, M.; Weissman, S.; Malik, M.I.; Jajja, A.A.; Khan, A.; Tabibian, J.H. The effects of liraglutide on liver enzymes and metabolic factors in patients with nonalcoholic steatohepatitis: A meta-analysis of randomized controlled trials. *Gastroenterol. Rev.* **2023**, *18*, 100–109. [CrossRef] [PubMed]
46. Sudha, M.; Rajkumar, D. Effect of glutathione in lipid profile in isoprenaline induced myocardial infarction in male albino rats. *MedPulse Int. J. Physiol.* **2019**, *11*, 45–48. [CrossRef]
47. Galal, O.; Mostafa, A.; Mohamed, H.; Ahmed, A.R.H.; Hashim, M.S.; Mohamed, N. Cardioprotective Effects of Nano-Vitamin D on Isoprenaline-Induced Myocardial Infarction Rat Model. *SVU-Int. J. Med. Sci.* **2022**, *5*, 136–151. [CrossRef]
48. Lan, T.; Zeng, Q.; Jiang, W.; Liu, T.; Xu, W.; Yao, P.; Lu, W. Metabolism disorder promotes isoproterenol-induced myocardial injury in mice with high temperature and high humidity and high-fat diet. *BMC Cardiovasc. Disord.* **2022**, *22*, 133. [CrossRef]
49. Ahsan, F.; Mahmood, T.; Wani, T.A.; Zargar, S.; Siddiqui, M.H.; Usmani, S.; Shamim, A.; Wahajuddin, M. Effectual Endeavors of Silk Protein Sericin against Isoproterenol Induced Cardiac Toxicity and Hypertrophy in Wistar Rats. *Life* **2022**, *12*, 1063. [CrossRef]
50. Nowrouzi-Sohrabi, P.; Soroush, N.; Tabrizi, R.; Shabani-Borujeni, M.; Rezaei, S.; Jafari, F.; Hosseini-Bensenjan, M.; Stricker, B.H.; van Hoek, M.; Ahmadizar, F. Effect of Liraglutide on Cardiometabolic Risk Profile in People with Coronary Artery Disease with or without Type 2 Diabetes: A Systematic Review and Meta-Analysis of Randomized Controlled Trials. *Front. Pharmacol.* **2021**, *12*, 618208. [CrossRef]

51. Aoki, K.; Kamiyama, H.; Takihata, M.; Taguri, M.; Shibata, E.; Shinoda, K.; Yoshii, T.; Nakajima, S.; Terauchi, Y. Effect of liraglutide on lipids in patients with type 2 diabetes: A pilot study. *Endocr. J.* **2020**, *67*, 957–962. [CrossRef] [PubMed]
52. Rankovic, M.; Draginic, N.; Jeremic, J.; Samanovic, A.M.; Stojkov, S.; Mitrovic, S.; Jeremic, N.; Radonjic, T.; Srejovic, I.; Bolevich, S.; et al. Protective Role of Vitamin B1 in Doxorubicin-Induced Cardiotoxicity in Rats: Focus on Hemodynamic, Redox, and Apoptotic Markers in Heart. *Front. Physiol.* **2021**, *12*, 690619. [CrossRef] [PubMed]
53. Bajic, Z.; Sobot, T.; Amidzic, L.; Vojinovic, N.; Jovicic, S.; Gajic Bojic, M.; Djuric, D.M.; Stojiljkovic, M.P.; Bolevich, S.; Skrbic, R. Liraglutide Protects Cardiomyocytes against Isoprenaline-Induced Apoptosis in Experimental Takotsubo Syndrome. *Biomedicines* **2024**, *12*, 1207. [CrossRef] [PubMed]
54. Fathiazad, F.; Tamarzadeh, N.; Alsos, D.; Garjani, A.; Vaez, H. The effect of astragaloside IV on isoproterenol-induced myocardial infarction in rats. *Pharm. Sci.* **2019**, *25*, 100–110. [CrossRef]
55. Zhang, L.; Li, C.; Zhu, Q.; Li, N.; Zhou, H. Liraglutide, a glucagon-like peptide-1 analog, inhibits high glucose-induced oxidative stress and apoptosis in neonatal rat cardiomyocytes. *Exp. Ther. Med.* **2019**, *17*, 3734–3740. [CrossRef]
56. El-Shafey, M.; El-Agawy, M.S.E.-d.; Eldosoky, M.; Ebrahim, H.A.; Elsherbini, D.M.A.; El-Sherbiny, M.; Asseri, S.M.; Elsherbiny, N.M. Role of Dapagliflozin and Liraglutide on Diabetes-Induced Cardiomyopathy in Rats: Implication of Oxidative Stress, Inflammation, and Apoptosis. *Front. Endocrinol.* **2022**, *13*, 862394. [CrossRef]
57. Konopelski, P.; Ufnal, M. Electrocardiography in rats: A comparison to human. *Physiol. Res.* **2016**, *65*, 717–725. [CrossRef]
58. Forte, E.; Panahi, M.; Baxan, N.; Ng, F.S.; Boyle, J.J.; Branca, J.; Bedard, O.; Hasham, M.G.; Benson, L.; Harding, S.E.; et al. Type 2 MI induced by a single high dose of isoproterenol in C57BL/6J mice triggers a persistent adaptive immune response against the heart. *J. Cell. Mol. Med.* **2021**, *25*, 229–243. [CrossRef]


**Disclaimer/Publisher's Note:** The statements, opinions and data contained in all publications are solely those of the individual author(s) and contributor(s) and not of MDPI and/or the editor(s). MDPI and/or the editor(s) disclaim responsibility for any injury to people or property resulting from any ideas, methods, instructions or products referred to in the content.

life

Review

# Perioperative Considerations of Novel Antidiabetic Agents in Heart Failure Patients Undergoing Cardiac Surgery

**Ashley Wang [1], Savannah Bitzas [2], Dilsa Perez [2], Jonathon Schwartz [1], Saleem Zaidi [1], Jonathan Oster [1] and Sergio D. Bergese [1,*]**

1 Department of Anesthesiology, Stony Brook University Hospital, Stony Brook, NY 11794, USA; ashley.wang@stonybrookmedicine.edu (A.W.); jonathon.schwartz@stonybrookmedicine.edu (J.S.); saleem.zaidi@stonybrookmedicine.edu (S.Z.); jonathan.oster@stonybrookmedicine.edu (J.O.)
2 Renaissance School of Medicine, Stony Brook University, Stony Brook, NY 11794, USA; savannah.bitzas@stonybrookmedicine.edu (S.B.); dilsa.perez@stonybrookmedicine.edu (D.P.)
* Correspondence: sergio.bergese@stonybrookmedicine.edu

**Abstract:** Diabetes mellitus (DM) is a major risk factor for cardiovascular disease, including heart failure (HF). A high proportion of DM patients eventually require cardiac surgery. While the traditional approach to DM therapy focuses on tight glucose control with insulin and oral hypoglycemic agents, novel antidiabetic drugs have emerged over the past two decades that offer not only improved glycemic control but also cardiovascular and renal protection, such as benefits in HF management. The aim of this review is to examine and evaluate the perioperative risk and benefits of novel antidiabetic agents in HF treatment for both DM and non-DM patients undergoing cardiac surgery. We specifically studied glucagon-like peptide-1 receptor agonists (GLP-1RAs), dipeptidyl peptidase-4 (DPP-4) inhibitors, and sodium–glucose cotransporter 2 inhibitors (SGLT2is). Although studies on novel antidiabetic therapy in cardiac surgeries were limited, the results showed all three agents to be safe for use in the perioperative period, with SLGT2i demonstrating the most benefits in HF management for those with or without DM and kidney impairment undergoing cardiac surgery. Future research on larger study populations and using a more rigorous study design is necessary in bridging current knowledge to improve patient outcomes.

**Keywords:** diabetes mellitus; heart failure; GLP-1 receptor agonist; DPP-4 inhibitors; SGLT2 inhibitors; cardiac surgery; cardiovascular disease; glycemic control; perioperative management

## 1. Introduction

Diabetes mellitus (DM) is a well-known risk factor for cardiovascular disease (CVD), which includes myocardial infarction (MI), strokes, and heart failure (HF). Among diabetics, CVD is one of the leading causes of mortality [1]. One hallmark of the DM-CVD interplay comes from the observation that the prevalence of HF in diabetics is between 9% to 22% in diabetic patients—four times higher than the general population [2]. Furthermore, among patients with HF, those with DM have a higher risk of hospitalization and worse health-related quality of life compared to those without [2]. As such, a comprehensive, multifactorial approach to the management of DM is essential to improved health outcomes in these patients.

Medical management for DM typically focuses on careful blood glucose (BG) control through insulin therapy, secretagogues, and oral hypoglycemic agents. However, this approach can be difficult to maintain given the challenges of frequent glucose monitoring, patient non-adherence, and adverse reactions from medications [3]. In addition, treating DM solely through tight blood sugar control does not adequately address the complexity of the disease across other organ systems such as the heart and kidneys. Given the need for new therapeutic approaches to DM management, several classes of novel antidiabetic agents have emerged over the past two decades for type 2 DM (T2DM) (Figure 1). Among these are glucagon-like peptide-1 (GLP-1) receptor agonists, dipeptidyl peptidase-4 (DPP-4) inhibitors, and sodium–glucose cotransporter 2 (SGLT-2) inhibitors. Besides providing improved BG control similar to traditional diabetic therapy, these novel agents have also demonstrated cardiovascular and renal protection, including benefits in HF management [3]. Approximately 20% of cardiac surgery patients have pre-existing diabetes mellitus, many of which require insulin therapy [4,5]. Because novel antidiabetic agents may confer organ protective effects separate from BG control, these agents may afford significant benefit in HF patients undergoing cardiac surgery, with or without DM.

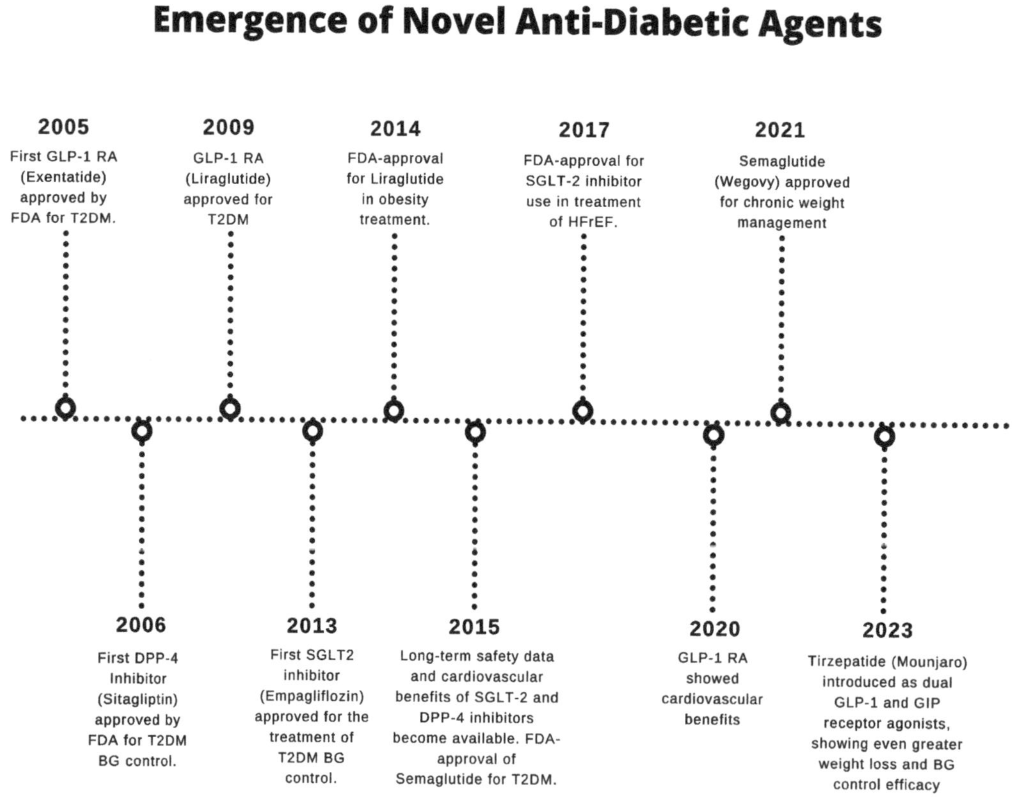


**Figure 1.** Timeline of emerging novel antidiabetic agents. GLP-1RA = Glucagon-like peptide-1 receptor agonists, FDA = Food and Drug Administration, T2DM = Type 2 diabetes mellitus, SGLT-2 = Sodium–glucose cotransporter 2, HFrEF = Heart failure with reduced ejection fraction, DPP-4 = Dipeptidyl peptidase-4, BG = Blood glucose, GIP = Glucose-dependent insulinotropic polypeptide.

Every year, an estimated 1 to 1.5 million cardiac surgeries are performed globally [6]. In coronary artery bypass grafting (CABG), the prevalence of DM ranges from 12% to 40% [7–10]. Despite the rise in popularity of novel antidiabetic therapy for managing DM and HF, guidelines addressing perioperative use of these medications in cardiac surgery are limited. Since HF is associated with poorer health outcomes and higher mortality rates following cardiac surgery, novel antidiabetic agents may have a role in improving perioperative outcomes, independent of diabetic status [11,12]. Therefore, the aim of this review is to examine and evaluate the risk and benefits of novel antidiabetic agents in HF treatment for patients undergoing cardiac surgery, with or without DM (Figure 2). The scope of this paper includes the use of novel antidiabetic agents independently, not as combination therapies, in HF patients undergoing cardiac surgeries, including, but not limited to, CABG, valvular surgery, and durable mechanical circulatory support. This review will focus on outcomes for cardiac surgery patients in the immediate postoperative period, i.e., from the time a patient exits the operating room after surgery to when he or she approaches readiness for discharge.

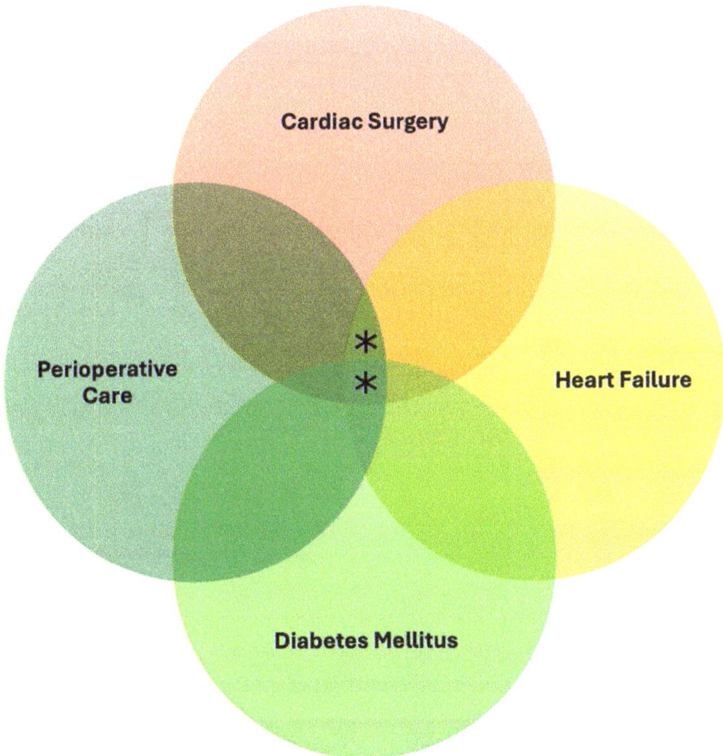


**Figure 2.** Venn diagram illustrating the various comorbidity and procedural features for the patient population of interest. The asterisks indicate the patient population of interest for the application of novel antidiabetic agents. Both heart failure and diabetes mellitus are common among cardiac surgery patients.

## 2. Overview of Novel Antidiabetic Agents

### *2.1. Glucagon-like Peptide-1 Receptor Agonists (GLP-1RAs)*

GLP-1 is a naturally occurring peptide produced from proglucagon within the intestinal mucosa, pancreatic islet alpha cells, and neurons in the nucleus of the solitary tract [13,14]. GLP-1 is an incretin hormone that regulates BG levels; it has a short duration of action as it is enzymatically degraded within 1 to 2 min by DPP-4. GLP-1 receptor is a G protein-coupled receptor with specific affinity for GLP-1 and is localized to the cellular membrane. GLP-1 receptor is involved in regulating insulin and glucagon secretion, maintaining glucose homeostasis [15,16]. GLP-1 receptor agonists (GLP-1RAs) are part of the new wave of antidiabetic agents that came to market, with Exenatide being the first GLP-1RA approved by the Food and Drug Administration (FDA) for T2DM in 2005 and Liraglutide approved by the FDA for obesity treatment in 2014. GLP-1RAs are GLP-1 analogs that stimulate insulin release and reduce glucagon production. GLP-1RAs, while structurally similar to GLP-1, include modifications to impede hydrolysis by DPP-4 to extend the half-life of the drug [15,16]. These GLP-1RAs have been shown to improve BG control in patients with T2DM and assist with weight loss in those experiencing obesity. This drug class should be considered in patients who have a contraindication to or intolerance of metformin, a glycated hemoglobin (HbA1c)—an indicator of long-term glycemic control—more than 1.5% over the target level, or those who cannot reach a target HbA1c within three months [17]. Minor side effects such as nausea, vomiting, and gastrointestinal (GI) upset have been reported [16]. Other effects include delayed gastric emptying and appetite suppression, which contribute to their success as a weight loss drug.

GLP-1RAs have shown a reduction in major adverse cardiac events (MACEs), all-cause mortality, and hospitalization for in the general population and those with T2DM [18,19]. These mortality benefits are evident in patients without baseline HF but absent in those with established HF [20].

Until recently, guidelines from the American Society of Anesthesiologists (ASA) recommended that GLP-1RAs be held on the day of surgery for those on a daily dosing schedule or the week prior to the surgery for those on a weekly dosing schedule, regardless of the indication for the drug (i.e., T2DM, weight loss) or the type of procedure/surgery [21]. This was based on the belief that withholding GLP-1RAs would lower the risk of delayed gastric emptying and aspiration. However, this approach did not fully account for the potential risks of stopping GLP-1RAs, including increasing blood sugar levels in DM patients [22]. As such, the ASA along with the American Gastroenterological Association, American Society for Metabolic and Bariatric Surgery, and others released an updated multisociety clinical practice guidance for the safe perioperative use of GLP-1RAs in October 2024 [23]. The new guidelines recommend that the use of GLP-1RAs in the perioperative period be based on shared decision-making of the patient with the procedural, anesthesia, and prescribing care teams. The guidance states GLP-1RA therapy may be continued preoperatively in patients without an elevated risk of delayed gastric emptying and aspiration [22,23].

On the other hand, GLP-1RA users considered at elevated risk include the following: (1) an escalation phase of GLP-1RAs—typically within 4 to 8 weeks of initiating therapy; (2) higher doses with a higher risk of GI side effects; (3) a weekly dosing schedule; (4) the presence of GI symptoms; and (5) medical conditions besides GLP-1RA usage, which may also delay gastric emptying, such as Parkinson's, gastroparesis, and bowl dysmotility [22,23]. For these high-risk patients, the risks and benefits of withholding GLP-1RA must be assessed. If the decision is made to stop GLP-1RAs before a procedure, the medication should be held one day vs. one week based on GLP-1RA dosing schedule, following the original ASA guidelines. In addition, the updated guidance recommends preoperative diet modification to liquid diet for at least 24 h for patients at elevated risk. It also encourages the use of point-of-care gastric ultrasound on the day of the procedure if there is clinical concern for retained gastric content [22,23]. To decrease aspiration risk during the procedure, rapid sequence induction (RSI) for tracheal intubation should be considered for airway protection in patients with symptoms of delayed gastric emptying (i.e., nausea, vomiting, and bloating), inadequate fasting time, emergency surgery, or other comorbid conditions (i.e., obesity and DM) that put them at an increased risk of aspiration [24]. When there is clinical concern for retained gastric contents, the anesthesia provider should engage patients in shared decision making while weighing the benefits and risks of rapid sequence induction for tracheal intubation in general anesthesia to reduce aspiration risk vs. procedure cancellation.

### 2.2. Dipeptidyl Peptidase-4 (DPP-4) Inhibitors

The catalytic glycoprotein DPP-4 (dipeptidyl peptidase-4), also known as CD26, is expressed in various cell types throughout the body, including hepatocytes, endothelial cells, and islet endocrine cells [25,26]. Incretin hormones such as GLP-1 and glucose-dependent insulinotropic polypeptide (GIP) are rapidly metabolized by DPP-4 to inactive forms [27]. DPP-4 inhibitors were developed to prevent the degradation of GLP-1 and GIP, and thereby extend the duration that incretin hormones stimulate insulin secretion. Satagliptin was the first DPP-4 inhibitor in the market to be approved by the FDA in 2006, shortly after the European Medicines Agency approved vidagliptin. Between 2006 and 2013, three additional DPP-4 inhibitors—alogliptin, saxagliptin, and linagliptin—were approved by the FDA for the treatment of T2DM [25]. The DPP-4 inhibitors have been found to effectively improve glycemic control by reducing mean HbA1c by 0.5–0.8% [28]. When compared to sulfonylurea, DPP-4 inhibitors had lower rates of hypoglycemia and less weight gain [29]. Side effects associated with DPP-4 inhibitors include headache, upper respiratory tract infections, and musculoskeletal pains [28]. DPP-4 inhibitors join GLP-1RAs in the new wave of antidiabetic agents brought to market. When comparing DPP-4 inhibitors to GLP-1RAs, the superiority of GLP-1RAs was based on their ability to decrease HbA1c by 1–1.2%, their long half-life, and their ability to increase GLP-1 concentrations more than DPP-4 inhibitors, despite having more adverse effects [25,28]. DPP-4 inhibitors offer benefits over traditional antidiabetic agents like sulfonylureas, but seem less favorable compared to GLP-1RAs. Guidelines for the discontinuation of DPP-4 inhibitors before surgery vary, with some stating they should be withheld on the day of surgery while others allow their continuation [30,31].

### 2.3. Sodium–Glucose Cotransporter 2 Inhibitors (SGLT2is)

On average, the human kidneys filter 120 to 180 g of glucose from the body daily, with less than 0.5 g excreted in the urine in large part due to the role of SGLT-2 [32]. The main site of glucose resorption, SGLT-2s are found on the apical membrane of the proximal convoluted tubules to facilitate the transportation of glucose into the epithelia driven via the sodium electrochemical potential gradient across the membrane [32,33]. The first SGLT-2 inhibitor (SGLT2i), phlorizin, or phloretin-2′-$\beta$-D-glucopyranoside, is an organic compound initially extracted from apple tree bark and discovered by French chemists De Koninck and Stas in 1835 [34,35]. It took nearly a century for studies to report that the intravenous administration of phlorizin completely inhibited the reabsorption of renally filtered glucose in humans [36] and another half-century to show that diabetic rats treated with the compound showed increased glucose excretion through urine by preventing resorption, lowered BG levels, and restored insulin sensitivity [37]. These findings inspired further research to target SGLT2 as potential therapy for T2DM, eventually leading to the development of the first FDA-approved SGLT2i drugs, including canagliflozin, dapagliflozin, empagliflozin, and more [38].

While the current guidelines from the American Diabetic Association (2022) recommend metformin plus comprehensive lifestyle modification as a first-line treatment for T2DM, other therapies (GLP-1RAs and SGLT2is) may be appropriate, with or without metformin, for T2DM patients at a high risk of developing atherosclerotic cardiovascular disease (ASCVD), HF, and/or chronic kidney disease (CKD) based on an individual's glycemic needs [39]. Whether used as a monotherapy or in combination with other glucose-lowering agents, SGLT2is have been shown to significantly lower HbA1c by 0.4 to 1.08%

in several randomized controlled trials (RCTs) of 3 to over 8 months, allowing patients to achieve HbA1c targets and lower fasting plasma glucose [40]. Additionally, SGLT2is have been shown to promote weight loss and modestly reduce systolic blood pressure through osmotic diuretic effects [40].

SGLT2is are considered efficacious and safe, with mostly mild and manageable adverse effects. The most common are genital and urinary tract infections (UTIs), particularly yeast infections, from extensive glycosuria [33,35]. Other adverse effects include volume depletion from mild diuresis, hypoglycemia, and rarely but, most seriously, euglycemic diabetic ketoacidosis (DKA) [33]. Euglycemic DKA is characterized by inappropriately low insulin levels and elevated glucagon levels in the presence of serum glucose less than 250 mg/dL, leading to ketosis and severe metabolic acidosis [41]. Patients may be especially vulnerable to this potentially life-threatening situation in the perioperative setting, since surgical stress increases counter-regulatory hormones (e.g., glucagon, cortisol, and epinephrine) to promote a catabolic state, while SGLT2is also reduce serum glucose and indirectly inhibit insulin release [41]. Consensus statements based on expert opinion recommend stopping SGLT2is at least 24 h before elective surgeries or planned invasive procedures, though supporting evidence from clinical data is limited [41,42]. The FDA went a step further to change their recommendations, calling for cessation of SLT2i at least three days prior to surgery given the drug's long half-life. Postoperatively, patients on SGLT2is should be observed closely for possible signs of adverse effects, continue insulin with dose adjustments made as required, and be monitored for acid/base status [41].

## 3. Novel Antidiabetic Agents in HF Management

Broadly speaking, heart failure (HF) is a complex condition characterized by the inability of the heart to pump blood effectively to meet the body's metabolic demands [43]. Based on a 2021 proposal by major global scientific bodies, HF is more precisely defined as a clinical syndrome with symptoms and/or signs caused by a structural and/or functional cardiac abnormality and corroborated by elevated natriuretic peptide levels and/or objective evidence of pulmonary or systemic congestion [44]. Common symptoms that arise with HF include dyspnea, fatigue, peripheral edema, and decreased exercise capacity. A growing global pandemic, HF affects an estimate of over 64 million individuals worldwide as of 2017 [45]. In the USA, between 2015 and 2018, around 6.0 million Americans aged 20 or older suffered from HF [46]. The condition also poses a tremendous economic burden on the healthcare system of the country, costing an estimated USD 30.7 billion in 2012 and a projected cost of USD 69.8 billion by 2030 [45]. Risk factors for HF development include HTN, CAD, valvular heart disease, cardiomyopathies, and DM [43]. HF is typically classified by left ventricular ejection fraction (LVEF) and can be categorized into the following three groups: HF with reduced EF (HFrEF) for symptomatic HF with LVEF $\leq$ 40%, HF with mildly reduced EF (HFmrEF) for symptomatic HF with LVEF 41–49%, and HF with preserved EF (HFpEF) for symptomatic HF with LVEF $\geq$ 50% [44].

Research models show a downregulation of certain metabolic processes and an upregulation of stress responses and profibrotic pathways during HF [47]. Factors that determine the treatment of HF include its underlying cause, symptoms, and ejection fraction. Current treatment options aim to strengthen the heart, decrease heart rate, lower blood pressure, reduce fluid retention, and alleviate heart failure symptoms [48]. The 2022 Guideline-Directed Medical Therapy (GDMT) for HF, as outlined by the American Heart Association, American College of Cardiology, and the Heart Failure Society of America, includes four classes of medications used in HFrEF [49]: (1) renin–angiotensin system inhibition, using angiotensin receptor–neprilysin inhibitors, angiotensin-converting enzyme inhibitors, or angiotensin

II receptor blockers; (2) beta-blockers; (3) mineralocorticoid receptor antagonists; and (4) sodium–glucose cotransporter-2 inhibitors (SGLT2is).

In a population-based retrospective cohort study, patients who underwent isolated primary CABG were found to have a higher prevalence of HFpEF in women [12]. This study also observed that both the operative and long-term mortality rates were higher in women with HFpEF [12]. At 30 days post-CABG, the proportion of deaths was highest in HF patients, specifically in those with HFrEF (5.1%; 244 of 4816 patients) [12]. Similarly, HFpEF was found to be highly associated with in-hospital mortality after CT surgery (hazard ratio [HR] 1.86, $p = 0.01$) [11]. Other outcomes, such as postoperative shock, occurred more frequently in HFpEF compared to control patients (17.8% vs. 6.7%, $p < 0.001$) [11]. HFpEF was also considered an independent risk factor of postoperative shock (adjusted odds ratio 2.9, $p < 0.001$) [11]. Overall, HF is a complex, multifactorial syndrome resulting in impaired ventricular filling and/or ejection [47,50]. The pathophysiology of HF involves signal transduction pathways affecting cardiomyocytes, fibroblasts, immune cells, microvascular endothelial cells, and lymphatic endothelial cells [51]. In HF, myocardial remodeling occurs in response to stress signals, which lead to cardiomyocyte hypertrophy or cell death [47,51].

### *3.1. GLP-1RAs in HF Management*

While the data for the use of GLP-1RAs in patients with HF are limited, research suggests that distinguishing between the type and chronicity of HF is important for assessing the potential benefits and harms of GLP-1RA use. In a meta-analysis performed by Ferreira et al., researchers found that GLP-1RAs reduced hospitalizations in patients with new onset HF, but not in those with HF at baseline [52]. Similarly, in the STEP-HFpEF trial, GLP-1RAs prevented hospitalization in patients with new onset-HF and reduced HF-associated symptoms in those with HFpEF [53]. HF patients receiving semaglutide showed greater improvement in exercise function and greater weight loss when compared to the placebo (−13.3% vs. −2.6% change in body weight after 1 year, respectively) [53]. Those in the semaglutide group had a significant reduction of 43.5% in the CRP level after 1 year compared to a 7.3% reduction in the placebo group [53]. These results may suggest an anti-inflammatory effect from GLP-1RA use in HF management. Most adverse events included GI upset, and semaglutide was associated with significantly less serious adverse events (death, arrhythmias, infection, etc.) when compared to the placebo [53]. Overall, there was a significant improvement in exercise function and weight loss in the semaglutide group compared to the placebo.

Alternatively, in the LIVE trial, GLP-1RAs resulted in either neutral or harmful effects in patients with known HFrEF with and without previously diagnosed T2DM [54]. While Liraglutide did not affect LV systolic function, it was significantly associated with an increased heart rate (six beats/min higher) and serious cardiac adverse events in HF patients when compared to the placebo [54]. Serious adverse events included death due to arrhythmia, aggravation of existing ischemic heart disease, and worsening of heart failure. Notedly, the group experiencing serious adverse events did not differ from the rest of the population when demographic and other health factors were accounted for [54].

In the EXSCEL (Exenatide Study of Cardiovascular Event Lowering) trial, there was no reduction in all-cause mortality in the HF subgroup (HR, 1.05), but mortality was reduced in the subgroup without HF (HR, 0.79, $p = 0.03$) [55]. Neves et al. performed a meta-analysis from the EXSCEL and FIGHT (Functional Impact of GLP-1 for Heart Failure Treatment) trials to investigate the risk of HF hospitalization with GLP-1RAs in patients with established HFrEF [56]. These authors found that GLP-1RAs increased the risk of HF hospitalizations in patients with an LVEF < 40%. The use of GLP-1RAs for other health conditions beyond T2DM has only recently been explored and more research is needed to identify the benefits and harms in patients with varying severity levels of HF.

*3.2. DPP-4 Inhibitors in HF Management*

After their FDA approval, four main clinical trials assessing the cardiovascular risk associated with DPP-4 inhibitors were conducted [25]. No significant difference in MACE, all-cause mortality, and heart failure was observed with DPP-4 inhibitors [25,57]. However, results from the SAVOR-TIMI 53 trial and the post hoc analysis of the EXAMINE trial indicated an increased hospitalization risk for heart failure associated with saxagliptin and alogliptin, respectively [57]. In 2016, the FDA issued a warning against two DPP-4 inhibitors (saxagliptin and alogliptin) regarding their role in increasing the risk of serious heart failure events. One possible mechanism to explain the worsening of heart failure in patients taking DPP-4 inhibitors is sympathetic overactivity through potentiation of endogenous stromal cell-derived factor 1, neuropeptide Y, and substance P [58]. These findings, however, are still controversial since subsequent studies have found mixed results with some studies stating no support has been found that DPP-4 inhibitors increase HF incidence [59].

As research continues to expand our understanding of these new antidiabetic agents, recent clinical guidelines have been modified by the American College of Physicians (ACP). The 2024 guidelines from the ACP recommended against the addition of DPP-4 inhibitors to metformin and lifestyle modification for the treatment of T2DM in patients with inadequate glycemic control to reduce morbidity and all-cause mortality [60]. Both GLP-1RAs and SGLT2is are preferred over DPP-4 inhibitors to reduce MACE, all-cause mortality, and heart failure in patients with T2DM based on the ACP guidelines. However, DPP-4 inhibitors have been found to provide some benefit in patients with diabetes and HFpEF. The use of DPP-4 inhibitors in DM patients with HFpEF, but not HFmrEF or HFrEF, was associated with a lower incidence of composite of cardiovascular death or HF hospitalization in these patients but not in HFmrEF or HFrEF [61]. Overall, DPP-4 inhibitors are less favored over the new antidiabetic agents (e.g., GLP-1RAs and SGLT2is), some benefits in HFmrEF are still limited by the data within the T2DM population.

*3.3. SGLT2is in HF Management*

A turning point for advancing treatment of cardiovascular complications in T2DM patients is the EMPA-REG OUTCOME trial (2015). A placebo-controlled RCT with over 7000 subjects, the landmark study was the first to show that a SGLT2i empagliflozin significantly lowered the risk of cardiovascular death (38% relative risk reduction) and HF hospitalization (35% relative risk reduction) for patients with T2DM and high cardiovascular risk [62]. The trial inspired a myriad of studies into SGLT2is as a potent agent for HF management in T2DM patients. The findings from these trials are summarized in Table 1.

A multinational double-blind, placebo-controlled RCT of over 17,000 patients, the DECLARE-TIMI 58 trial (2019) specifically looked at the effect of dapagliflozin in individuals with T2DM who have either established ASCVD (defined as clinically evident ischemic heart disease, ischemic cerebrovascular disease, or peripheral artery disease) or multiple risk factors for ASCVD (men age $\geq$ 55 and women age $\geq$ 60 with one or more traditional risk factors, including hypertension, dyslipidemia, or tobacco use) [63]. The study found that while dapagliflozin did not result in a higher or lower rate of MACE, it did lead to a lower rate of cardiovascular death or hospitalization for HF compared to placebo (4.9% for dapagliflozin vs. 5.8% for placebo). The advantage of SGLT2i use in T2DM patients for HF therapy was once again highlighted in the SOLOIST-WHF trial (2020), in which diabetic patients recently hospitalized for worsening HF were randomly assigned to receive sotagliflozin or placebo and followed up for 9 months [64]. The results showed that those started on sotagliflozin therapy before or shortly after discharge had a significantly lower total number of deaths from cardiovascular causes, as well as lower hospitalizations and urgent visits for HF (HR 0.67). Taken together, the remarkable cardiovascular benefits of SGLT2is, even in those without established CVD, allowed for the wider clinical application of the antidiabetic in HF management.

**Table 1.** Clinical trials on SGLT2is for heart failure management in type 2 diabetes mellitus patients.

| Clinical Trial | SGLT2i | Subjects | T2DM | HF | MACE | Target Population | Outcome |
|---|---|---|---|---|---|---|---|
| DECLARE-TIMI 58 (2018) | Dapagliflozin | 17,160 | + | ↓ | ND | Patients with T2DM and established atherosclerotic CV disease or multiple risk factors for CV disease | * SGLT2is did not result in a higher or lower rate of MACE, but did result in a lower rate of CV death or hospitalization for HF |
| DAPA-HF (2019) | Dapagliflozin | 4744 | − | ↓ | ↓ | NYHA II/III/IV HF and EF ≤40% | Lower risk of worsening HF or CV deaths, regardless of DM status |
| SOLOIST-WHF (2020) | Sotagliflozin | 1222 | + | ↓ | ↓ | T2DM patients recently hospitalized for worsening HF | Lower worsening HF and lower CV deaths |
| EMPEROR-Reduced (2020) | Empagliflozin | 3730 | − | ↓ | NA | NYHA II/III/IV HF and EF ≤ 40% | Lower risk and total number of inpatient and outpatient worsening HF at 12 days after starting SGLT2is |
| EMPULSE (2022) | Empagliflozin | 530 | − | NA | ↓ | Acute HF (both de novo and decompensated chronic HF with reduced or preserved EF, and with or without T2DM) | Improved symptoms, lesser physical limitations, and better quality of life as early as 15 days after starting SGLT2is and maintained through 90 days |
| DELIVER (2022) | Dapagliflozin | 6263 | − | ↓ | ↓ | Chronic HF and LVEF > 40%, i.e., preserved or mildly reduced | Lower combined risk of worsening HF or CV deaths |
| EMPEROR-Preserved (2022) | Empagliflozin | 5988 | +/− | ↓ | ↓ | Symptomatic HF and EF > 40%, elevated natriuretic peptide levels, and evidence of cardiac changes or previous HF hospitalization | Improvement in worsening HF outcomes; also slowed decline in kidney function—regardless of T2DM status |

SGLT2i = Sodium-glucose cotransporter 2 inhibitor,T2DM = type 2 diabetes mellitus, + = patients with T2DM, − = patients without T2DM, HF = heart failure, ↓ = statistically significant reduction, MACE = major adverse cardiovascular event, NA = data not available, ND = no difference, CV = cardiovascular, NYHA = New York Heart Association functional classification, EF = Ejection fraction, LVEF = Left ventricular ejection fraction. * Worsening HF generally defined as hospitalization or urgent visits for HF.

Subsequent RCTs on SGLT2is for HF treatment have specifically examined HFpEF and HFrEF patients regardless of DM status. Looking at subjects with HFpEF and a LVEF > 40%, the DELIVER trial (2022) demonstrated that dapagliflozin reduced the combined risk of worsening HF or cardiovascular death (16.4% in dapagliflozin vs. 19.5% in placebo) [65]. The EMPEROR-Preserved trial (2022) confirmed similar outcomes, noting a reduced rate of first hospitalization for HF or cardiovascular death in HFpEF patients with LVEF > 50% with or without T2DM. Furthermore, EMPEROR-Preserved also observed a slower rate of estimated glomerular filtration rate (GFR) decline in SGLT2i-treated HFpEF patients; this effect appears more pronounced in patients with DM [66]. These benefits are also extended to HFrEF patients with LVEF $\leq$ 40%, as demonstrated in the DAPA-HF (2019) and EMPEROR-Reduced (2022) trials. The DAPA-HF trial showed a lower risk of worsening HF (defined as hospitalization or urgent visit resulting in IV therapy for HF) or death from cardiovascular causes in the dapagliflozin group (16.3%) compared to placebo (21.2%) [67], whereas the EMPEROR-Reduced study found a reduced risk and total number of inpatients and outpatient worsening HF events, with early and sustained duration of effects [68]. Finally, the EMPULSE trial (2022) found that clinical benefits, along with improved symptoms, physical limitations, and quality of life, can be observed as early as 15 days and maintained through 90 days after initiating empagliflozin in patients hospitalized for acute HF, regardless of the degree of symptomatic impairment at baseline [69]. Overall, SGLT2i use in HF therapy appears beneficial across a wide range of HF severities and DM comorbidities.

## 4. Perioperative Considerations of Novel Antidiabetic Use in Cardiac Surgeries

A summary of the following studies presented on the use of antidiabetic agents in cardiac surgeries can be found in Table 2.

### *4.1. GLP-1RAs in Cardiac Surgeries*

The use of novel antidiabetic agents in patients undergoing cardiac surgery has increased due to the rise in popularity of these drugs in recent years. While GLP-1RAs have cardioprotective effects, its use in those undergoing cardiac surgery must also be explored as individuals on this drug often have cardiac-related comorbidities. Current research primarily compares the insulin requirements, BG levels, and glycemic variability of patients on GLP-1RAs to those on standard insulin who are undergoing cardiac surgery. Sindhvananda et al. found that the BG levels of those on Liraglutide with insulin were significantly lower than before, during, and after the operation as compared to insulin-only controls among patients with established T2DM undergoing cardiac surgery [70]. The perioperative mean difference of BG levels was 15.9 mg/dL, and those receiving Liraglutide with insulin had significantly less hyperglycemic episodes [70]. The study found that on postoperative day 0, the Liraglutide group had fewer patients who had BG > 180 mg/dL compared to the placebo (43.75% vs. 67.85%, $p$ = 0.061). On postoperative day 2, the Liraglutide group demonstrated less glycemic variability compared to the placebo (SD 23.65 vs. 32.79 mg/dL, $p$ = 0.018) [70].

**Table 2.** Summary of studies on the use of antidiabetic agents in cardiac surgeries.

| Study: Author (Year), Type | Antidiabetic Agent | Subjects (n) | T2DM (n) | HF (n) | Others | Target Population and Cardiac Surgery Type | Outcomes |
|---|---|---|---|---|---|---|---|
| Sindhvananda et al. (2023) [70] RCT | GLP-1RA (Liraglutide) | 56 | Yes (56) | No | | T2DM patients undergoing CABG | Significantly lower BG levels in patients on Liraglutide and insulin before, during, and after CABG compared to insulin-only controls. |
| Hulst et al. (2020) RCT [71] | GLP-1RA (Liraglutide) | 278 | Yes (43) | No | | Patients with or without T2DM undergoing elective cardiac surgery | Significantly lower total intraoperative insulin doses and a significantly lower number of insulin administrations, as well as better postoperative BG control in the Liraglutide treatment group compared to the placebo control group. |
| Makino et al. (2019) [72] RCT | GLP-1RA (Liraglutide) | 70 | Yes (70) | No | | T2DM patients undergoing CABG | Significantly lower M values (proximity index of target glucose level) in the Liraglutide treatment group compared to the insulin-only control group, suggestive of better glycemic control. |
| Oosterom-Eijmael et al. (2024) [73] Prospective cohort | GLP-1RA (Liraglutide) | 25 | Yes (3) | No | | Patients with or without T2DM undergoing elective cardiac surgery | The Liraglutide treatment group had increased glycemic time in range compared to the placebo control group. |
| Hulst et al. (2020) [74] Secondary analysis | GLP-1RA (Liraglutide) | 261 | Yes (42) | No | | Postoperative patients with or without T2DM after elective cardiac surgery | The Liraglutide group had a lower ICU admission rate and higher rates of normal LV systolic function postoperatively compared to the control group. |
| Cardona et al. (2021) [75] RCT | DPP-4 inhibitor (Sitagliptin) | 182 | Yes (182) | No | | T2DM patients undergoing CABG | No differences in hypoglycemia rate, mean daily glucose, hospital stay, or readmissions after discharge in the DPP-4 inhibitor group compared to placebo. Lower insulin requirement in the DPP-4 inhibitor group upon transfer from ICU to wards. |

**Table 2.** *Cont.*

| Study: Author (Year), Type | Antidiabetic Agent | Subjects (n) | T2DM (n) | HF (n) | Others | Target Population and Cardiac Surgery Type | Outcomes |
|---|---|---|---|---|---|---|---|
| Sardu et al. (2021) [76] Prospective cohort | SGLT2i | 648 | Yes (188) | No | Yes, IHD (188) | IHD patients undergoing CABG via MiECC | Patients without T2DM had lower levels of inflammatory markers postoperatively. Among T2DM patients, those treated with SGLT2is had lower levels of inflammatory markers compared to the non-SGLT2i group after surgery. |
| Al Namat et al. (2023) [77] Prospective cohort | SGLT2i (Dapagliflozin) | 120 | Yes (65) | Yes (87) | Yes, CKD (35) | Age $\geq$ 40 with clinical indication for CABG surgery | All patients underwent post-CABG rehabilitation and SGLT2i treatment. Regardless of cardiac statuses, rehabilitation and SGLT2i treatment led to improved mean EF, glycemic status, and renal function in patients with or without T2DM and with or without CKD. |
| Cagliostro et al. (2022) [78] Retrospective cohort | SGLT2i | 34 | Yes (34) | Yes (17) | Yes, CKD (16) | T2DM patients undergoing LVAD implantation | Lower BUN levels at 180-day follow-up with SGLT2i treatment but no significant change in BMI, HbA1c, or diuretic dose. |
| Fardman et al. (2023) [79] Retrospective cohort | SGTL2i | 29 | Yes (23) | Yes (29) | | Patients undergoing LVAD implantation initiated on SGLT2i postoperatively | SGLT2i initiation after LVAD placement associated with decreased daily furosemide dose, weight, and sPAP but possibly higher RV dysfunction rate. No change in LVAD parameters. |

T2DM = Type 2 diabetes mellitus, HF = Heart failure, RCT = Randomized controlled trial, GLP-1RA = Glucagon-like peptide-1 receptor agonist, CABG = Coronary artery bypass grafting, BG = Blood glucose, ICU = Intensive care unit, LV = Left ventricle, DPP-4 = Dipeptidyl peptidase-4, SGLT2i = Sodium-glucose cotransporter 2 inhibitor, IHD = Ischemic heart disease, MiECC = Minimally invasive extracorporeal circulation, EF = Ejection fraction, CKD = Chronic kidney disease, BUN = Blood urea nitrogen, LVAD = Left ventricular assist device, BMI = Body mass index, HbA1c = Glycated hemoglobin, sPAP = Systolic pulmonary artery pressure, RV = Right ventricule.

These results are consistent with the findings of Hulst et al., who showed that those on Liraglutide required significantly lower total intraoperative insulin doses and a significantly lower number of insulin administrations compared to the placebo group. The mean intraoperative BG level in the Liraglutide group was 11.89 mg/dL lower than the placebo group [71]. Within the study, 16% of patients with previously diagnosed T2DM were evenly distributed between the intervention and placebo group, and, overall, these patients required more insulin and had higher perioperative BG levels; however, the results remained similar for those with or without T2DM and it did not result in a different effect on perioperative insulin. Postoperatively, the mean BG levels for the Liraglutide and placebo group were 8.8 $\pm$ 1.4 and 9.2 $\pm$ 1.4 ($p = 0.006$), respectively [71].

Makino et al. investigated the use of Liraglutide with insulin compared to insulin alone in patients with established T2DM undergoing cardiac surgery (2/3 CABG cases and 1/3 valve replacement cases), finding that the M values (indicative of proximity index of the target glucose level from day 1–10) were significantly lower in the Liraglutide group (5.8 vs. 12.3, respectively). These authors also found that the Liraglutide group required a significantly lower frequency of insulin dose modification and had a lower frequency of hypoglycemia [72]. Similarly, Oosterom-Eijmael et al. conducted a triple-blind randomized controlled trial comparing preoperative Liraglutide treatment to placebo in patients with or without established T2DM undergoing cardiac surgery, monitoring the effect on BG via Dexacom (continuous BG monitor); they found that Liraglutide increased the glycemic time in range by 72% compared to 47% in the control group [73]. These investigators also found that the peak mean glucose concentration occurred approximately 14–16 h postoperatively, with the Liraglutide group blood glucose peaking at approximately 8.2 mmol/L and the placebo group peaking at approximately 9.4 mmol/L [73].

Hulst et al. further explored the impact of Liraglutide on myocardial function after cardiac surgery in patients with or without previously diagnosed T2DM, finding that the effects on Liraglutide had lower intensive care unit (ICU) admittance [74]. They also found that despite left ventricular (LV) systolic function being comparable between the Liraglutide and placebo groups preoperatively, patients in the Liraglutide group had significantly higher rates of normal LV systolic function postoperatively [74]. While the Liraglutide group had a significantly higher heart rate (83 $\pm$ 11 beats/min) compared to the placebo group (77 $\pm$ 11 beats/min), there was no significant difference in mean arterial pressure or vasoactive/inotropic support needed throughout the postoperative course [74].

### 4.2. DPP-4 Inhibitors in Cardiac Surgeries

An investigation into the use of DPP-4 inhibitors in patients undergoing cardiac surgery is necessary due to the increased use of these drugs in the recent decades and its controversial effects on heart failure. Research on DPP-4 inhibitors used in cardiac surgery is limited. In Cardona et al. [75], the use of sitagliptin in patients with T2DM undergoing CABG surgery was investigated for its ability to prevent and treat perioperative hyperglycemia. A total of 182 participants undergoing CABG were divided into two groups (sitagliptin or placebo). Patient characteristics included HbA1c 7.6% $\pm$ 1.5%. HF was not a clinical characteristic considered for this study. Sitagliptin or a placebo was given once daily, starting the day before surgery, and this continued until hospital discharge or for up to 10 days. The findings determined no differences in frequency of hypoglycemia or in mean daily glucose during the hospital stay, the duration of surgery, the duration of ICU or hospital length of stay, the need for vasopressors, perioperative complications, surgical reinterventions, or readmissions after hospital discharge. The study did find that lower insulin requirement was found in the sitagliptin group upon transfer from the ICU to the wards [75].

### 4.3. SGLT2is in Cardiac Surgeries

Given the significant outcome improvement SGLT2i offers in HF management, it is possible that the novel antidiabetic agent may provide similar benefits in HF patients undergoing cardiac surgery. While limited, there have been studies exploring the perioperative use of SGLT2is in CABG and LVAD procedures. In a multi-center prospective cohort study, Sardu et al. recruited patients with ischemic heart disease (IHD) receiving CABG via minimally invasive extracorporeal circulation (MiECC) and examined the inflammatory burden (as measured by inflammatory markers such as leukocyte counts, CRP, IL-1, IL-6, and TNF-α), clinical events (namely any cause of death, cardiac death, non-fatal MI, stroke, and revascularization), and quality of life 5 years after surgery [76]. Out of the 648 subjects, 188 had preexisting T2DM, with 64 of those being SGLT2i users. The results found that patients without T2DM had a lower expression of inflammatory markers after the follow-up compared to those with T2DM. However, among T2DM patients, SGLT2i users had lower levels of inflammatory markers compared to the non-SGLT2i cohort. Similar trends were reflected in terms of clinical events; the non-SGLT2i cohort was found to have the highest rate of adverse outcomes compared to the non-T2DM and SGLT2i user cohorts at the 5-year follow-up [76]. Limitations of the study include the small sample size of the SGLT2i cohort, the lack of comparison with CABG via conventional extracorporeal circulation, and the lack of randomization in study design. But, overall, the study suggests that while T2DM might be a risk factor for worse prognosis in those receiving CABG via MiECC, treatment with SGLT2is for T2DM patients may confer some level of long-term anti-inflammatory protection to lower the rate of adverse clinical events. Of note, the article did not put focus on HF patients; rather, the authors recruited patients with IHD who qualify for CABG via MiECC.

Another prospective study by Al Namat et al. also investigated SGLT2i use in the setting of CABG surgeries, specifically assessing outcomes related to cardiac ischemia, glycemic status, and renal function at 6 months after surgery [77]. All patients were enrolled in a 6-month cardiac rehabilitation program with daily dapagliflozin treatment. The 120 subjects were split into four subgroups: T2DM patients with CKD, T2DM without CKD, prediabetes with CKD, and prediabetes without CKD. Of note, 87 out of the 120 patients (72.5%) were previously diagnosed with HF. The results showed an increase in mean EF by 8.43% across all patients, with more significant improvement in the prediabetes group compared to the T2DM group (10.14% vs. 6.98). For all patients, ischemic markers such as heart-type fatty-acid-binding protein (H-FABP) levels returned to normal at follow-up, while and troponin levels were significantly decreased (44,458 ng/L overall), particularly in CKD patients regardless of T2DM status (73,294 to 82,500 ng/L) [77]. Unsurprisingly, HbA1c levels improved in both the prediabetes and T2DM groups regardless of CKD status. Finally, there was an overall increase of 11.51 in the GFR for all patients, notably in the CKD with the T2DM cohort (18.93 increase) and the prediabetes group (14.89 increase) [77]. It should be noted that the study did not include a control group of patients not receiving SGLT2is given the largely established benefits of the drug in treating the pathologies. Other limitations include a disproportionately male study pool (less than 25% female) and the exclusion of CABG recipients with adequate glycemic control (i.e., without established diabetes or signs of prediabetes). Nevertheless, the analysis by Al Namat et al. demonstrated that regardless of one's cardiac status (e.g., previous history of HF), treatment with SGLT2i dapagliflozin for CABG recipients significantly reduced ischemic risk, increased mean EF, enhanced glycemic status, and improved renal function across all patients regardless of T2DM and/or CKD status, which may prove especially beneficial for those with complex comorbidities.

The number of studies assessing the safety and efficacy of SGLT2is in patients receiving durable mechanical support such as left ventricular assist devices (LVADs) is also growing. In a retrospective cohort study, Cagliostro et al. followed T2DM patients placed on LVAD support to examine the rates of SGLT2i use among the population, as well as subsequent changes in body mass index (BMI), HbA1c, diuretic dose (furosemide equivalent), and renal function over time. Out of the 509 T2DM patients on LVAD support, only 34 (6.7%) were treated with SGLT2is, and 17 of these patients (50%) had diagnosed HF characterized as ischemic cardiomyopathy (ICM) [78]. Cagliostro et al. reported that among the SGLT2i-treated cohort, there was no significant change in the BMI, HbA1c, or diuretic dose at 30-, 60-, and 180-day follow-ups. The only difference noted was a decrease in blood urea nitrogen (BUN) at 180 days. Potential SGLT2i-related adverse events such as genitourinary infections, acute kidney injury, limb amputations, and driveline infections occurred, though it is hard to know whether these were caused by SGLT2is or chance events given their nonspecific nature. No episodes of DKA, volume depletion, fracture, or hypersensitivity reactions were reported. Cagliostro et al. advocated for further research on the safety and impact of SGLT2is for LVAD patients [78].

In another retrospective study that also investigated SGLT2is in the setting of LVAD implantation, 29 out of 138 patients (21%) were started on SGLT2i therapy after LVAD placement, with a mean time of 108 days from LVAD placement to SGLT2i initiation [79]. Fardman et al. found a significant decrease in daily furosemide dose (23.5 mg/day) and weight loss (2.50 kg average weight loss) in patients started on SGLT2is. In addition, there was a significant reduction in systolic pulmonary artery pressure (sPAP, 5.6 mm Hg reduction) among a subgroup of 11 patients who underwent right heart catheterization during follow-up. Echocardiographic evaluation showed a higher prevalence of right ventricular (RV) dysfunction after SGLT2i initiation, though none of the patients with severe RV dysfunction required HF hospitalization during the study. Finally, there was no significant difference in LVAD parameters before or after SGLT2i initiation [79]. The study focused on outcome measures related to HF rather than DM and glycemic control (e.g., HbA1c, mean BG, and fasting BG). Overall, no SGLT2i-related adverse effects were reported. Although the study is limited in generalizability due to its small sample size and lack of comparison with a control group not treated with SGLT2is, it suggested that certain clinical benefits may come from initiating SGLT2is after LVAD placement.

## 5. Discussion and Future Directions

Our comprehensive review of the three classes of novel antidiabetic agents showed potential benefits in the perioperative setting for cardiac surgeries in HF patients, particularly for BG control and certain organ protective effects. These findings are summarized in Table 3. GLP-1RAs are safe for perioperative use and improve BG control, decrease insulin requirements, and support postoperative cardiac function. They do not increase the risk of hypoglycemic episodes or adverse effects when compared to insulin. Based on current guidelines, the case of whether or not GLP-1RAs should be stopped for surgery depends on clinical team's judgment of patients' aspiration risk. If a patient is deemed low-risk, GLP-1RAs may be continued until surgery. However, if the risk of aspiration is high and a decision is made to hold GLP-1RAs for surgery, the medication should be held on the day of surgery if the patient is on a daily dosing schedule or the week prior to surgery if the patient is on a weekly dosing schedule. Point-of-care gastric ultrasound can be used on the day of the procedure if there is clinical concern for retained gastric content [21–23]. After surgery, if the patient can safely tolerate oral intake, GLP-1RAs can be resumed the day after surgery if daily dosing or the next week if weekly dosing, although the current literature on when to resume this medication after surgery is limited. Within HF, GLP-1RAs reduce hospitalizations for new-onset HF and improves symptoms in HFpEF. However, GLP-1RAs generally do not improve health outcomes in patients with HFrEF and may even be harmful in those with a LVEF < 40% [52,56,58]. Overall, GLP-1RAs are beneficial in cardiovascular and renal outcomes within the general population and those in diabetes, but there are limited data available for these benefits within the HF population.

While studies on perioperative use of DPP-4 inhibitors in cardiac surgery are limited, they are generally safe without causing serious adverse effects, including hypoglycemia and weight gain, which are seen in DPP-4 inhibitor use [29]. The use of DPP-4 inhibitors led to lower mean daily insulin requirements in patients with T2DM undergoing CABG surgery [75]. However, saxagliptin and alogliptin were noted to increase hospitalization risk in HF patients [67], whereas DPP-4 inhibitors for HFpEF and DM were associated with lower rates of cardiovascular death or HF hospitalization [61]. Published recommendations on the discontinuation of DPP-4 inhibitors before surgery are less well established compared to those for SGLT2is and GLP-1RAs. In conclusion, DPP-4 inhibitors are generally safe but offer limited clinical benefits, with potential risks in heart failure patients and some benefit in HFpEF.

Out of the three novel antidiabetic agents discussed, SGLT2is showed the most promising perioperative benefits for cardiac surgeries. Not only does SGLT2is significantly lower HbA1c and fasting plasma glucose for T2DM patients, especially those at high risk for ASCVD, HF, and/or CKD, it also promotes weight loss and a reduction in high blood pressure [39,40]. Several RCTs established the remarkable benefits of SGLT2is in HF therapy, from a lower risk of worsening HF or cardiovascular deaths and slowing decline in kidney function to an improvement in symptoms, physical activity, and quality of life (Table 1). One study suggests that SGLT2is offer certain anti-inflammatory protective effects that reduce the rate of adverse clinical events in T2DM patients undergoing CABG via MiECC [76], while another demonstrated a lower ischemic risk, a higher mean EF, and an improved HbA1c, as well as renal function, in both T2DM and/or CKD patients undergoing CABG [77]. However, decisions on SGLT2i use in LVAD surgeries are mixed: one study showed no significant change in BMI, HbA1c, or diuretic dose but an increased risk of adverse effects (e.g., genitourinary infections, acute kidney injury, limb amputations, and driveline infections) [78], while the other noted a significant reduction in daily diuretic requirements, weight reduction, and sPAP reduction with no change in LVAD settings [79]. Based on current guidelines, stopping SGLT2is three to four days prior to cardiac surgery may be appropriate to minimize the risk of hypovolemia, hypoglycemia, and in extreme cases like euglycemia DKA. Only after careful postoperative monitoring of patients' blood glucose and acid/base status, as well as ensuring adequate hydration and nutrition, should SGLT2is be resumed. In summary, SGLT2is provide the most advantages in HF management for those with or without T2DM and/or CKD in cardiac surgeries, as reflected in improved mean EF, reduced HbA1c, and lower inflammatory burden.

**Table 3.** Summary of novel antidiabetic agents and their effects.

| | Antidiabetic Class | | |
|---|---|---|---|
| | **GLP-1RAs** | **DPP-4 Inhibitors** | **SGLT2is** |
| Glycemic control | Significant reduction in HbA1c by ~1–1.2%. | Moderate reduction in HbA1c (0.5–0.8%). | Significant reduction in HbA1c (0.4–1.08%) and lower fasting plasma glucose as monotherapy or combined use with other agents. |
| HF with T2DM | Lower incidence of hospitalization for new-onset HFpEF but not in patients with established HF at baseline.<br>Neutral or harmful in HFrEF. | Lower incidence of hospitalization and composite of cardiovascular death in HFpEF. | Improved outcomes (less worsening HF, hospitalization and/or urgent visits for HF, and quality of life) for HFpEF, HFmrEF, and HFrEF. |
| Cardiac surgery outcomes | Improved perioperative BG control with lower intraoperative insulin requirements. | Limited studies: No differences in frequency of hypoglycemia, mean daily glucose, hospital length of stay, surgical reinterventions, or readmissions after discharge in the DPP-4 inhibitor group compared to placebo. Lower insulin requirement in the DPP-4 inhibitor group upon transfer from ICU to wards. | CABG: Significant decrease in ischemic risk, improved mean EF, glycemic status, and renal function with or without T2DM, with or without CKD in the SGLT2i treatment group compared to the control. Lower-level inflammatory markers and ameliorated clinical outcomes at the 5-year postop point via MiECC.<br>LVAD: Reduction in BUN and sPAP. Questionable reduction in weight/BMI and daily diuretic requirements. Possible higher RV dysfunction prevalence. No change in HbA1c or LVAD parameters. |
| Adverse events | GI upset (nausea/vomiting), delayed gastric emptying, appetite suppression, renal dysfunction, arrhythmias, and worsening of existing ischemic heart disease. | Upper respiratory tract infection, nasopharyngitis, headache, UTI, and arthralgia. | Volume depletion, UTI/yeast infection, hypoglycemia, and euglycemic DKA. |

**Table 3.** *Cont.*

| | Antidiabetic Class | | |
|---|---|---|---|
| | **GLP-1RAs** | **DPP-4 Inhibitors** | **SGLT2is** |
| Perioperative recommendations | If the risk of delayed gastric emptying/aspiration is low, continue before surgery.<br>If the risk of delayed gastric emptying/aspiration is high, hold GLP-1RAs on the day of surgery if on a daily dosing schedule or the week prior to surgery if on a weekly dosing schedule, as well as a 24 hr preoperative liquid diet<br>Resume GLP-1RAs after surgery if patient is able to safely tolerate oral intake. | Continue DPP-4 inhibitor use or withhold on day of surgery.<br>May resume DPP-4 inhibitor use immediately after surgery. | Hold SGLT2is at least 3 days before surgery.<br>Monitor closely for glucose level and acid/base status after surgery and resume SGLT2is if able to tolerate oral intake and maintain adequate hydration. |

GLP-1RA = Glucagon-like peptide-1 receptor agonist, DPP-4 = Dipeptidyl peptidase-4, SGLT2i = Sodium-glucose cotransporter 2 inhibitor, HbA1c = Glycated hemoglobin, HF = Heart failure, T2DM = Type 2 diabetes mellitus, HFpEF = Heart failure with preserved ejection fraction, HFrEF = Heart failure with reduced ejection fraction, HFmrEF = Heart failure with mildly reduced ejection fraction, BG = Blood glucose, ICU = Intensive care unit, CABG = Coronary artery bypass grafting, EF = Ejection fraction, CKD = Chronic kidney disease, MiECC = Minimally invasive extracorporeal circulation, LVAD = Left ventricular assist device, BUN = Blood urea nitrogen, sPAP = Systolic pulmonary artery pressure, BMI = Body mass index, RV = Right ventricle, GI = Gastrointestinal, UTI = Urinary tract infection, DKA = Diabetic ketoacidosis.

Given the many potential benefits that novel antidiabetic agents can offer in patients undergoing cardiac surgery, further research and studies are critical in bridging current knowledge and improving outcomes for all future patients. For one, most studies on the use of novel antidiabetic agents in cardiac surgeries presented in this review are small cohort studies with limited power. Larger study populations with a more rigorous study design would enhance validity and generalizability of findings. Also, a direct comparison of the three antidiabetic agents in cardiac surgeries proved to be challenging given that the studies presented highlighted different outcome measures. Future studies with consistent and standardized measures would allow for more rigorous comparison. While discussions on novel antidiabetic agents are focused on T2DM patients, there is room to investigate the use of these agents in those with type 1 DM. Additionally, investigation into combination therapy of two novel antidiabetic agents (such as GLP1-RAs and SGLT2is) may reveal new, potentially synergistic effects in treating patients with complex comorbidities. Finally, the majority of studies focused on the immediate postoperative period from the end of surgery to patient readiness to discharge. Further research on novel antidiabetic agents in the late postoperative period weeks, months, or even years after surgery would help guide chronic medication in future patients.

## 6. Conclusions

While studies on the use of novel antidiabetic agents in the setting of cardiac surgeries are limited at the moment, our review of the current literature suggests that all three agents (GLP-1RAs, DPP-4 inhibitors, and SGLT2is) are safe for use in the perioperative period, with SLGT2i showing the most benefits in HF management and other organ protection for those with or without DM undergoing cardiac surgery.

**Author Contributions:** Conceptualization, J.O., S.Z. and J.S.; literature review, A.W., S.B., D.P., J.S. and S.Z.; writing—original draft preparation, A.W., S.B. and D.P.; writing—review and editing, A.W., J.S., S.Z., J.O. and S.D.B.; visualization, A.W., S.B. and J.S.; supervision, J.S., S.Z., J.O. and S.D.B. All authors have read and agreed to the published version of the manuscript.

**Funding:** This research received no external funding.

**Acknowledgments:** The authors are grateful for Alina Razak for her assistance in assembling the team and facilitating the publication process.

**Conflicts of Interest:** The authors declare no conflicts of interest.

## References

1. Yun, J.-S.; Ko, S.-H. Current Trends in Epidemiology of Cardiovascular Disease and Cardiovascular Risk Management in Type 2 Diabetes. *Metabolism* **2021**, *123*, 154838. [CrossRef]
2. Dunlay, S.M.; Givertz, M.M.; Aguilar, D.; Allen, L.A.; Chan, M.; Desai, A.S.; Deswal, A.; Dickson, V.V.; Kosiborod, M.N.; Lekavich, C.L.; et al. Type 2 Diabetes Mellitus and Heart Failure: A Scientific Statement from the American Heart Association and the Heart Failure Society of America. *Circulation* **2019**, *140*, E294–E324. [CrossRef] [PubMed]
3. Olanrewaju, O.A.; Sheeba, F.; Kumar, A.; Ahmad, S.; Blank, N.; Kumari, R.; Kumari, K.; Salame, T.; Khalid, A.; Varrassi, G.; et al. Novel Therapies in Diabetes: A Comprehensive Narrative Review of GLP-1 Receptor Agonists, SGLT2 Inhibitors, and Beyond. *Cureus* **2023**, *15*, e51151. [CrossRef] [PubMed]
4. Greco, G.; Ferket, B.S.; D'Alessandro, D.A.; Shi, W.; Horvath, K.A.; Rosen, A.; Welsh, S.; Bagiella, E.; Neill, A.E.; Williams, D.L.; et al. Diabetes and the Association of Postoperative Hyperglycemia with Clinical and Economic Outcomes in Cardiac Surgery. *Diabetes Care* **2016**, *39*, 408–417. [CrossRef] [PubMed]
5. Lazar, H.L.; McDonnell, M.; Chipkin, S.R.; Furnary, A.P.; Engelman, R.M.; Sadhu, A.R.; Bridges, C.R.; Haan, C.K.; Svedjeholm, R.; Taegtmeyer, H.; et al. The Society of Thoracic Surgeons Practice Guideline Series: Blood Glucose Management During Adult Cardiac Surgery. *The Annals of Thoracic Surgery* **2009**, *87*, 663–669. [CrossRef]
6. Vervoort, D.; Meuris, B.; Meyns, B.; Verbrugghe, P. Global cardiac surgery: Access to cardiac surgical care around the world. *J. Thorac. Cardiovasc. Surg.* **2020**, *159*, 987–996.e6. [CrossRef]

7. van Straten, A.H.; Soliman Hamad, M.A.; van Zundert, A.A.; Martens, E.J.; Schönberger, J.P.; ter Woorst, J.F.; de Wolf, A.M. Diabetes and Survival after Coronary Artery Bypass Grafting: Comparison with an Age- and Sex-Matched Population. *Eur. J. Cardiothorac. Surg.* **2010**, *37*, 1068–1074. [CrossRef]
8. Leavitt, B.J. Effect of Diabetes and Associated Conditions on Long-Term Survival after Coronary Artery Bypass Graft Surgery. *Circulation* **2004**, *110* (Suppl. S1), II-41. [CrossRef]
9. Barsness, G.W.; Peterson, E.D.; Ohman, E.M.; Nelson, C.L.; DeLong, E.R.; Reves, J.G.; Smith, P.K.; Anderson, R.D.; Jones, R.H.; Mark, D.B.; et al. Relationship between Diabetes Mellitus and Long-Term Survival after Coronary Bypass and Angioplasty. *Circulation* **1997**, *96*, 2551–2556. [CrossRef]
10. Santos, K.A.Q.; Berto, B.; Sousa, A.G.; Costa, F.A.A.D. Prognosis and Complications of Diabetic Patients Undergoing Isolated Coronary Artery Bypass Surgery. *Braz. J. Cardiovasc. Surg.* **2015**, *31*, 7–14. [CrossRef]
11. Nguyen, L.S.; Baudinaud, P.; Brusset, A.; Nicot, F.; Pechmajou, L.; Salem, J.E.; Estagnasie, P.; Squara, P. Heart failure with preserved ejection fraction as an independent risk factor of mortality after cardiothoracic surgery. *J. Thorac. Cardiovasc. Surg.* **2018**, *156*, 188–193.e2. [CrossRef] [PubMed]
12. Sun, L.Y.; Tu, J.V.; Eddeen, A.B.; Liu, P.P. Prevalence and Long-Term Survival after Coronary Artery Bypass Grafting in Women and Men with Heart Failure and Preserved versus Reduced Ejection Fraction. *J. Am. Heart Assoc.* **2018**, *7*, e008902. [CrossRef] [PubMed]
13. MacDonald, P.E.; El-kholy, W.; Riedel, M.J.; Salapatek, A.M.F.; Light, P.E.; Wheeler, M.B. The Multiple Actions of GLP-1 on the Process of Glucose-Stimulated Insulin Secretion. *Diabetes* **2002**, *51* (Suppl. S3), S434–S442. [CrossRef]
14. Bu, T.; Sun, Z.; Pan, Y.; Deng, X.; Yuan, G. Glucagon-like Peptide-1: New Regulator in Lipid Metabolism. *Diabetes Metab. J.* **2024**, *48*, 354–372. [CrossRef] [PubMed]
15. Collins, L.; Costello, R.A. Glucagon-like Peptide-1 Receptor Agonists. StatPearls. Available online: https://www.ncbi.nlm.nih.gov/books/NBK551568/ (accessed on 16 November 2024).
16. Zheng, Z.; Zong, Y.; Ma, Y.; Tian, Y.; Pang, Y.; Zhang, C.; Gao, J. Glucagon-like Peptide-1 Receptor: Mechanisms and Advances in Therapy. *Signal Transduct. Target. Ther.* **2024**, *9*, 234. [CrossRef]
17. American Diabetes Association. Pharmacologic Approaches to Glycemic Treatment: Standards of Medical Care in Diabetes—2019. *Diabetes Care* **2018**, *42* (Suppl. S1), S90–S102. [CrossRef]
18. Parab, P.; Chaudhary, P.; Mukhtar, S.; Moradi, A.; Kodali, A.; Okoye, C.; Klein, D.; Mohamoud, I.; Olanisa, O.O.; Hamid, P. Role of Glucagon-like Peptide-1 (GLP-1) Receptor Agonists in Cardiovascular Risk Management in Patients with Type 2 Diabetes Mellitus: A Systematic Review. *Cureus* **2023**, *15*, e45487. [CrossRef]
19. Rivera, F.B.; Cruz, L.L.A.; Magalong, J.V.; Ruyeras, J.M.M.J.; Aparece, J.P.; Bantayan, N.R.B.; Lara-Breitinger, K.; Gulati, M. Cardiovascular and Renal Outcomes of Glucagon-like Peptide 1 Receptor Agonists among Patients with and without Type 2 Diabetes Mellitus: A Meta-Analysis of Randomized Placebo-Controlled Trials. *Am. J. Prev. Cardiol.* **2024**, *18*, 100679. [CrossRef]
20. Khan, M.S.; Fonarow, G.C.; McGuire, D.K.; Hernandez, A.F.; Vaduganathan, M.; Rosenstock, J.; Handelsman, Y.; Verma, S.; Anker, S.D.; McMurray, J.J.V.; et al. Glucagon-like Peptide 1 Receptor Agonists and Heart Failure. *Circulation* **2020**, *142*, 1205–1218. [CrossRef]
21. Joshi, G.; Abdelmalak, B.; Weigel, W.; Soriano, S.; Harbell, M.; Kuo, C.; Stricker, P.; Domino, K. *American Society of Anesthesiologists Consensus-Based Guidance on Preoperative Management of Patients (Adults and Children) on Glucagon-like Peptide-1 (GLP-1) Receptor Agonists*; American Society of Anesthesiologists (ASA); Volume 2023, Available online: https://www.asahq.org/about-asa/newsroom/news-releases/2023/06/american-society-of-anesthesiologists-consensus-based-guidance-on-preoperative (accessed on 20 November 2024).
22. *Most Patients Can Continue Diabetes, Weight Loss GLP-1 Drugs Before Surgery, Those at Highest Risk for GI Problems Should Follow Liquid Diet Before Procedure*; American Society of Anesthesiologists (ASA), 2024; Available online: https://www.asahq.org/about-asa/newsroom/news-releases/2024/10/new-multi-society-glp-1-guidance (accessed on 30 November 2024).
23. Kindel, T.L.; Wang, A.Y.; Wadhwa, A.; Schulman, A.R.; Sharaiha, R.Z.; Kroh, M.; Ghanem, O.M.; Levy, S.; Joshi, G.P.; LaMasters, T.L.; et al. Multisociety clinical practice guidance for the safe use of glucagon-like peptide-1 receptor agonists in the perioperative period. *Surg. Obes. Relat. Dis.* **2024**, *20*, 1183–1186. [CrossRef]
24. Robinson, M.; Davidson, A. Aspiration under Anaesthesia: Risk Assessment and Decision-Making. *Contin. Educ. Anaesth. Crit. Care Pain* **2014**, *14*, 171–175. [CrossRef]
25. Ahrén, B. DPP-4 Inhibition and the Path to Clinical Proof. *Front. Endocrinol.* **2019**, *10*, 376. [CrossRef] [PubMed]
26. Nistala, R.; Savin, V. Diabetes, Hypertension, and Chronic Kidney Disease Progression: Role of DPP-4. *Am. J. Physiol. Ren. Physiol.* **2017**, *312*, F661–F670. [CrossRef] [PubMed]
27. Godinho, R.; Mega, C.; Teixeira-de-Lemos, E.; Carvalho, E.; Teixeira, F.; Fernandes, R.; Reis, F. The Place of Dipeptidyl Peptidase-4 Inhibitors in Type 2 Diabetes Therapeutics: A "Me Too" or "the Special One" Antidiabetic Class? *J. Diabetes Res.* **2015**, *2015*, 806979. [CrossRef] [PubMed]

28. Gilbert, M.P.; Pratley, R.E. GLP-1 Analogs and DPP-4 Inhibitors in Type 2 Diabetes Therapy: Review of Head-to-Head Clinical Trials. *Front. Endocrinol.* **2020**, *11*, 178. [CrossRef] [PubMed]
29. Zhang, Y.; Hong, J.; Chi, J.; Gu, W.; Ning, G.; Wang, W. Head-to-Head Comparison of Dipeptidyl Peptidase-IV Inhibitors and Sulfonylureas—A Meta-Analysis from Randomized Clinical Trials. *Diabetes Metab. Res. Rev.* **2014**, *30*, 241–256. [CrossRef]
30. Crowley, K.; Scanaill, P.; Hermanides, J.; Buggy, D.J. Current Practice in the Perioperative Management of Patients with Diabetes Mellitus: A Narrative Review. *Br. J. Anaesth.* **2023**, *131*, 242–252. [CrossRef]
31. Kirk, J.K.; Gonzales, C.F. Preoperative Considerations for Patients with Diabetes. *Expert Rev. Endocrinol. Metab.* **2023**, *18*, 503–512. [CrossRef]
32. Wright, E.M. SGLT2 inhibitors: Physiology and Pharmacology. *Kidney360* **2021**, *2*, 2027–2037. [CrossRef]
33. Boutsikos, I.; Beltsios, E.; Schmack, B.; Pantazopoulos, I.; Chatzis, D.G. Sodium glucose Co-Transporter 2 inhibitors and the cardiovascular System: Current knowledge and future expectations. *Heart Int.* **2023**, *17*, 12. [CrossRef]
34. Ehrenkranz, J.R.L.; Lewis, N.G.; Kahn, C.R.; Roth, J. Phlorizin: A review. *Diabetes/Metab. Res. Rev.* **2004**, *21*, 31–38. [CrossRef] [PubMed]
35. Chan, J.C.H.; Chan, M.C.Y. SGLT2 inhibitors: The next blockbuster multifaceted drug? *Medicina* **2023**, *59*, 388. [CrossRef] [PubMed]
36. Chasis, H.; Jolliffe, N.; Smith, H.W. The action of phlorizin on the excretion of glucose, xylose, sucrose, creatinine and urea by man. *J. Clin. Investig.* **1933**, *12*, 1083–1090. [CrossRef] [PubMed]
37. Rossetti, L.; Smith, D.; Shulman, G.I.; Papachristou, D.; DeFronzo, R.A. Correction of hyperglycemia with phlorizin normalizes tissue sensitivity to insulin in diabetic rats. *J. Clin. Investig.* **1987**, *79*, 1510–1515. [CrossRef]
38. Story of Discovery: SGLT2 Inhibitors: Harnessing the Kidneys to Help Treat Diabetes; National Institute of Diabetes and Digestive and Kidney Diseases: 2020. Available online: https://www.niddk.nih.gov/news/archive/2016/story-discovery-sglt2-inhibitors-harnessing-kidneys-help-treat-diabetes#:~:text=The%20first%20SGLT2%20inhibitor%20to,Jardiance%C2%AE)%20in%20August%202014 (accessed on 15 November 2024).
39. American Diabetes Association. Pharmacologic Approaches to Glycemic Treatment: Standards of Medical Care in Diabetes—2022. *Diabetes Care* **2021**, *45* (Suppl. S1), S125–S143. [CrossRef]
40. Scheen, A.J. Pharmacodynamics, efficacy and safety of Sodium–Glucose Co-Transporter Type 2 (SGLT2) inhibitors for the treatment of Type 2 diabetes mellitus. *Drugs* **2014**, *75*, 33–59. [CrossRef]
41. Madhok, J.; Vanneman, M.W. SGLT-2 inhibitors: Proliferating indications and perioperative pitfalls. *J. Cardiothorac. Vasc. Anesth.* **2022**, *36*, 1815–1819. [CrossRef]
42. Handelsman, Y.; Henry, R.R.; Bloomgarden, Z.T.; Dagogo-Jack, S.; DeFronzo, R.A.; Einhorn, D.; Ferrannini, E.; Fonseca, V.A.; Garber, A.J.; Grunberger, G.; et al. American Association of Clinical Endocrinologists and American College of Endocrinology Position Statement on the Association of SGLT-2 Inhibitors and Diabetic Ketoacidosis. *Endocr. Pract.* **2016**, *22*, 753–762. [CrossRef]
43. Elendu, C.; Amaechi, D.C.; Elendu, T.C.; Fiemotonghan, B.-E.; Okoye, O.K.; Agu-Ben, C.M.; Onyekweli, S.O.; Amapu, D.A.; Ikpegbu, R.; Asekhauno, M.; et al. A comprehensive review of heart failure: Unraveling the etiology, decoding pathophysiological mechanisms, navigating diagnostic modalities, exploring pharmacological interventions, advocating lifestyle modifications, and charting the horizon of emerging therapies in the complex landscape of chronic cardiac dysfunction. *Medicine* **2024**, *103*, e36895. [CrossRef]
44. Bozkurt, B.; Coats, A.J.S.; Tsutsui, H.; Abdelhamid, C.M.; Adamopoulos, S.; Albert, N.; Anker, S.D.; Atherton, J.; Böhm, M.; Butler, J.; et al. Universal definition and classification of heart failure: A report of the Heart Failure Society of America, Heart Failure Association of the European Society of Cardiology, Japanese Heart Failure Society and Writing Committee of the Universal Definition of Heart Failure. *Eur. J. Heart Fail.* **2021**, *23*, 352–380. [CrossRef]
45. Savarese, G.; Becher, P.M.; Lund, L.H.; Seferovic, P.; Rosano, G.M.C.; Coats, A.J.S. Global burden of heart failure: A comprehensive and updated review of epidemiology. *Cardiovasc. Res.* **2022**, *118*, 3272–3287. [CrossRef] [PubMed]
46. Heidenreich, P.A.; Bozkurt, B.; Aguilar, D.; Allen, L.A.; Byun, J.J.; Colvin, M.M.; Deswal, A.; Drazner, M.H.; Dunlay, S.M.; Evers, L.R.; et al. 2022 AHA/ACC/HFSA Guideline for the Management of Heart Failure. *J. Am. Coll. Cardiol.* **2022**, *79*, e263–e421. [CrossRef]
47. Gao, Z.; Barth, A.S.; DiSilvestre, D.; Akar, F.G.; Tian, Y.; Tanskanen, A.; Kass, D.A.; Winslow, R.L.; Tomaselli, G.F. Key pathways associated with heart failure development revealed by gene networks correlated with cardiac remodeling. *Physiol. Genom.* **2008**, *35*, 222–230. [CrossRef] [PubMed]
48. Baman, J.R.; Ahmad, F.S. Heart failure. *JAMA* **2020**, *324*, 1015. [CrossRef]
49. Heidenreich, P.A.; Bozkurt, B.; Aguilar, D.; Allen, L.A.; Byun, J.J.; Colvin, M.M.; Deswal, A.; Drazner, M.H.; Dunlay, S.M.; Evers, L.R.; et al. 2022 AHA/ACC/HFSA guideline for the management of heart failure: A report of the American College of Cardiology/American Heart Association Joint Committee on Clinical Practice Guidelines. *Circulation* **2022**, *145*, e895–e1032. [CrossRef] [PubMed]

50. Reina-Couto, M.; Pereira-Terra, P.; Quelhas-Santos, J.; Silva-Pereira, C.; Albino-Teixeira, A.; Sousa, T. Inflammation in human heart failure: Major mediators and therapeutic targets. *Front. Physiol.* **2021**, *12*, 746494. [CrossRef]
51. He, X.; Du, T.; Long, T.; Liao, X.; Dong, Y.; Huang, Z.P. Signaling cascades in the failing heart and emerging therapeutic strategies. *Signal Transduct. Target. Ther.* **2022**, *7*, 134. [CrossRef]
52. Ferreira, J.P.; Saraiva, F.; Sharma, A.; Vasques-Nóvoa, F.; Angélico-Gonçalves, A.; Leite, A.R.; Borges-Canha, M.; Carvalho, D.; Packer, M.; Zannad, F.; et al. Glucagon-like Peptide 1 Receptor Agonists in Patients with Type 2 Diabetes with and without Chronic Heart Failure: A Meta-Analysis of Randomized Placebo-Controlled Outcome Trials. *Diabetes Obes. Metab.* **2023**, *25*, 1495–1502. [CrossRef]
53. Kosiborod, M.N.; Abildstrøm, S.Z.; Borlaug, B.A.; Butler, J.; Rasmussen, S.; Davies, M.J.; Hovingh, G.K.; Kitzman, D.W.; Lindegaard, M.L.; Møller, D.V.; et al. Semaglutide in Patients with Heart Failure with Preserved Ejection Fraction and Obesity. *N. Engl. J. Med.* **2023**, *389*, 1069–1084. [CrossRef]
54. Jorsal, A.; Kistorp, C.; Holmager, P.; Tougaard, R.S.; Nielsen, R.; Hänselmann, A.; Nilsson, B.; Møller, J.E.; Hjort, J.; Rasmussen, J.; et al. Effect of Liraglutide, a Glucagon-like Peptide-1 Analogue, on Left Ventricular Function in Stable Chronic Heart Failure Patients with and without Diabetes ( LIVE )—A Multicentre, Double-Blind, Randomised, Placebo-Controlled Trial. *Eur. J. Heart Fail.* **2016**, *19*, 69–77. [CrossRef]
55. Fudim, M.; White, J.; Pagidipati, N.J.; Lokhnygina, Y.; Wainstein, J.; Murin, J.; Iqbal, N.; Öhman, P.; Lopes, R.D.; Reicher, B.; et al. Effect of Once-Weekly Exenatide in Patients with Type 2 Diabetes Mellitus with and without Heart Failure and Heart Failure–Related Outcomes. *Circulation* **2019**, *140*, 1613–1622. [CrossRef] [PubMed]
56. Neves, J.S.; Packer, M.; Ferreira, J.P. Increased Risk of Heart Failure Hospitalization with GLP-1 Receptor Agonists in Patients with Reduced Ejection Fraction: A Meta-Analysis of the EXSCEL and FIGHT Trials. *J. Card. Failure* **2023**. [CrossRef]
57. Mannucci, E.; Nreu, B.; Montereggi, C.; Ragghianti, B.; Gallo, M.; Giaccari, A.; Monami, M. Cardiovascular Events and All-Cause Mortality in Patients with Type 2 Diabetes Treated with Dipeptidyl Peptidase-4 Inhibitors: An Extensive Meta-Analysis of Randomized Controlled Trials. *Nutr. Metab. Cardiovasc. Dis.* **2021**, *31*, 2745–2755. [CrossRef]
58. Packer, M. Do DPP-4 Inhibitors Cause Heart Failure Events by Promoting Adrenergically Mediated Cardiotoxicity? Clues from Laboratory Models and Clinical Trials. *Circ. Res.* **2018**, *122*, 928–932. [CrossRef]
59. Li, L.; Li, S.; Deng, K.; Liu, J.; Vandvik, P.O.; Zhao, P.; Zhang, L.; Shen, J.; Bala, M.M.; Sohani, Z.N.; et al. Dipeptidyl Peptidase-4 Inhibitors and Risk of Heart Failure in Type 2 Diabetes: Systematic Review and Meta-analysis of Randomised and Observational Studies. *BMJ* **2016**, *352*, i610. [CrossRef] [PubMed]
60. Qaseem, A.; Obley, A.J.; Shamliyan, T.; Hicks, L.A.; Harrod, C.S.; Crandall, C.J. Newer Pharmacologic Treatments in Adults with Type 2 Diabetes: A Clinical Guideline from the American College of Physicians. *Ann. Intern. Med.* **2024**, *177*, 658–666. [CrossRef]
61. Enzan, N.; Matsushima, S.; Kaku, H.; Tohyama, T.; Nagata, T.; Ide, T.; Tsutsui, H. Beneficial Effects of Dipeptidyl Peptidase-4 Inhibitors on Heart Failure with Preserved Ejection Fraction and Diabetes. *JACC Asia* **2023**, *3*, 93–104. [CrossRef] [PubMed]
62. Zinman, B.; Wanner, C.; Lachin, J.M.; Fitchett, D.; Bluhmki, E.; Hantel, S.; Mattheus, M.; Devins, T.; Johansen, O.E.; Woerle, H.J.; et al. Empagliflozin, Cardiovascular Outcomes, and Mortality in Type 2 Diabetes. *N. Engl. J. Med.* **2015**, *373*, 2117–2128. [CrossRef] [PubMed]
63. Wiviott, S.D.; Raz, I.; Bonaca, M.P.; Mosenzon, O.; Kato, E.T.; Cahn, A.; Silverman, M.G.; Zelniker, T.A.; Kuder, J.F.; Murphy, S.A.; et al. Dapagliflozin and cardiovascular outcomes in type 2 diabetes. *N. Engl. J. Med.* **2018**, *380*, 347–357. [CrossRef]
64. Bhatt, D.L.; Szarek, M.; Steg, P.G.; Cannon, C.P.; Leiter, L.A.; McGuire, D.K.; Lewis, J.B.; Riddle, M.C.; Voors, A.A.; Metra, M.; et al. Sotagliflozin in Patients with Diabetes and Recent Worsening Heart Failure. *N. Engl. J. Med.* **2020**, *384*, 117–128. [CrossRef]
65. Solomon, S.D.; McMurray, J.J.V.; Claggett, B.; De Boer, R.A.; DeMets, D.; Hernandez, A.F.; Inzucchi, S.E.; Kosiborod, M.N.; Lam, C.S.P.; Martinez, F.; et al. Dapagliflozin in Heart Failure with Mildly Reduced or Preserved Ejection Fraction. *N. Engl. J. Med.* **2022**, *387*, 1089–1098. [CrossRef] [PubMed]
66. Filippatos, G.; Butler, J.; Farmakis, D.; Zannad, F.; Ofstad, A.P.; Ferreira, J.P.; Green, J.B.; Rosenstock, J.; Schnaidt, S.; Brueckmann, M.; et al. Empagliflozin for heart failure with preserved left ventricular ejection fraction with and without diabetes. *Circulation* **2022**, *146*, 676–686. [CrossRef]
67. McMurray, J.J.V.; Solomon, S.D.; Inzucchi, S.E.; Køber, L.; Kosiborod, M.N.; Martinez, F.A.; Ponikowski, P.; Sabatine, M.S.; Anand, I.S.; Bělohlávek, J.; et al. Dapagliflozin in Patients with Heart Failure and Reduced Ejection Fraction. *N. Engl. J. Med.* **2019**, *381*, 1995–2008. [CrossRef]
68. Packer, M.; Anker, S.D.; Butler, J.; Filippatos, G.; Ferreira, J.P.; Pocock, S.J.; Carson, P.; Anand, I.; Doehner, W.; Haass, M.; et al. Effect of empagliflozin on the clinical stability of patients with heart failure and a reduced ejection fraction. *Circulation* **2020**, *143*, 326–336. [CrossRef]
69. Kosiborod, M.N.; Angermann, C.E.; Collins, S.P.; Teerlink, J.R.; Ponikowski, P.; Biegus, J.; Comin-Colet, J.; Ferreira, J.P.; Mentz, R.J.; Nassif, M.E.; et al. Effects of empagliflozin on symptoms, physical limitations, and quality of life in patients hospitalized for acute heart failure: Results from the EMPULSE trial. *Circulation* **2022**, *146*, 279–288. [CrossRef]

70. Sindhvananda, W.; Poopuangpairoj, W.; Jaiprasat, T.; Ongcharit, P. Comparison of Glucose Control by Added Liraglutide to Only Insulin Infusion in Diabetic Patient Undergoing Cardiac Surgery: A Preliminary Randomized-Controlled Trial. *Ann. Card. Anaesth.* **2023**, *26*, 63–71. [CrossRef] [PubMed]
71. Hulst, A.H.; Visscher, M.J.; Godfried, M.B.; Thiel, B.; Gerritse, B.M.; Scohy, T.V.; Bouwman, R.A.; Willemsen, M.G.A.; Hollmann, M.W.; Preckel, B.; et al. Liraglutide for Perioperative Management of Hyperglycaemia in Cardiac Surgery Patients: A Multicentre Randomized Superiority Trial. *Diabetes Obes. Metab.* **2019**, *22*, 557–565. [CrossRef] [PubMed]
72. Makino, H.; Tanaka, A.; Asakura, K.; Koezuka, R.; Tochiya, M.; Ohata, Y.; Tamanaha, T.; Son, C.; Shimabara, Y.; Fujita, T.; et al. Addition of Low-Dose Liraglutide to Insulin Therapy Is Useful for Glycaemic Control during the Peri-Operative Period: Effect of Glucagon-like Peptide-1 Receptor Agonist Therapy on Glycaemic Control in Patients Undergoing Cardiac Surgery (GLOLIA Study). *Diabet. Med.* **2019**, *36*, 1621–1628. [CrossRef]
73. Oosterom-Eijmael, M.J.P.; Hermanides, J.; van Raalte, D.H.; Kouw, I.W.K.; DeVries, J.H.; Hulst, A.H. Continuous Glucose Monitoring and the Effect of Liraglutide in Cardiac Surgery Patients: A Sub-Study of the Randomized Controlled GLOBE Trial. *J. Cardiothorac. Vasc. Anesth.* **2024**, *38*, 1965–1971. [CrossRef]
74. Hulst, A.H.; Visscher, M.J.; Cherpanath, T.G.V.; van de Wouw, L.; Godfried, M.B.; Thiel, B.; Gerritse, B.M.; Scohy, T.V.; Bouwman, R.A.; Willemsen, M.G.A.; et al. Effects of Liraglutide on Myocardial Function after Cardiac Surgery: A Secondary Analysis of the Randomised Controlled GLOBE Trial. *J. Clin. Med.* **2020**, *9*, 673. [CrossRef]
75. Cardona, S.; Tsegka, K.; Pasquel, F.J.; Jacobs, S.; Halkos, M.; Keeling, W.B.; Davis, G.M.; Fayfman, M.; Albury, B.; Urrutia, M.A.; et al. Sitagliptin for the Prevention and Treatment of Perioperative Hyperglycemia in Patients with Type 2 Diabetes Undergoing Cardiac Surgery: A Randomized Controlled Trial. *Diabetes Obes. Metab.* **2021**, *23*, 480–488. [CrossRef] [PubMed]
76. Sardu, C.; Massetti, M.; Testa, N.; Di Martino, L.; Castellano, G.; Turriziani, F.; Sasso, F.C.; Torella, M.; De Feo, M.; Santulli, G.; et al. Effects of Sodium-Glucose Transporter 2 Inhibitors (SGLT2-I) in Patients with Ischemic Heart Disease (IHD) Treated by Coronary Artery Bypass Grafting via MiECC: Inflammatory Burden, and Clinical Outcomes at 5 Years of Follow-Up. *Front. Pharmacol.* **2021**, *12*. [CrossRef] [PubMed]
77. Al Namat, R.; Duceac, L.D.; Chelaru, L.; Dabija, M.G.; Guțu, C.; Marcu, C.; Popa, M.V.; Popa, F.; Goroftei, E.R.B.; Țarcă, E. Post-Coronary Artery Bypass Grafting Outcomes of Patients with/without Type-2 Diabetes Mellitus and Chronic Kidney Disease Treated with SGLT2 Inhibitor Dapagliflozin: A Single-Center Experience Analysis. *Diagnostics* **2023**, *14*, 16. [CrossRef] [PubMed]
78. Cagliostro, M.; Hundal, P.; Ting, P.; Patel, S.; Sudarshan, S.; Thomas, J.; Morris, K.; Mancini, D.M.; Moss, N.; Lala, A.; et al. Safety and effects of SGLT-2 inhibitor use among LVAD patients with type 2 diabetes mellitus. *Am. Heart J. Plus Cardiol. Res. Pract.* **2022**, *18*, 100154. [CrossRef]
79. Fardman, A.; Kodesh, A.; Siegel, A.J.; Segev, A.; Regev, E.; Maor, E.; Berkovitch, A.; Kuperstein, R.; Morgan, A.; Nahum, E.; et al. The safety of sodium glucose transporter 2 inhibitors and trends in clinical and hemodynamic parameters in patients with left ventricular assist devices. *Artif. Organs* **2024**, *48*, 902–911. [CrossRef]


**Disclaimer/Publisher's Note:** The statements, opinions and data contained in all publications are solely those of the individual author(s) and contributor(s) and not of MDPI and/or the editor(s). MDPI and/or the editor(s) disclaim responsibility for any injury to people or property resulting from any ideas, methods, instructions or products referred to in the content.

life

MDPI

*Review*

# Left Atrial Strain in Patients with Chronic Heart Failure with Preserved Ejection Fraction: A Narrative Review

**Dana Emilia Man [1,2], Alexandru Catalin Motofelea [3,*], Valentina Buda [4], Dana Emilia Velimirovici [1,2], Olivia Bodea [1], Daniel Marius Duda-Seiman [1,2], Constantin Tudor Luca [2,5] and Simona-Ruxanda Dragan [1,2]**

1 University Clinic of Internal Medicine and Ambulatory Care, Prevention and Cardiovascular Recovery, Department VI—Cardiology, "Victor Babes" University of Medicine and Pharmacy, 3000041 Timisoara, Romania; man.dana@umft.ro (D.E.M.); dana.velimirovici@umft.ro (D.E.V.); olivia-maria.bodea@umft.ro (O.B.); daniel.duda-seiman@umft.ro (D.M.D.-S.); simona.dragan@umft.ro (S.-R.D.)
2 Research Centre of Timisoara Institute of Cardiovascular Diseases, "Victor Babes" University of Medicine and Pharmacy, 3000041 Timisoara, Romania; constantin.luca@umft.ro
3 Center for Molecular Research in Nephrology and Vascular Disease, Faculty of Medicine, "Victor Babes" University of Medicine and Pharmacy, 300041 Timisoara, Romania
4 University Clinic of Clinical Pharmacy, Communication in Pharmacy, Pharmaceutical Care, Department I, Faculty of Pharmacy, "Victor Babeş" University of Medicine and Pharmacy, 2 Eftimie Murgu Square, 300041 Timisoara, Romania; buda.valentina@umft.ro
5 University Clinic of Cardiology II, Department VI—Cardiology, "Victor Babes" University of Medicine and Pharmacy, 3000041 Timisoara, Romania
* Correspondence: alexandru.motofelea@umft.ro

**Abstract:** Background: Heart failure with preserved ejection fraction (HFpEF) represents a significant portion of heart failure cases, but diagnosis is challenging due to its diverse presentation and the limitations of traditional echocardiographic parameters. Left atrial (LA) strain provides valuable insights into LA function and is increasingly used to evaluate cardiac function, including left ventricular (LV) diastolic function. LA strain, particularly reservoir strain, is considered a reliable indicator of LV diastolic function and can be used to grade diastolic function and estimate LV filling pressure. Unlike traditional LA measurements, LA strain offers detailed insights into LA function, conduit, and booster-pump phases, making it crucial for evaluating both structural and functional cardiac performance, especially in HFpEF. HFpEF diagnosis currently relies on a combination of echocardiographic parameters, clinical symptoms, and natriuretic peptide levels, encompassing various pathophysiological entities and complicating standardized management. Precise characterization of cardiac pathologies in HFpEF patients is essential. This review assesses global longitudinal strain (GLS) and left atrial strain (LAS) as echocardiographic biomarkers for diagnosing and characterizing HFpEF. Strain imaging, particularly speckle tracking echocardiography, offers a refined assessment of myocardial deformation, providing detailed insights into left heart function beyond traditional measures. Normal ranges for GLS and LAS are discussed, acknowledging demographic and technical influences. Clinical studies confirm the prognostic value of GLS and LAS in HFpEF, especially for predicting cardiovascular outcomes and distinguishing HFpEF from other dyspnea causes. However, variability in strain measurements and false-negative risks necessitate cautious clinical interpretation. The HFA-PEFF scoring system includes these biomarkers but does not fully cover the HFpEF pathology spectrum. Combining GLS and LAS shows promise in defining HFpEF phenogroups, potentially guiding individualized treatments. Global longitudinal strain (GLS) and left atrial strain (LAS) are central to non-invasive HFpEF diagnosis and stratification, with potential for more tailored therapies. Integration of these biomarkers into standard diagnostic practice requires an organized approach, and future guidelines should recommend their combined use for comprehensive HFpEF assessment.

**Keywords:** left atrial strain; speckle tracking echocardiography; diastolic dysfunction; diastolic function; HFpEF; left atrium; heart failure; biomarkers; diagnosis; echocardiography; exercise echocardiography; natriuretic peptides

## 1. Introduction

More than half of all heart failure (HF) cases are classified as heart failure with preserved ejection fraction (HFpEF) [1]. In patients presenting with HF symptoms, assessment of left ventricular (LV) function is typically conducted through transthoracic echocardiography (TTE), the primary imaging tool in clinical cardiology. Many HF patients with elevated or high-normal natriuretic peptide levels show a preserved or normal LV ejection fraction (LVEF) above 50% are currently categorized as HFpEF. However, HFpEF should be viewed not as a distinct diagnosis but rather as a syndrome. This phenotype, labeled "HFpEF", can arise from multiple pathological entities, each with unique comorbidities and varied prognoses. Therefore, the true diagnostic objective of TTE in these patients extends beyond measuring LVEF; it is to identify underlying cardiac pathologies and achieve a precise diagnosis [2].

The term "diastolic HF" was originally defined as "an increased resistance to filling in one or both ventricles, causing symptoms of pulmonary congestion due to an abnormal upward shift in the diastolic pressure-volume relation". This was later redefined as "HFpEF" [1]. Recent diagnostic algorithms classify patients with preserved LVEF and heart failure symptoms under the broad diagnosis of "HFpEF", despite varying underlying pathologies, treatment options, and prognoses. These HFpEF algorithms rely on clinical symptoms, lab results, echocardiographic data, and/or invasive hemodynamic measurements, which often fall short of identifying the specific underlying diagnosis. When identifiable cardiac conditions such as valvular diseases, significant coronary artery disease, or pericardial constriction are found, they are classified as "HFpEF masqueraders" and should be excluded. Arrhythmias, often stemming from specific cardiac conditions, are also seen as HFpEF masqueraders, with the exception of atrial fibrillation (AF), which is frequently associated with HFpEF symptoms [2,3]. Ultimately, excluding HFpEF masqueraders may lead only to a diagnosis of HFpEF of unknown origin. Non-cardiac conditions—such as pulmonary diseases, anemia, diabetes, systemic infections, cancer, obesity, and frailty—add to the multifactorial complexity of HFpEF as a diagnosis [4,5]. In a study conducted by Shah A.M. et al. [6], it was documented that elevated right and left pressures, left ventricular hypertrophy, as well as right ventricular enlargement, all play a crucial role in outcome estimation. A recent study by Duchnowski et al. identified hs-TnT and NT-proBNP as independent predictors of postoperative cardiogenic shock requiring MCS in heart valve surgery patients. Given NT-proBNP's role in HFpEF, these findings highlight the importance of hemodynamic monitoring and biomarker evaluation in HF risk stratification, linking myocardial stress and hemodynamic instability to both post-surgical outcomes and HFpEF [7].

The aim of this study was to analyze clinical, echocardiographic, and hemodynamic characteristics in HFpEF patients, focusing on parameters such as elevated right and left pressures, left ventricular hypertrophy, and right ventricular enlargement to identify key predictors of prognosis and refine diagnostic approaches.

## 2. Materials and Methods

From the beginning, the present review was designed to be a narrative review, with the main focus stipulated in the title of the present article (the clinical utility of left arterial strain in HFpEF patients). Two researchers conducted the literature research independently on two electronic databases (PubMed and Scopus) from June 2014 to September 2024. The search included different keyword combinations, such as "left arterial strain"/"speckle tracking echocardiography" AND "HFpEF"/"heart failure with preserved ejection fraction"/"diastolic function"/"diastolic dysfunction" AND "diagnosis"/"biomarkers". Strain measurements were performed using vendor-independent software (Version 4.6, TomTec Imaging Systems GmbH, Unterschleißheim, Germany). A third researcher removed the duplicates using an Microsoft Excel (Microsoft Corporation, Redmond, WA, USA; Version: Microsoft 365) based on article title, author names, and year of publication. Moreover, the three researchers also screened the relevant review articles for additional references that may have been overlooked in the initial search.

### 2.1. Inclusion Criteria

The review included studies focusing on patients with chronic heart failure with preserved ejection fraction (HFpEF) and those with documented left atrial (LA) strain measurements using 2D speckle tracking echocardiography. Eligible study designs encompassed original research, meta-analyses, systematic reviews, and prospective and retrospective cohort studies. Only studies providing detailed insights into the relationship between left atrial strain (LAS), global longitudinal strain (GLS), and cardiac function were included. Outcomes of interest involved the evaluation of LA strain in the diagnosis, phenotyping, prognosis, or treatment response for HFpEF. Additionally, studies had to report echocardiographic parameters, left ventricular diastolic function, or predictive value for cardiovascular outcomes, such as major adverse cardiovascular events or atrial fibrillation. The review focused on studies utilizing 2D speckle tracking echocardiography as the primary method for assessing LA strain.

### 2.2. Exclusion Criteria

The review excluded studies that focused exclusively on heart failure with reduced ejection fraction (HFrEF) or other cardiac conditions without a specific emphasis on HFpEF. Pediatric or non-adult population studies were also excluded. Case reports, editorials, and narrative commentaries without primary data or comprehensive reviews were not included. Studies lacking quantitative analysis of LA strain or GLS were excluded. Articles that did not provide sufficient data on the role of LA strain in HFpEF or presented ambiguous or inconsistent strain values and thresholds were deemed ineligible. Studies using imaging techniques other than 2D speckle tracking echocardiography or those employing outdated or experimental imaging software without vendor-independent validation were excluded. Methodologically flawed studies, those with small sample sizes (fewer than 30 patients), or those providing low-quality evidence were omitted. Articles not published in English or those without accessible full texts were also excluded.

## 3. Discussion

Different stages and severities of heart failure (HF) present a wide range of echocardiographic findings, characterized by diverse functional analyses and varying strain thresholds. Among these, left atrial (LA) strain and left ventricular (LV) strain have emerged as critical early indicators of diastolic dysfunction and contractile impairment, often becoming evident before structural changes occur. LA strain reflects the atrium's reservoir, conduit, and booster-pump functions, offering insights into atrial stiffness, elevated left ventricular filling pressures (LVFP), and early diastolic dysfunction [8,9]. Similarly, global longitudinal strain (GLS) of the LV is a sensitive marker for detecting subtle systolic dysfunction that may not be captured by traditional ejection fraction (EF) measurements. Together, these strain parameters play a crucial role in refining the phenotyping of HF, improving the identification of subclinical dysfunction, and guiding appropriate clinical management [8,9].

LA strain, in particular, has gained recognition as a valuable and increasingly reliable tool for assessing cardiac function, especially in the context of left ventricular diastolic dysfunction (LVDD) and heart failure with preserved ejection fraction (HFpEF) [8–10]. Its reliability stems from its capacity to provide detailed insights into left atrial function, which is intricately linked to LVFP. Studies have demonstrated that LA strain offers independent predictive value for elevated LV pressures [8,9] and serves as a sensitive marker for early diastolic dysfunction. Furthermore, it is non-invasive and reproducible, making it practical for routine clinical application. The use of 2D speckle tracking echocardiography (STE) to measure LA strain allows for real-time evaluation of myocardial deformation, offering a comprehensive view of atrial mechanics [10].

The strengths and weaknesses of LA strain are summarized in Table 1. Among its strengths, LA strain can detect subtle atrial dysfunction earlier than conventional parameters, such as LA volume, and provides significant prognostic value for heart failure progression, atrial fibrillation (AF), and valvular diseases. Additionally, it is a non-invasive and practical method that aids in risk stratification and tracking disease progression over time. However, LA strain is limited by technical variability across imaging platforms, dependence on image quality, and the lack of standardized cut-off values. Furthermore, irregular rhythms, such as atrial fibrillation, and significant mitral valve disease can impair strain measurement accuracy. Acute changes in loading conditions and variability in operator expertise can further complicate its application [10,11].

**Table 1.** Strengths and weaknesses of LA strain.

| Strengths | Bibliography | Weaknesses | Bibliography |
|---|---|---|---|
| Early Detection of Dysfunction: LA strain can detect subtle left atrial dysfunction even before structural changes occur. | Aung et al., 2017 [12]; Nagueh and Khan, 2022 [13] | Technical Variability: Different imaging techniques, software platforms, and vendor-specific algorithms can produce inconsistent results, making comparisons challenging. | Khan et al., 2020 [14] Nagueh and Khan, 2022 [13]; |
| Prognostic Value: Provides significant prognostic information for heart failure, atrial fibrillation (AF), and valvular diseases. | Kagami et al., 2024 [10]; Reddy et al., 2020 [11]; Shin et al., 2021 [15] | Image Quality: Poor echocardiographic windows, especially in obese patients or those with lung disease, can reduce the accuracy of LA strain measurements. | Aung et al., 2017 [12]; Nagueh and Khan, 2022 [13] |
| Sensitive Marker for LA Function: More sensitive than conventional parameters (e.g., LA size) in identifying reduced LA function. | Aung et al., 2017 [12] | Dependence on Heart Rhythm: Irregular rhythms, such as atrial fibrillation, can impair strain analysis and limit the reproducibility of results. | Reddy et al., 2020 [11] |
| Non-invasive: Offers a non-invasive way to assess atrial mechanics. | Ye et al., 2020 [16] | Mitral Valve Disease: The presence of significant mitral valve disease (e.g., stenosis, regurgitation, or annular calcification) can interfere with LA function, complicating strain interpretation. | Pournazari et al., 2022 [17] |

**Table 1.** *Cont.*

| Strengths | Bibliography | Weaknesses | Bibliography |
|---|---|---|---|
| Valuable for Risk Stratification: Helps identify high-risk patients in AF, heart failure, and post-surgery cases. | Maffeis et al., 2022 [18] | Load Dependence: LA strain is influenced by preload and afterload conditions, which may affect its reliability as a measure of intrinsic LA function. | Pournazari et al., 2022 [17]; Nagueh and Khan, 2022 [13] |
| Utility in Monitoring: Useful for tracking disease progression and treatment response over time. | Aung et al., 2017 [12]; Ye et al., 2020 [16] | Lack of Standardized Cut-Offs: There is no universally accepted threshold for differentiating normal and pathological LA strain values, leading to ambiguity in clinical practice. | Nagueh and Khan, 2022 [13] |
| Strong Correlation with Outcomes: LA strain correlates well with clinical outcomes like AF recurrence and cardiovascular events. | Jasic-Szpak et al., 2021 [19]; Shin et al., 2021 [15] | Limited Longitudinal Data: The prognostic value of LA strain over time and its role in disease progression remain areas of ongoing research. | Khan et al., 2020 [14]; Fauchier et al., 2023 [20] |

Despite its limitations, the strong correlation between LA strain and adverse cardiovascular outcomes, such as heart failure progression and atrial fibrillation recurrence, underscores its clinical utility. Research suggests that reduced LA strain is associated with worse prognoses, emphasizing its value as a prognostic marker [8–10].

LA strain is measured using 2D speckle tracking echocardiography, a non-invasive imaging technique that evaluates myocardial deformation by tracking the movement of acoustic markers within the echocardiographic image frame by frame. The process involves capturing high-quality echocardiographic images and analyzing them with software that calculates strain parameters. This method provides quantitative data on atrial mechanics, enabling clinicians to assess left atrial function and LV diastolic pressures with precision [10]. Although its reliability depends on operator expertise and technical consistency, LA strain remains a powerful tool for evaluating LVDD and HFpEF, particularly when integrated with other echocardiographic parameters [11]. With growing evidence supporting its prognostic value, LA strain is increasingly recognized as a cornerstone of advanced echocardiographic assessment, despite the need for further standardization and longitudinal research [8–11].

### *3.1. Characteristics of an Optimal Index for LV Diastolic Function*

In patients with myocardial disease, there is often impaired left ventricular (LV) relaxation and increased LV chamber stiffness. An ideal index for assessing LV diastolic function should clarify whether it primarily reflects LV relaxation, LV chamber stiffness, or both. Although these two hemodynamic abnormalities frequently coexist, an optimal noninvasive index would primarily indicate one of these aspects while accurately representing the underlying abnormality it aims to measure, allowing for effective tracking of changes in either LV relaxation or stiffness over time [16].

To ensure reliability, this ideal index would minimize the influence of extraneous variables such as heart rate, LV systolic properties, and right ventricular–LV interactions. While it is challenging to develop a noninvasive measure that meets all these criteria, these attributes provide essential guidelines for evaluating potential indices of LV diastolic function. For example, some echocardiographic measures, like peak tricuspid regurgitation velocity, are not directly related to LV relaxation or stiffness. In contrast, indices such as myocardial velocities via tissue Doppler imaging (reflecting LV relaxation), myocardial diastolic strain rate (also reflecting LV relaxation), and shear wave propagation velocity (indicating myocardial stiffness) are directly impacted by LV diastolic function [14].

### 3.2. Measuring Left Atrial (LA) Strain

LA strain was initially measured using tissue Doppler imaging and is now primarily assessed with speckle tracking. The current guidelines recommend measuring LA strain in the apical four-chamber view, with the QRS complex as the reference point. Although LA strain can also be measured in the apical two-chamber view, which includes additional LA segments, there is no strong evidence suggesting this view provides added diagnostic or prognostic value [21].

In practice, achieving clear imaging of the LA roof can be challenging, and significant variation in LA strain measurements may occur between the interatrial septum and the LA free wall. It remains unclear if the fewer segments captured in the apical four-chamber view yield comparable results to a comprehensive view with all segments, particularly in evaluating diastolic function [12] (Figures 1 and 2).

Left atrial strain curve analysis: The right upper panel displays the left atrial (LA) strain curves from a normal subject. The LA strain curve consists of a positive peak during end-systole (reservoir phase), followed by two descending phases: one during early diastole (passive emptying) and the other during late diastole (active emptying). In the right lower panel, LA dyssynchrony is quantified as the maximum difference in time-to-peak regional LA strain, adjusted for the RR interval (referred to as LA time-diff). LA: left atrium; GLS: global longitudinal strain.

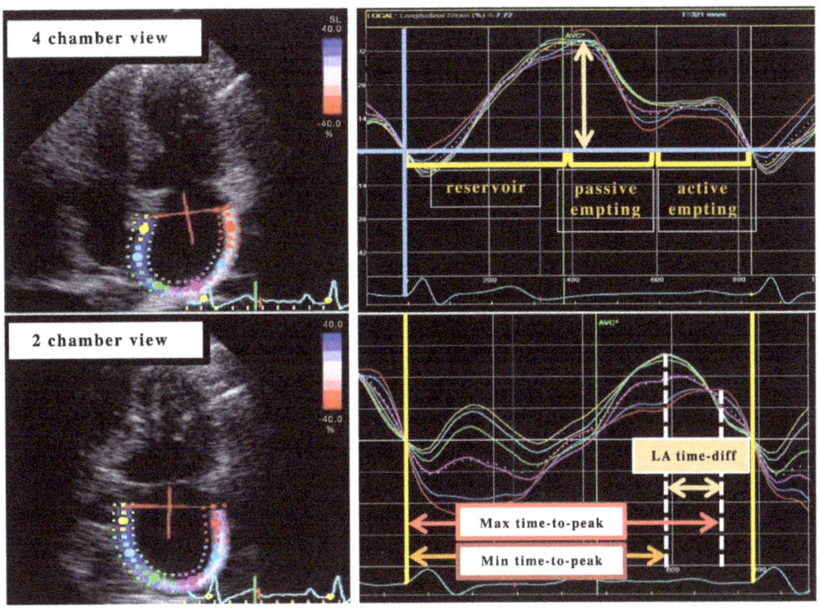


**Figure 1.** Echocardiographic analysis of left atrial (LA) strain: Phases of atrial function and dyssynchrony assessment.

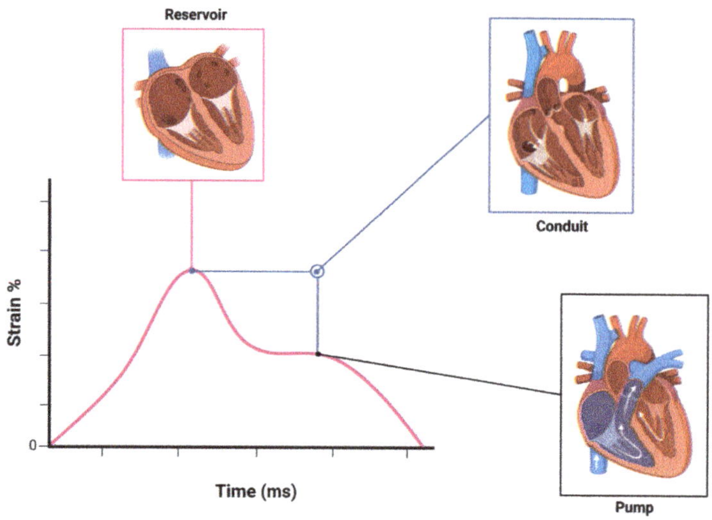


**Figure 2.** Phases of left atrial strain in HFpEF.

### 3.3. Normal Values of LA Strain

A recent important study that included 1765 normal subjects reported on the normal values of LA strain. There were 402 subjects older than 65 years of age, with 864 women. In this sample, 38.4% were White, 39.9% were Asian, and 9.7% were Black [13]. Strain measurements were performed by a vendor of independent software (Version 4.6, TomTec, Unterschleißheim, Germany). As noted, there is a wide range for normal LA strain values for all age groups and for both sexes. A study published by Singh et al. [22] is very important from our perspective because it includes both normal patients and patients with type 2 diastolic dysfunction, subjects from several countries, with a wide age range; here, central analysis was carried out in a core laboratory and using a software that is vendor independent. All these attributes are important, and as a result, when looking at normal values, we believe that the data from the report by Singh et al. [22] supersede findings based on single-center studies or meta-analysis that did not take into account the impact of the specific vendor software used to analyze LA strain. Importantly, other large and multicenter studies that reported on normal values of LA strain have shown similar findings with respect to lower limits of normal values for left atrial reservoir strain (LARS) [23].

### 3.4. Hemodynamic Influences on Left Atrial Reservoir Strain (LARS)

While there is strong interest in using LARS as an indicator of left ventricular diastolic function, data on its hemodynamic determinants remain limited. LARS, which occurs during systole, is influenced by various factors due to its association with left atrial (LA) filling. As LA strain reflects filling during systole, its relation to early systolic LA relaxation is crucial. Efficient LA relaxation, which occurs early in systole, reduces LA pressure, promoting forward pulmonary venous flow and increasing LA expansion [1].

Another key factor affecting LARS is the descent of the mitral annulus during systole, which is influenced by LV systolic function, especially the longitudinal function associated with sub endocardial fibers [2]. This movement can be quantified through LV global longitudinal strain (GLS). Additionally, LA chamber stiffness plays a critical role, as greater stiffness restricts LA expansion, raises LA V-wave pressure, and reduces the pressure gradient from the pulmonary veins to the LA, thus lowering LARS. Consequently, the relationship between LARS and LA pressures is indirect and modified by other hemodynamic factors [1] (Figure 3).

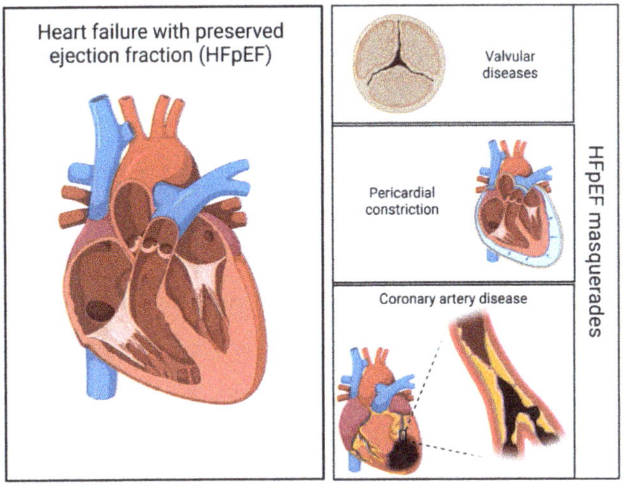


**Figure 3.** Alternative diagnoses mimicking HFpEF: key considerations for differential diagnosis.

In studies involving patients undergoing cardiac catheterization, LARS showed a direct relationship with LA pump strain and LV GLS [2]. However, the association of LARS with mean pulmonary capillary wedge pressure and LV pre-A-wave pressure was significantly affected by LV systolic function. For patients with normal LV ejection fraction (LVEF), LARS proved less accurate in estimating LV filling pressure, and in patients with GLS $\geq$ 18%, no significant relation between LARS and LV filling pressure was observed. This may be due to an interaction where enhanced LA contractility supports faster LA relaxation, as evidenced by the relationship between LA reservoir and pump strain [18].

Further evidence of LA relaxation's effects on LARS comes from a study by Pournazari et al. [17], which involved patients with primary mitral regurgitation undergoing transcatheter mitral valve repair. Here, LA relaxation was calculated as the pressure difference between peak A-wave and X-wave pressures relative to the time interval, showing that faster LA relaxation correlated with a more substantial pressure drop over a shorter time. This study confirmed a strong relationship between LA relaxation and LARS both before and after the procedure. Moreover, the study highlighted the influence of LA chamber stiffness on LARS, noting an inverse relationship between LA stiffness and LARS [24].

Through multiple regression analyses, LA relaxation, LV GLS, and LA chamber stiffness emerged as independent determinants of LARS before and after transcatheter mitral repair, although LARS variability post-repair was substantial [15,25].

### 3.5. Hemodynamic Influences on LA Conduit Strain and Pump Strain

While left atrial reservoir strain is often highlighted as a key indicator of LV diastolic function, less attention has been given to LA conduit and pump strain. Typically, impaired LV relaxation with normal LA pressure corresponds with reduced LA conduit strain and elevated LA pump strain. However, research in this area remains limited [15].

One study involving patients with hypertrophic cardiomyopathy found that LA conduit strain directly correlated with early diastolic mitral annulus velocity (e′). Conversely, LA conduit strain showed a significant inverse relationship with the myocardial extracellular volume fraction (measured by cardiac magnetic resonance) and with an index of

LV end-diastolic pressure (LVEDP), namely, the time difference between atrial velocity in pulmonary vein flow and peak atrial mitral inflow (Ar-A duration) [26,27].

Thus, LA conduit strain appears to depend on both LV relaxation, as indicated by e′, and on LV interstitial fibrosis, as suggested by extracellular volume fraction, which impacts LV chamber stiffness (Table 2).

**Table 2.** Hemodynamic reference values for LA conduit and pump strain in hypertrophic cardiomyopathy.

| Reference | Patient Population | LA Conduit Strain (%) | LA Pump Strain (%) | Methodology | Key Findings |
|---|---|---|---|---|---|
| [15] | Hypertrophic cardiomyopathy patients | Reduced | Elevated | Speckle tracking echocardiography, echocardiographic indices | Impaired LV relaxation with normal LA pressure results in reduced LA conduit strain and elevated LA pump strain. |
| [26] | Hypertrophic cardiomyopathy patients | Correlated with e′ | Not specified | Mitral annulus velocity (e′), cardiac magnetic resonance for fibrosis | Positive correlation of LA conduit strain with early diastolic mitral annulus velocity (e′); inverse relationship with myocardial extracellular volume fraction. |
| [27] | Hypertrophic cardiomyopathy patients | Inversely related | Not specified | Ar-A duration (time difference between atrial velocity in pulmonary vein flow and peak atrial mitral inflow) | LA conduit strain showed a significant inverse relationship with Ar-A duration, an index of LV end-diastolic pressure (LVEDP). |

### 3.6. Determinants of LA Pump Strain

LA pump strain, occurring at end diastole, is influenced by LA systolic function and afterload, primarily reflecting LV late diastolic pressures. Early studies established a strong correlation between LA pump strain and LV filling pressures, a finding reaffirmed by recent research. Tayal et al. [28] demonstrated a direct relationship between LA pump strain and LA systolic function markers, including late diastolic mitral inflow peak velocity (A), mitral annulus late diastolic velocity (a′), and LA ejection force [29]. An inverse correlation exists between LA pump strain and Doppler-derived LV end-diastolic pressure (LVEDP), as represented by the Ar-A duration. Furthermore, LA pump strain correlates with LV late diastolic stiffness, measured via A-wave transit time. Increased LV stiffness shortens A-wave transit time, reducing LA pump strain due to elevated LV diastolic pressures [19].

### 3.7. Determinants of Left Atrial (LA) Pump Strain: HFpEF vs. HFrEF

LA pump strain reflects atrial contractile function and differs between heart failure with preserved ejection fraction (HFpEF) and reduced ejection fraction (HFrEF), influencing strain curve patterns and clinical interpretation.

HFpEF: LA enlargement and fibrosis from chronically elevated LV filling pressures increase atrial stiffness, reducing reservoir function. The booster pump phase compensates early, but progressive dysfunction decreases LA pump strain. A cut-off value <7–9% indicates significant dysfunction.

HFrEF: LA dilation results from LV systolic dysfunction and volume overload, leading to impaired contractility and remodeling. LA pump strain is markedly reduced, with a flatter strain curve reflecting severe dysfunction. A cut-off < 6–7% suggests advanced impairment (Table 3).

**Table 3.** Comparison of LA strain patterns in HFpEF vs. HFrEF [27].

| Parameter | HFpEF | HFrEF |
|---|---|---|
| LA Reservoir Strain | Mild to moderately reduced | Severely reduced |
| LA Conduit Strain | Reduced (due to increased stiffness) | Reduced (due to LV dysfunction) |
| LA Pump Strain | Preserved initially, reduced later | Significantly reduced |
| Adaptation | LA compensates via active contraction | LA fails due to contractile dysfunction |
| Typical Cut-Off | LA pump strain < 7–9% | LA pump strain < 6–7% |

Clinically, LA pump strain serves as a marker of increased LA stiffness and subclinical dysfunction in HFpEF, while in HFrEF, it highlights advanced atrial remodeling and poor contractility. Disease-specific strain thresholds enhance heart failure phenotyping and management [27].

### 3.8. Correlation with LV Filling Pressure (PAWP)

Left atrial (LA) strain serves as a valuable non-invasive marker for assessing left ventricular (LV) filling pressures, commonly represented by pulmonary artery wedge pressure (PAWP). Abnormalities in LA strain, particularly during the reservoir phase, have consistently shown a strong correlation with elevated LV filling pressures, making it a useful tool for diagnosing and monitoring patients with HFpEF. A decrease in LV filling pressures is typically accompanied by a reduction in LA volumes, although complete normalization is rare. Importantly, there is a strong correlation between reduced LV filling pressures and improved LA function, as reflected by enhanced LA strain. This relationship is particularly significant, as elevated filling pressures are a hallmark of HFpEF and contribute to its clinical manifestations [30].

### 3.9. Association with Major Adverse Cardiovascular Events (MACE)

Left atrial (LA) strain has shown significant predictive value for major adverse cardiovascular events (MACE) in patients with HFpEF. Reduced LA strain is linked to worse cardiovascular outcomes, including all-cause mortality, cardiovascular mortality, and heart failure hospitalizations. The decline in LA function, as indicated by impaired strain, underscores the complex relationship between LA dysfunction and the progression of HFpEF. Consequently, LA strain serves as a valuable prognostic tool, helping clinicians in risk stratification and identifying patients at increased risk of cardiovascular events [31].

### 3.10. Risk of Atrial Fibrillation (AF)

Atrial fibrillation (AF) is highly prevalent among HFpEF patients and is associated with increased morbidity and mortality. Left atrial (LA) strain has emerged as a valuable predictor of AF development in this population. Reduced LA strain reflects impaired LA function, which is linked to atrial remodeling and electrical disturbances that facilitate the onset and maintenance of AF. As such, LA strain not only provides insight into the current status of HFpEF but also serves as a potential marker for identifying individuals at higher risk of developing AF [13].

In this context, left atrial (LA) strain plays a crucial role in the management of HFpEF by providing valuable insights into left ventricular (LV) filling pressures, predicting major adverse cardiovascular events, and identifying patients at risk for atrial fibrillation. As a key element of advanced echocardiographic assessment, LA strain has proven to be the most reliable imaging marker for distinguishing HFpEF from non-cardiac causes of dyspnea. Furthermore, abnormalities in LA strain are more strongly associated with adverse outcomes than those in LV function [20].

Abnormalities in left ventricular longitudinal strain have emerged as a valuable marker for identifying a distinct phenogroup within the heterogeneous HFpEF syndrome. This phenogroup, characterized by reduced global longitudinal strain (HFpEF-rLS), reflects the presence of contractile dysfunction, myocardial fibrosis, maladaptive hypertrophy, and other underlying myocardial disorders [19] (Table 4).

**Table 4.** Articles published about left atrial strain.

| Title | Authors | Year | Pts No | Study Type | Conclusion |
|---|---|---|---|---|---|
| Impaired Left Atrial Reserve Function in Heart Failure With Preserved Ejection Fraction [10] | Kagami, K.; Harada, T.; Yuasa, N.; Saito, Y.; Sorimachi, H.; Murakami, F.; Naito, A.; Tani, Y.; Kato, T.; Wada, N.; et al. | 2024 | 240 | Original research | Reduced left atrial (LA) reservoir function during exercise in heart failure with preserved ejection fraction (HFpEF) is linked to biventricular reserve limitations, exercise intolerance, and a higher risk of heart failure events. |
| Atrial Dysfunction in Patients With Heart Failure With Preserved Ejection Fraction and Atrial Fibrillation [11] | Reddy, Y.N.V.; Obokata, M.; Verbrugge, F.H.; Lin, G.; Borlaug, B.A. | 2020 | 278 | Original research | Left atrial (LA) compliance and mechanics progressively deteriorate as atrial fibrillation (AF) burden increases in HFpEF, elevating the risk of new-onset AF and the progression of existing AF. |
| Left Atrial Strain in Evaluation of Heart Failure with Preserved Ejection Fraction [16] | Ye, Z.; Miranda, W.R.; Yeung, D.F.; Kane, G.C.; Oh, J.K. | 2020 | 450 | Original research | Left atrial strain during the reservoir phase (LASreservoir) has the potential to identify patients with intermediate HFpEF scores who may exhibit elevated left ventricular filling pressures during exercise (LVFP-ex) only. Thus, it serves as a promising diagnostic alternative when exercise testing is not feasible. |
| Left atrial function in heart failure with preserved ejection fraction: a systematic review and meta-analysis [14] | Khan, M.S.; Memon, M.M.; Murad, M.H.; Vaduganathan, M.; Greene, S.J.; Hall, M.; Triposkiadis, F.; Lam, C.S.P.; Shah, A.M.; Butler, J.; et al. | 2020 | 2725 | Meta-analysis | Although impaired left atrial (LA) function shows potential diagnostic and prognostic value in HFpEF, its ability to significantly enhance diagnostic or prognostic accuracy has yet to be fully established. |

**Table 4.** *Cont.*

| Title | Authors | Year | Pts No | Study Type | Conclusion |
|---|---|---|---|---|---|
| Left atrial structure and function in heart failure with reduced (HFrEF) versus preserved ejection fraction (HFpEF): systematic review and meta-analysis [21] | Jin, X.; Nauta, J.F.; Hung, C.L.; Ouwerkerk, W.; Teng, T.K.; Voors, A.A.; Lam, C.S.; van Melle, J.P. | 2022 | 18.734 | Meta-analysis | While left atrial (LA) abnormalities have been proposed as a hallmark of HFpEF, our findings indicate that LA structure and function are more impaired in patients with HFrEF than in those with HFpEF. Therefore, the role of intrinsic LA myopathy as a key pathophysiological feature should be equally emphasized in both HFrEF and HFpEF populations. |
| Left atrial strain in heart failure with preserved ejection fraction [12] | Aung, S.M.; Güler, A.; Güler, Y.; Huraibat, A.; Karabay, C.Y.; Akdemir, I | 2017 | 83 | Prospective single-center cohort study | Left atrial (LA) function, as evaluated by 2D speckle-tracking echocardiography (2D-STE), is impaired in patients with HFpEF. A global left atrial strain during the reservoir phase (GLAs-res) value of <17.5% may serve as a useful diagnostic marker for HFpEF. |
| Left Atrial Strain for Assessment of Left Ventricular Diastolic Function: Focus on Populations With Normal LVEF [13] | Nagueh, S.F.; Khan, S.U. | 2022 | | | Left atrial (LA) strain is a valuable metric for assessing the mechanical properties of the LA, providing insight into its reservoir, conduit, and pump functions. |
| Heart Failure With Preserved Ejection Fraction: Do You Know Your Left Atrial Strain? [23] | Jellis, C.L.; Klein, A.L. | 2016 | | Editorial | Beyond serving as an alternative prognostic marker in HFpEF, left atrial (LA) strain holds promise for tracking disease severity or treatment response over time. This could minimize the need for repeated comprehensive assessments of diastolic parameters during follow-up. |
| Left atrial strain predicts exercise capacity in heart failure independently of left ventricular ejection fraction [18] | Maffeis, C.; Rossi, A.; Cannata, L.; Zocco, C.; Belyavskiy, E.; Radhakrishnan, A.K.; Feuerstein, A.; Morris, D.A.; Pieske-Kraigher, E.; Pieske, B.; et al. | 2022 | 171 | Prospective single-center cohort study | In patients with chronic heart failure (CHF), impaired left atrial (LA) reservoir function is independently associated with significantly reduced peak oxygen consumption ($pVO_2$). LA dysfunction serves as a marker of poor prognosis regardless of left ventricular ejection fraction (LVEF) classification within the CHF population. |

Table 4. *Cont.*

| Title | Authors | Year | Pts No | Study Type | Conclusion |
| --- | --- | --- | --- | --- | --- |
| Left atrial strain evaluation to assess left ventricle diastolic dysfunction and heart failure with preserved ejection fraction: a guide to clinical practice [24] | Reiber, J.H. | 2023 | | Editorial | As highlighted in the authors' summary, left atrial (LA) function plays a critical role in overall cardiac performance by modulating left ventricular (LV) filling through its three primary functions: reservoir, conduit, and booster pump. Due to the close interdependence between the LA and LV, LA size and/or function are often used as surrogate markers for LV diastolic function. |
| The novel left atrial strain parameters in diagnosing of heart failure with preserved ejection fraction [25] | Ma, C.S.; Liao, Y.P.; Fan, J.L.; Zhao, X.; Su, B.; Zhou, B.Y. | 2022 | 389 | Prospective single-center cohort study | The novel left atrial (LA) parameters could be valuable in estimating left ventricular filling pressure (LVFP) and, if integrated into the 2016 EACVI/ASE criteria, may enhance diagnostic efficiency. These parameters might also improve the ability to differentiate HFpEF patients from those with risk factors for HFpEF, increasing diagnostic accuracy. |
| Prognostic Value of Minimal Left Atrial Volume in Heart Failure With Preserved Ejection Fraction [15] | Shin, S.H.; Claggett, B.; Inciardi, R.M.; Santos, A.B.S.; Shah, S.J.; Zile, M.R.; Pfeffer, M.A.; Shah, A.M.; Solomon, S.D. | 2021 | 347 | Research article | In patients with heart failure with preserved ejection fraction (HFpEF), minimum left atrial volume index (LAVImin) was a stronger predictor of cardiovascular outcomes than indexed maximal LA volume. This suggests that LAVImin may be more physiologically relevant and better at identifying patients at high risk for cardiovascular events. Additionally, left atrial functional parameters offer prognostic information that is independent of LAVImin. |
| Prognostic Implications of Left Atrial Stiffness Index in Heart Failure Patients With Preserved Ejection Fraction [27] | Kim, D.; Seo, J.H.; Choi, K.H.; Lee, S.H.; Choi, J.O.; Jeon, E.S.; Yang, J.H. | 2023 | 307 | Retrospective single-center cohort | In patients with HFpEF, increased left atrial (LA) stiffness was associated with a higher risk of all-cause mortality and heart-failure-related hospitalizations. Moreover, its prognostic value exceeded that of traditional markers of left ventricular filling pressure. |
| Prediction of AF in Heart Failure With Preserved Ejection Fraction: Incremental Value of Left Atrial Strain [19] | Jasic-Szpak, E.; Marwick, T.H.; Donal, E.; Przewlocka-Kosmala, M.; Huynh, Q.; Gozdzik, A.; Woznicka, A.K.; Jankowska, E.A.; Ponikowski, P.; Kosmala, W. | 2021 | 170 | Original research | Peak atrial contraction strain (PACS) and peak atrial longitudinal strain (PALS) have predictive value for incident atrial fibrillation (AF) in HFpEF, beyond established clinical and echocardiographic predictors. Combining atrial remodeling markers, such as left atrial (LA) deformation and size, may provide a sensitive tool for screening AF risk in this population. |

## 4. Future Directions

In patients with HFpEF-pLS and reduced LAS, there is a disproportionate impairment of left atrial (LA) function due to atrial cardiomyopathy, positioning the LA as a central mechanical hub in the disease's pathophysiology. This perspective represents a relatively new concept in cardiology, as traditional understanding of diastology has primarily viewed LA dysfunction as a secondary consequence of advanced left ventricular (LV) diastolic dysfunction and chronically elevated LV end-diastolic pressure [32].

The development of left atrial (LA) strain imaging has highlighted its potential role in evaluating left ventricular (LV) diastolic function, providing additional insights beyond conventional echocardiographic indices. Strain analysis has demonstrated a strong association between reduced LV filling pressure and subsequent LA reverse remodeling with improved function, suggesting its future utility in clinical practice.

Numerous studies have explored the role of atrial strain imaging in heart failure, particularly in clarifying specific HFpEF subtypes where traditional diagnostic methods fall short. LA strain analysis may also prove valuable in assessing the effects of pharmacological interventions on atrial remodeling in heart failure patients. Additionally, the assessment of LA strain in coronary patients and hemodialysis patients with associated cardiac diseases could provide valuable insights into the broader applicability of this technique. In coronary patients, LA strain may help identify subclinical diastolic dysfunction, while in hemodialysis patients, it could offer unique perspectives on atrial remodeling under the influence of volume overload and chronic systemic inflammation. These patient populations represent critical areas for future research to extend the diagnostic and prognostic utility of LA strain imaging.

The implementation of LA strain imaging in the research and clinical management of atrial fibrillation (AF) is growing. Increasing evidence supports its utility in evaluating atrial remodeling, predicting thromboembolic risk, assessing the success of AF ablation, and identifying the likelihood of arrhythmia recurrence. However, larger studies are needed to validate these findings and determine whether strain analysis can reliably identify at-risk patients in routine clinical practice.

Additionally, efforts are underway to standardize atrial strain analysis across different imaging platforms and to develop new algorithms that are vendor independent.

By combining traditional HFpEF scores (HFA-PEFF, H2FPEF) with advanced imaging techniques (LA strain, GLS, cardiac MRI), stress testing, and biomarkers, clinicians can achieve a more detailed and accurate phenotyping of HFpEF. This multimodal approach improves diagnostic precision and aids in tailored treatment strategies.

## 5. Limitations

This study has several limitations that warrant consideration. As a narrative review, it does not follow the systematic approach of a meta-analysis, which could introduce selection bias and affect the generalizability of the findings. Additionally, there is considerable variability in the methodologies of the included studies, particularly in the techniques used to measure strain, such as vendor-specific software and imaging platforms. This inconsistency may lead to challenges in interpreting and comparing results across different studies.

A notable limitation is the lack of standardized cut-offs and reference values for left atrial strain (LAS) and global longitudinal strain (GLS), which complicates their clinical application. The patient populations across the reviewed studies are diverse, with varying comorbidities, demographics, and disease severities, further complicating the comparability of findings. The review also focuses primarily on echocardiographic assessments, largely excluding other imaging modalities like cardiac MRI, which might offer complementary or more detailed insights in certain cases.

There is also a risk of publication bias due to the restriction to English-language studies and the exclusion of gray literature, which may result in an overrepresentation of studies with positive findings. Moreover, the majority of studies included are cross-sectional or have short follow-up durations, limiting the ability to draw conclusions about the long-term prognostic value of LAS and GLS in heart failure with preserved ejection fraction (HFpEF).

The sensitivity of LAS and GLS measurements to loading conditions such as preload and afterload adds another layer of complexity, as these can vary significantly across clinical settings and patient populations. Operator dependency is also a concern, as the accuracy of strain imaging is influenced by the expertise of the operator and the quality of image acquisition. Furthermore, by excluding pediatric and younger adult populations, the study's findings may not be applicable to these groups.

While some studies included in the review integrate biomarkers like NT-proBNP, the overall lack of extensive integration between strain imaging findings and biomarker data limits the potential for combined diagnostic or prognostic insights. Finally, the practical application of LAS and GLS in routine clinical practice has not been validated in large, multicenter prospective studies, leaving questions about their widespread feasibility and utility. Addressing these limitations in future research will be crucial to enhancing the clinical impact of strain imaging in HFpEF.

## 6. Conclusions

This review underscores the clinical utility of left atrial strain (LAS) as a precise and sensitive marker for evaluating left atrial function in patients with chronic heart failure with preserved ejection fraction (HFpEF). Evidence indicates that LAS correlates strongly with left ventricular filling pressures and diastolic dysfunction, offering a more nuanced assessment than conventional echocardiographic parameters. By providing early insights into atrial remodeling and dysfunction, LAS facilitates improved HFpEF phenotyping, which may ultimately guide targeted therapeutic strategies. Future research should concentrate on standardizing LAS measurement protocols and validating its prognostic value in large, multicenter cohorts, thereby enhancing its integration into routine HFpEF management.

**Author Contributions:** Conceptualization: D.E.M. and A.C.M.; collecting data and resources: V.B., D.M.D.-S., O.B. and D.E.V.; literature analysis and concluding: D.E.M., C.T.L. and S.-R.D.; writing—original draft: A.C.M. and D.M.D.-S.; reviewing and editing: D.M.D.-S., D.E.V. and S.-R.D.; project administration: C.T.L., S.-R.D. and A.C.M. All authors have read and agreed to the published version of the manuscript.

**Funding:** We would like to acknowledge "Victor Babes" University of Medicine and Pharmacy Timisoara, Romania, for their support in covering the publication costs for this review article.

**Conflicts of Interest:** The authors declare no conflict of interest.

## References

1. Pieske, B.; Tschöpe, C.; de Boer, R.A.; Fraser, A.G.; Anker, S.D.; Donal, E.; Edelmann, F.; Fu, M.; Guazzi, M.; Lam, C.S.P.; et al. How to Diagnose Heart Failure with Preserved Ejection Fraction: The HFA-PEFF Diagnostic Algorithm: A Consensus Recommendation from the Heart Failure Association (HFA) of the European Society of Cardiology (ESC). *Eur. Heart J.* **2019**, *40*, 3297–3317. [CrossRef] [PubMed]
2. Litwin, S.E.; Komtebedde, J.; Hu, M.; Burkhoff, D.; Hasenfuß, G.; Borlaug, B.A.; Solomon, S.D.; Zile, M.R.; Mohan, R.C.; Khawash, R.; et al. Exercise-Induced Left Atrial Hypertension in Heart Failure with Preserved Ejection Fraction. *JACC Heart Fail.* **2023**, *11*, 1103–1117. [CrossRef] [PubMed]
3. Beladan, C.C.; Gual-Capllonch, F.; Popescu, A.C.; Popescu, B.A. Diagnosing Diastolic Dysfunction and Heart Failure with Preserved Ejection Fraction in Patients with Atrial Fibrillation: A Clinical Challenge. *Eur. Heart J. Cardiovasc. Imaging* **2024**, *25*, 1546–1553. [CrossRef] [PubMed]
4. Palazzuoli, A.; Buono, M.G.D.; Ruocco, G.; Caravita, S.; Abbate, A.; Lavie, C.J. The Conundrum of HFpEF Definition: Non-Invasive Assessment Uncertainties and Alternative Diagnostic Strategies. *Curr. Probl. Cardiol.* **2023**, *48*, 101433. [CrossRef]
5. Shinzato, M.H.; Santos, N.; Nishida, G.; Moriya, H.; Assef, J.; Feres, F.; Hortegal, R.A. Left Ventricular and Atrial Myocardial Strain in Heart Failure with Preserved Ejection Fraction: The Evidence so Far and Prospects for Phenotyping Strategy. *Cardiovasc. Ultrasound* **2024**, *22*, 4. [CrossRef]

6. Shah, A.M.; Cikes, M.; Prasad, N.; Li, G.; Getchevski, S.; Claggett, B.; Rizkala, A.; Lukashevich, I.; O'Meara, E.; Ryan, J.J.; et al. Echocardiographic Features of Patients with Heart Failure and Preserved Left Ventricular Ejection Fraction. *J. Am. Coll. Cardiol.* **2019**, *74*, 2858–2873. [CrossRef]
7. Duchnowski, P.; Śmigielski, W. Usefulness of Myocardial Damage Biomarkers in Predicting Cardiogenic Shock in Patients Undergoing Heart Valve Surgery. *Pol. Heart J. Kardiol. Pol.* **2024**, *82*, 423–426. [CrossRef]
8. Călburean, P.-A.; Lupu, S.; Huțanu, A.; Oprica, M.; Opriș, D.R.; Stan, A.; Scurtu, A.-C.; Aniței, D.; Harpa, M.; Brînzaniuc, K.; et al. Natriuretic Peptides and Soluble ST2 Improves Echocardiographic Diagnosis of Elevated Left Ventricular Filling Pressures. *Sci. Rep.* **2024**, *14*, 22171. [CrossRef]
9. Ovchinnikov, A.G.; Potekhina, A.; Belyavskiy, E.; Gvozdeva, A.; Ageev, F. Left Atrial Dysfunction as the Major Driver of Heart Failure with Preserved Ejection Fraction Syndrome. *J. Clin. Ultrasound JCU* **2022**, *50*, 1073–1083. [CrossRef]
10. Kagami, K.; Harada, T.; Yuasa, N.; Saito, Y.; Sorimachi, H.; Murakami, F.; Naito, A.; Tani, Y.; Kato, T.; Wada, N.; et al. Impaired Left Atrial Reserve Function in Heart Failure with Preserved Ejection Fraction. *Circ. Cardiovasc. Imaging* **2024**, *17*, e016549. [CrossRef]
11. Reddy, Y.N.V.; Obokata, M.; Verbrugge, F.H.; Lin, G.; Borlaug, B.A. Atrial Dysfunction in Patients with Heart Failure with Preserved Ejection Fraction and Atrial Fibrillation. *J. Am. Coll. Cardiol.* **2020**, *76*, 1051–1064. [CrossRef] [PubMed]
12. Aung, S.M.; Güler, A.; Güler, Y.; Huraibat, A.; Karabay, C.Y.; Akdemir, I. Left Atrial Strain in Heart Failure with Preserved Ejection Fraction. *Herz* **2017**, *42*, 194–199. [CrossRef] [PubMed]
13. Nagueh, S.F.; Khan, S.U. Left Atrial Strain for Assessment of Left Ventricular Diastolic Function: Focus on Populations with Normal LVEF. *JACC Cardiovasc. Imaging* **2023**, *16*, 691–707. [CrossRef]
14. Khan, M.S.; Memon, M.M.; Murad, M.H.; Vaduganathan, M.; Greene, S.J.; Hall, M.; Triposkiadis, F.; Lam, C.S.P.; Shah, A.M.; Butler, J.; et al. Left Atrial Function in Heart Failure with Preserved Ejection Fraction: A Systematic Review and Meta-Analysis. *Eur. J. Heart Fail.* **2020**, *22*, 472–485. [CrossRef]
15. Shin, S.-H.; Claggett, B.; Inciardi, R.M.; Santos, A.B.S.; Shah, S.J.; Zile, M.R.; Pfeffer, M.A.; Shah, A.M.; Solomon, S.D. Prognostic Value of Minimal Left Atrial Volume in Heart Failure with Preserved Ejection Fraction. *J. Am. Heart Assoc.* **2021**, *10*, e019545. [CrossRef]
16. Ye, Z.; Miranda, W.R.; Yeung, D.F.; Kane, G.C.; Oh, J.K. Left Atrial Strain in Evaluation of Heart Failure with Preserved Ejection Fraction. *J. Am. Soc. Echocardiogr. Off. Publ. Am. Soc. Echocardiogr.* **2020**, *33*, 1490–1499. [CrossRef]
17. Pournazari, P.; Faza, N.N.; Goel, S.S.; Islam, M.U.; Little, S.H.; Nagueh, S.F. Hemodynamic Determinants of Left Atrial Strain in Symptomatic Patients with Significant Primary Mitral Regurgitation. *Circ. Cardiovasc. Imaging* **2022**, *15*, e013836. [CrossRef]
18. Maffeis, C.; Rossi, A.; Cannata, L.; Zocco, C.; Belyavskiy, E.; Radhakrishnan, A.K.; Feuerstein, A.; Morris, D.A.; Pieske-Kraigher, E.; Pieske, B.; et al. Left Atrial Strain Predicts Exercise Capacity in Heart Failure Independently of Left Ventricular Ejection Fraction. *ESC Heart Fail.* **2022**, *9*, 842–852. [CrossRef]
19. Jasic-Szpak, E.; Marwick, T.H.; Donal, E.; Przewlocka-Kosmala, M.; Huynh, Q.; Gozdzik, A.; Woznicka, A.K.; Jankowska, E.A.; Ponikowski, P.; Kosmala, W. Prediction of AF in Heart Failure With Preserved Ejection Fraction: Incremental Value of Left Atrial Strain. *JACC Cardiovasc. Imaging* **2021**, *14*, 131–144. [CrossRef]
20. Fauchier, L.; Bisson, A.; Bodin, A. Heart Failure with Preserved Ejection Fraction and Atrial Fibrillation: Recent Advances and Open Questions. *BMC Med.* **2023**, *21*, 54. [CrossRef]
21. Jin, X.; Nauta, J.F.; Hung, C.-L.; Ouwerkerk, W.; Teng, T.-H.K.; Voors, A.A.; Lam, C.S.; van Melle, J.P. Left Atrial Structure and Function in Heart Failure with Reduced (HFrEF) versus Preserved Ejection Fraction (HFpEF): Systematic Review and Meta-Analysis. *Heart Fail. Rev.* **2022**, *27*, 1933–1955. [CrossRef] [PubMed]
22. Smiseth, O.A.; Rider, O.; Cvijic, M.; Valkovič, L.; Remme, E.W.; Voigt, J.-U. Myocardial Strain Imaging. *JACC Cardiovasc. Imaging* **2024**. *online ahead of print*. [CrossRef] [PubMed]
23. Jellis, C.L.; Klein, A.L. Heart Failure with Preserved Ejection Fraction: Do You Know Your Left Atrial Strain? *Circ. Cardiovasc. Imaging* **2016**, *9*, e004521. [CrossRef] [PubMed]
24. Reiber, J. Editor's Choice to the June 2023 Issue: Left Atrial Strain Evaluation to Assess Left Ventricle Diastolic Dysfunction and Heart Failure with Preserved Ejection Fraction: A Guide to Clinical Practice. *Int. J. Cardiovasc. Imaging* **2023**, *39*, 1081–1082. [CrossRef] [PubMed]
25. Ma, C.-S.; Liao, Y.-P.; Fan, J.-L.; Zhao, X.; Su, B.; Zhou, B.-Y. The Novel Left Atrial Strain Parameters in Diagnosing of Heart Failure with Preserved Ejection Fraction. *Echocardiography* **2022**, *39*, 416–425. [CrossRef]
26. Shi, R.; Shi, K.; Huang, S.; Li, X.; Xia, C.-C.; Li, Y.; He, S.; Li, Z.-L.; He, Y.; Guo, Y.-K.; et al. Association Between Heart Failure with Preserved Left Ventricular Ejection Fraction and Impaired Left Atrial Phasic Function in Hypertrophic Cardiomyopathy: Evaluation by Cardiac MRI Feature Tracking. *J. Magn. Reson. Imaging JMRI* **2022**, *56*, 248–259. [CrossRef]
27. Kim, D.; Seo, J.H.; Choi, K.H.; Lee, S.H.; Choi, J.-O.; Jeon, E.-S.; Yang, J.H. Prognostic Implications of Left Atrial Stiffness Index in Heart Failure Patients With Preserved Ejection Fraction. *JACC Cardiovasc. Imaging* **2023**, *16*, 435–445. [CrossRef]
28. Tayal, B.; Malahfji, M.; Buergler, J.M.; Shah, D.J.; Nagueh, S.F. Hemodynamic Determinants of Left Atrial Strain in Patients with Hypertrophic Cardiomyopathy: A Combined Echocardiography and CMR Study. *PLoS ONE* **2021**, *16*, e0245934. [CrossRef]

29. Omote, K.; Sorimachi, H.; Obokata, M.; Verbrugge, F.H.; Omar, M.; Popovic, D.; Reddy, Y.N.V.; Pislaru, S.V.; Pellikka, P.A.; Borlaug, B.A. Biatrial Myopathy in Heart Failure with Preserved Ejection Fraction. *Eur. J. Heart Fail.* **2024**, *26*, 288–298. [CrossRef]
30. Donal, E.; Galli, E.; Schnell, F. Left Atrial Strain: A Must or a Plus for Routine Clinical Practice? *Circ. Cardiovasc. Imaging* **2017**, *10*, e007023. [CrossRef]
31. Patel, R.B.; Lam, C.S.P.; Svedlund, S.; Saraste, A.; Hage, C.; Tan, R.-S.; Beussink-Nelson, L.; Tromp, J.; Sanchez, C.; Njoroge, J.; et al. Disproportionate Left Atrial Myopathy in Heart Failure with Preserved Ejection Fraction among Participants of the PROMIS-HFpEF Study. *Sci. Rep.* **2021**, *11*, 4885. [CrossRef]
32. Bouwmeester, S.; van der Stam, J.A.; van Loon, S.L.M.; van Riel, N.A.W.; Boer, A.-K.; Dekker, L.R.; Scharnhorst, V.; Houthuizen, P. Left Atrial Reservoir Strain as a Predictor of Cardiac Outcome in Patients with Heart Failure: The HaFaC Cohort Study. *BMC Cardiovasc. Disord.* **2022**, *22*, 104. [CrossRef]


**Disclaimer/Publisher's Note:** The statements, opinions and data contained in all publications are solely those of the individual author(s) and contributor(s) and not of MDPI and/or the editor(s). MDPI and/or the editor(s) disclaim responsibility for any injury to people or property resulting from any ideas, methods, instructions or products referred to in the content.

life

MDPI

*Article*

# High and Low Adherence to Mediterranean and DASH Diet Patterns and the Risk of Heart Failure: A Meta-Analysis of Observational Studies †

**Mehmet Emin Arayici [1,2,*], Mustafa Eray Kilic [3] and Mehmet Birhan Yilmaz [3]**

1 Department of Biostatistics and Medical Informatics, Faculty of Medicine, Dokuz Eylül University, 35340 İzmir, Türkiye
2 Department of Public Health, Faculty of Medicine, Dokuz Eylül University, 35340 İzmir, Türkiye
3 Department of Cardiology, Faculty of Medicine, Dokuz Eylül University, 35340 İzmir, Türkiye; mustafaeraykilic@gmail.com (M.E.K.); prof.dr.mbyilmaz@gmail.com (M.B.Y.)
* Correspondence: mehmet.e.arayici@gmail.com; Tel.: +90-532-576-1965

† This study was presented as an oral presentation during the Plant-Based Diets: Health and Well-Being season at the 4th International Electronic Conference on Nutrients on 16–18 October 2024.

**Abstract:** Background. The relationship between heart failure (HF) and Mediterranean and DASH diets is not well delineated. This meta-analysis aimed to assess the effectiveness of high adherence to Mediterranean and DASH diets compared to low adherence in reducing the risk of incident HF (primary prevention of HF) and reducing all-cause mortality in patients with HF (secondary prevention of HF). Methods. The reporting stages of this meta-analysis closely adhered to the PRISMA guidelines. A comprehensive literature search was undertaken for published papers in PubMed, Embase, EBSCO, ICTRP, and the NIH clinical trials databases. Results. A total of 16 reports from 14 studies were included in this paper. A significant inverse association was identified between high adherence to the Mediterranean diet model (compared to low adherence) and the risk of incident HF (OR = 0.77, 95% CI: 0.63–0.93, $p = 0.007$) among patients without previous diagnosis of HF. Similarly, there was a significant and inverse relationship between high adherence to the DASH diet (compared to low adherence) and the risk of incident HF (OR = 0.83, 95% CI: 0.70–0.98, $p = 0.03$) among patients without previous diagnosis of HF. High adherence to the Mediterranean diet model (compared to low adherence) was associated with lower all-cause mortality (OR = 0.88, 95% CI: 0.78–0.99, $p = 0.03$) among patients with HF. Conclusions. This paper demonstrated that high adherence to Mediterranean and DASH diets significantly reduced the risk of incident HF among individuals without a previous diagnosis of HF, whereas only high adherence to the Mediterranean diet was associated with lower all-cause mortality among patients with HF.

**Keywords:** heart failure; Mediterranean diet; DASH diet; meta-analysis

## 1. Introduction

It is well-established that heart failure (HF) presents a complex medical challenge, impacting approximately 1–2% of the global adult population [1,2]. The prevalence of HF increases with age and has a significant adverse impact on public health. The prevalence of HF is expected to increase by 46% from 2012 to 2030, elevating the overall HF prevalence from 2.4% to 3.0% [3]. The lifetime risk of HF in the general population varies between 20% and 46% at 45 years of age, with particularly higher rates among individuals with hypertension and a high body mass index (BMI) [4].

According to the World Health Organization (WHO), lifestyle modifications targeted at the prevention and management of risk factors have the potential to reduce approximately 75% of cardiovascular disease (CVD)-related deaths. Unhealthy eating habits, lack of physical activity, smoking, and excessive alcohol consumption were identified as the primary behavioral risk factors associated with cardiovascular disease and stroke [5,6]. Cost-effective interventions are required to improve outcomes in HF. One potential approach may involve nutritional interventions as patients with HF can experience nutritional imbalances and malnutrition, which could contribute to higher morbidity and mortality rates [5]. Previous research including Diet and Reinfarction Trial (DART), Dietary Approaches to Stop Hypertension (DASH), and Prevención con Dieta Mediterránea (PREDIMED) have highlighted the substantial influence of dietary intake on the incidence and severity of CVD [7].

The most beneficial dietary regimen for CVD risk reduction emphasizes the consumption of whole grains, fruits, vegetables, legumes, nuts, fish, poultry, moderate dairy products, and heart-healthy vegetable oils [8]. The Mediterranean diet, which prioritizes plant-based foods and sources of plant protein, stands out as an established favorable dietary pattern for mitigating CVD risk. Meanwhile, the DASH diet, comprising fruits, vegetables, whole grains [9], poultry, fish, nuts, and low-fat dairy items, has gained prominence owing to its capacity to lower blood pressure and potentially prevent left ventricular dysfunction, a common complication associated with hypertension [10–12].

The importance of diet in managing HF is increasingly recognized, and the Mediterranean and DASH diets are usable as potential research and intervention strategies for HF in the future [13]. These diets, which are affordable, accessible, and long-term nutritional treatments, may have effects associated with both HF risk and mortality in patients with HF. However, the growing evidence base on the subject has suggested contradictory results for both the Mediterranean diet model [14–16] and the DASH diet pattern [17–19]. Therefore, the relationship between HF and associated dietary patterns is not clearly understood. The purpose of this review-based study employing systematic and meta-analytic approaches was to comprehensively assess and enlighten the influence of high adherence to Mediterranean and DASH diets compared to low adherence on HF-related outcomes using a meta-analysis method.

## 2. Methods

All reporting stages of this review-based study employing systematic and meta-analytic approaches were carried out in accordance with PRISMA (Preferred Reporting Items for Systematic Reviews and Meta-Analyses) guidelines [20]. The meta-analysis protocol was officially registered with the International Prospective Register of Systematic Reviews (PROSPERO) with the registration number CRD42023427976. The PRISMA checklist has been related to Supplementary Table S1, serving as an essential tool to validate adherence to PRISMA guidelines, ensuring the thoroughness and reporting accuracy of the study.

PICOS framework related to meta-analysis was defined as follows: Population: healthy individuals for HF risk or patients diagnosed with HF for mortality; Intervention: adherence to Mediterranean and DASH diets; Comparison: levels of adherence (high adherence vs. low adherence); Outcomes: reduction in risk of HF, and all-cause mortality in patients with HF; Study Design: cohort or case–control studies.

### 2.1. Information Sources, Search Strategy, and Study Selection Process

Comprehensive literature searches were executed in PubMed/Medline, Embase, EBSCO Academic Search Ultimate, International Clinical Trials Registry Platform (ICTRP), and NIH clinical trials databases. The search strategy was formulated by utilizing Medical Subject Headings (MeSH) and free-text terms that incorporated "HF", "Mediterranean diet", "DASH diet", "hospitalization", and "mortality". Boolean operators (AND/OR) were used to combine related keywords. Originally, the search strategy was developed in PubMed and subsequently applied to other databases. Detailed search strategies were documented in Supplemental Table S2. In August 2024, an initial comprehensive literature search was performed, and an update was conducted in October 2024.

### 2.2. Eligibility Criteria

Papers were included if they focused on adults aged 18 years or older who were healthy individuals or who were diagnosed with HF, either systolic and/or diastolic, for this study. To meet the inclusion criteria, the studies had to assess the comparison of adherence to Mediterranean and DASH diets across different quantiles (high and low) and report results for at least one of the following outcomes: HF-related risk or all-cause mortality in patients with HF. Inclusion criteria were limited to studies published in the English language. Papers published in other languages were directly excluded from the study. Studies that met any of the following exclusion criteria were not considered: (i) those with insufficient data or lacking key outcome reporting; (ii) articles categorized as case reports, case series, editorials, comments, or expert opinions; (iii) studies involving animal or in vitro research; and (iv) studies utilizing overlapping or duplicate data sets.

### 2.3. Data Collection Process

Two independent researchers (MEA and MEK) extracted data from the primary papers obtained from relevant databases and recorded it in a predefined Microsoft Excel® spreadsheet. Data extracted covered a variety of parameters, including first author name, publication date, study design, study name, type of diet, sample size, mean or median age, follow-up time, effect size, 95% confidence intervals (CI), $p$-values, and adjusted covariates/confounders. In studies where more than one result was reported, data in the highest quarter/category and the lowest quarter/category were considered, and a multivariate-adjusted model was selected (the latest model with the most factors included). If data were missing or unclear on some topics, we made an effort to contact the corresponding authors of the original articles through email for clarification. To ensure accuracy, both investigators cross-verified all the extracted data and arrived at a consensus.

### 2.4. Quality Assessment in Individual Studies

The methodological quality and risk of bias for the included studies were assessed using standardized tools. For cohort and case–control studies, the Newcastle–Ottawa Scale (NOS) [21] was employed. The NOS scores between 6 and 9 indicated a moderate-to-high quality of the studies involved. Studies with lower scores that were not within this range were excluded from the pooled analysis. To maintain the reliability of this evaluation, both reviewers conducted these assessments independently. If discrepancies arose, discussions were held to reach a consensus, and if required, a third investigator was consulted for mediation.

### 2.5. Statistical Analysis

The statistical analyses were carried out using R software version 4.2.3, employing the "*metafor*" package [22], The Review Manager version 5.4 (The Nordic Cochran Centre, Copenhagen, Denmark) [23], and ProMeta3® meta-analysis software version 3.0 [24]. Effect size (ES) was computed as the odds ratio (OR) for risk of HF and all-cause mortality in patients with HF. The level of heterogeneity among the included studies was quantified using $I^2$ statistics or the chi-squared ($\chi 2$) test. The $I^2$ statistic represents the proportion of variance between studies attributed to heterogeneity rather than random sampling error. Significant heterogeneity was confirmed with a $p$-value of less than 0.05 in the chi-squared ($\chi2$) test and an $I^2$ quantitative estimation value exceeding 50%. In the case of low to moderate heterogeneity, fixed effect models were used, whereas random effect models were utilized for high heterogeneity. To assess the potential for bias, Egger's linear regression test, Begg and Mazumdar's rank correlation test, as well as funnel plot visualizations, were conducted [25]. Statistical significance was depicted as a two-tailed $p$-value less than 0.05 in all tests performed.

In order to thoroughly investigate the connection between individual dietary components of the Mediterranean and DASH diets and cardiovascular outcomes, with a particular focus on HF risk and all-cause mortality in patients with HF, we conducted a subgroup analysis. To address potential statistical heterogeneity among the included studies, we employed both fixed effects and random effects models with restricted maximum likelihood estimation.

To evaluate the robustness of our results, sensitivity analyses were conducted. This involved reassessing the effect size (ES) by sequentially omitting each study from the pooled analysis, thereby estimating the influence of individual studies on the overall findings.

## 3. Results

### 3.1. Literature Search

The initial search was operated across multiple databases, including PubMed/Medline ($n$ = 341), Embase ($n$ = 177), EBSCO ($n$ = 578), ICTRP ($n$ = 9), and NIH clinical trials ($n$ = 13), yielding a total of 1118 papers. Out of the total 1118 records identified, 483 of these were found to be duplicates and were subsequently eliminated from consideration. The remaining 635 records underwent a relevance screening process, which involved reviewing the titles and abstracts of each record. Out of these, 41 papers were considered suitable for comprehensive full-text evaluation. Throughout this evaluation, 15 studies were excluded due to unsuitable study designs, and 12 were excluded for the absence of data related to HF mortality or incidence. In the final analysis, a total of 16 reports derived from 14 papers [14–19,26–33] met the predefined inclusion criteria and were integrated into the meta-analysis. A flowchart representation of the literature search and study selection process in accordance with PRISMA guidelines is provided in Figure 1.

### 3.2. Baseline Characteristics of Included Studies

This meta-analysis included 16 reports from 14 observational studies [14–19,26–33] and a total of 424,502 participants. The studies were conducted in several countries, including Spain, the United States, Sweden, Germany, Italy, and the Netherlands, and they were published between 2014 and 2022. The ages of the participants in all studies were generally middle-aged and older. The majority of studies consisted of population-based and prospective cohort studies. Multiple dietary adherence scores have been utilized across these studies, including the 14-point Mediterranean diet adherence score, the DASH score, the MeDi Score, and the aMed scoring system. Among the studies included were MEDIT-AHF (Mediterranean DieT in Acute HF) [17], Women's Health Initiative [14], Cohort of Swedish Men [32,33], Swedish Mammography Cohort [16,18], EPIC (European Prospective Investigation into Cancer and Nutrition) [15,31], REGARDS (REasons for Geographic and Racial Differences in Stroke) [19], MESA (The Multi-Ethnic Study of Atherosclerosis) [29], Cardiovascular Health Study [26], SCCS (Southern Community Cohort Study) [30], and NHANES (National Health and Nutrition Examination Survey) [27,28].

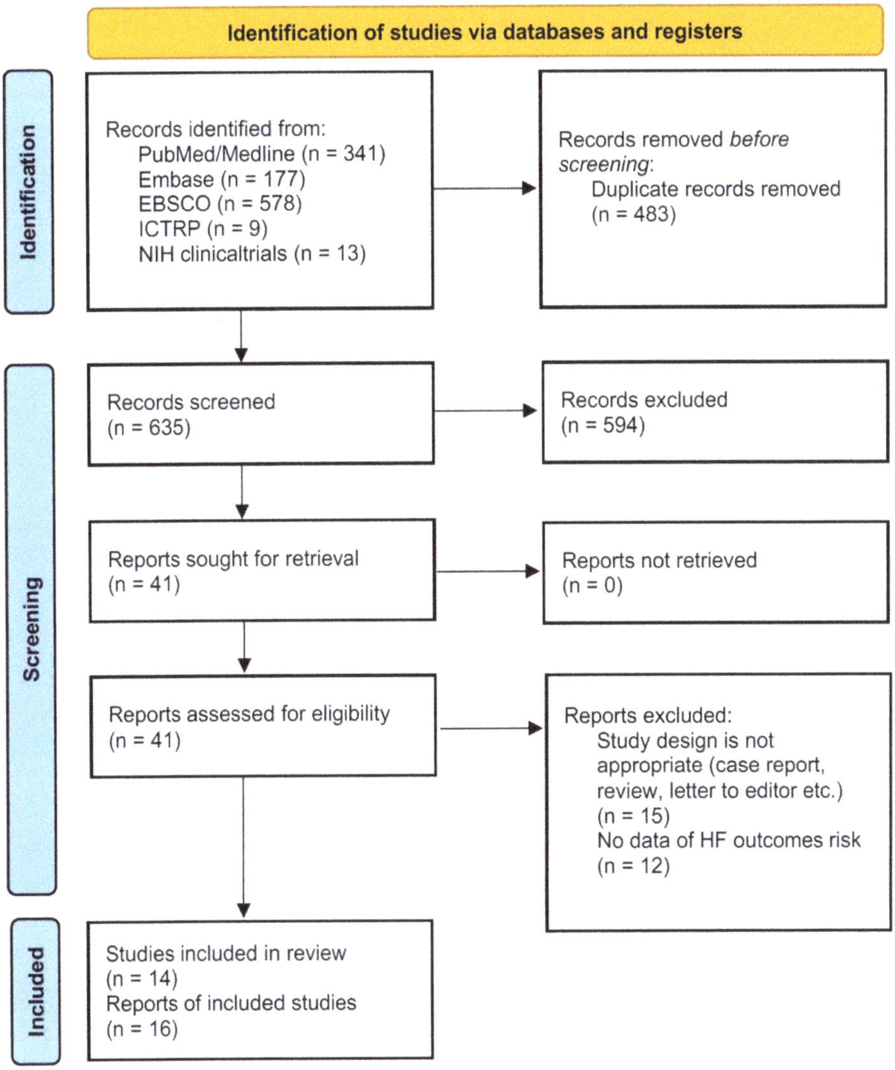


**Figure 1.** Flow chart for the selection of studies included in the systematic review and the meta-analysis.

The follow-up periods in the included studies ranged from 2.1 years in the MEDIT-AHF study to 21.5 years in the Cardiovascular Health Study, with an overall average of 8.9 years. The two main dietary therapies studied in these trials were the Mediterranean and DASH diets. Diet adherence was frequently assessed using a variety of scoring techniques, with people with poorer adherence scores serving as comparator groups. In general, in the DASH diet scoring, food groups including fruits, vegetables, whole grains, nuts, legumes, and low-fat dairy products are scored positively. Red and processed meats, sweetened beverages, and sodium were listed as negative food groups and reverse scored [14,18,26,29,33]. Yielding considerable clinical heterogeneity was emerging between studies regarding dietary scoring. In some studies, dietary adherence was divided into four groups or five quantiles [14,18,29,33], while in another study, diet compliance was divided into two groups [27]. In studies related to the Mediterranean diet pattern, participants consumed moderate amounts of alcohol (10–25 g/day for men and 5–15 g/day for women), seafood, whole grains, legumes, monounsaturated fat + polyunsaturated fat/saturated fat ratio, nuts, fruits, and vegetables were determined as positive foods. Consumption of red and processed meat, dairy, and more than moderate amounts of alcohol were scored negatively. Diet adherence was assessed utilizing different scoring scales in some studies, divided into two groups [17,18], and in some studies, divided into three or four categories [15,16,31]. These studies scrutinized outcomes such as HF-related hospitalizations, HF risk, and all-cause deaths or cardiovascular deaths. The baseline characteristics and study designs of the included investigations are associated with Table 1.

The adherence to DASH and Mediterranean diets has been assessed using diverse methodological approaches across the included studies, contributing to clinical heterogeneity in evaluating dietary impacts. Self-administered FFQs were frequently employed, as seen in Levitan et al. [14,18,33] and Del Gobbo et al. [26], focusing on DASH components like fruits, vegetables, and sodium intake. Modified block FFQs, used in the Women's Health Initiative studies [14], included both DASH and Mediterranean dietary patterns, adapting for regional food availability. For the Mediterranean diet, adherence was assessed using tools like the PREDIMED questionnaire, modified Mediterranean Diet Score (mMED), and traditional Mediterranean Diet Score (MeDi) [16,17,34]. Semi-quantitative FFQs were common in Mediterranean diet assessments, as applied in studies like Wirth et al. [15] and Tektonidis et al. [16,32], highlighting core components such as olive oil, fish, and nuts. The PREDIMED questionnaire, a specialized tool for Mediterranean dietary patterns, was used by Miro et al. (2018) [17], emphasizing the diet's unique elements like extra virgin olive oil and nuts. Other studies, such as Chang et al. (2022) [28] and Chou et al. (2022) [27], relied on 24 h dietary recall interviews to provide detailed dietary intake data, albeit with increased reliance on participant memory. Campos et al. [29] and Goyal et al. [19] employed extended FFQs, offering comprehensive dietary analysis.

The NOS scores for the included 14 observational studies varied between 6 and 9, indicating a moderate-to-high quality of the studies involved. A detailed quality assessment is summarized in Supplementary Table S3.

### 3.3. Results of the Meta-Analysis

A meta-analysis was executed that yielded data from eight reports on the Mediterranean diet and eight studies on the DASH diet. Among the Mediterranean diet, five reports from four studies focused on evaluating the risk of HF [15,16,31,32], while three studies focused on assessing all-cause mortality in patients with HF [14,17,28]. In the DASH diet, six studies reported results related to the risk of HF [18,19,26,29,30,33], while two studies reported results related to mortality in patients with HF [14,27].

### 3.4. Outcomes of the Meta-Analysis on Incident Heart Failure Risk

In the pooled meta-analysis utilizing a random effects model, a significant inverse association was identified between high adherence to the Mediterranean diet model (compared to low adherence) and the risk of incident HF among patients without a previous diagnosis of HF (OR = 0.77, 95% CI: 0.63–0.93, $p = 0.007$) (Figure 2). Moderate and significant heterogeneity was observed in the studies assessing the Mediterranean diet and the risk of incident HF ($Tau^2 = 0.03$, $Chi^2 = 11.15$, $I^2 = 64\%$, $p = 0.02$). The analyses conducted showed no significant evidence of bias. This outcome was confirmed by the results of Egger's test (Intercept = $-1.01$, t = $-0.50$, $p = 0.65$) and Begg and Mazumdar's rank correlation test (z = $-0.49$, $p = 0.62$). The visualization of the funnel plot is illustrated in Supplemental Figure S1.

**Table 1.** Baseline characteristics of studies included in the systematic review and meta-analysis.

| First Author/Year | Study Type | Study Name | Sample Size (*n*) | Age Range (Years) | Events (*n*) | Event of Death (*n*) | Questionnaire | Type of Diet | Follow-Up Time (Years) | Outcome |
|---|---|---|---|---|---|---|---|---|---|---|
| Levitan et al., 2009 [33] | Cohort | Cohort of Swedish Men | 38,987 | 45–79 | 710 | 97 | Self-administered FFQ | DASH | 9 | Incidence |
| Levitan et al., 2009 [18] | Cohort | Swedish Mammography Cohort | 36,019 | 48–83 | 415 | 28 | Self-administered FFQ | DASH | 7 | Incidence |
| Levitan et al., 2013 [14] | Cohort | Women's Health Initiative | 161,808 | 50–79 | 3215 | 1385 | Modified block FFQ | MED | 4.6 | All-cause mortality |
| Levitan et al., 2013 [14] | Cohort | Women's Health Initiative | 161,808 | 50–79 | 3215 | 1385 | Modified block FFQ | DASH | 4.6 | All-cause mortality |
| Del Gobbo et al., 2015 [26] | Cohort | Cardiovascular Health Study | 5201 | ≥65 | 1380 | N/A | 99-item FFQ | DASH | 21.5 | Incidence |
| Tektonidis et al., 2015 [16] | Population based cohort | Swedish Mammography Cohort | 32,921 | 48–83 | 1648 | N/A | FFQ | MED | 10.4 | Incidence |
| Wirth et al., 2016 [15] | Prospective population-based cohort | EPIC | 24,008 | 35–65 | 209 | N/A | Semi-quantitative, self-administered FFQ | MED | 8.2 | Incidence |
| Tektonidis et al., 2016 [32] | Population-based cohort | Cohort of Swedish Men | 37,308 | 45–79 | 1269 | 146 | 96-item semi-quantitative, self-administered FFQ | MED | 10.9 | Incidence |
| Miro et al., 2018 [17] | Prospective cohort study | MEDIT-AHF | 991 | N/A | N/A | 569 | PREDIMED questionnaire | MED | 2.1 | All-cause mortality |
| Campos et al., 2019 [29] | Cohort | MESA | 4478 | 45–84 | 179 | N/A | 120-item FFQ | DASH | 13 | Incidence |
| Strengers et al., 2021 (a) [31] | Cohort | EPIC-NL | 9316 | 21–64 | 144 | N/A | Semi-quantitative FFQ | MED | 15 | Incidence |
| Strengers et al., 2021 (b) [31] | Cohort | EPIC-NL | 27,645 | 40–70 | 489 | N/A | Semi-quantitative FFQ | MED | 15 | Incidence |
| Goyal et al., 2021 [19] | Cohort | REGARDS | 18,856 | ≥45 | 767 | 111 | FFQ | DASH | 10.1 | Incidence |
| Chang et al., 2022 [28] | Population-based cohort | NHANES | 832 | ≥18 | 832 | 319 | 24 h dietary recall interview | MED | 4.7 | All-cause mortality |
| Chang et al., 2022 [30] | Prospective cohort study | SCCS | 25,300 | 40–79 | 7045 | N/A | 89 food items 24 h dietary recall questionnaires | DASH | 11 | Incidence |
| Chou et al., 2022 [27] | Population-based cohort | NHANES | 832 | ≥18 | 832 | 319 | 24 h dietary recall interview | DASH | 4.7 | All-cause mortality |

DASH The Dietary Approaches to Stop Hypertension, N/A not available, FFQ food frequency questionnaire, EPIC European Prospective Investigation into Cancer and Nutrition, MED Mediterranean diet, MEDIT-AHF Mediterranean DieT in Acute Heart Failure, PREDIMED Prevención con Dieta Mediterránea, MESA Multi-Ethnic Study of Atherosclerosis, NL Netherlands, (a) male, (b) female, REGARDS REasons for Geographic And Racial Differences in Stroke, NHANES National Health and Nutrition Examination Survey, SCCS Southern Community Cohort Study.

| Study or Subgroup | log[Odds Ratio] | SE | Weight | Odds Ratio IV, Random, 95% CI |
|---|---|---|---|---|
| **1.1.1 Mediterranean diet** | | | | |
| Strengers 2021 (female) | 0.0702 | 0.1248 | 22.5% | 1.07 [0.84, 1.37] |
| Strengers 2021 (male) | −0.6297 | 0.2444 | 11.2% | 0.53 [0.33, 0.86] |
| Tektonidis 2015 | −0.2345 | 0.0771 | 28.9% | 0.79 [0.68, 0.92] |
| Tektonidis 2016 | −0.3742 | 0.0959 | 26.3% | 0.69 [0.57, 0.83] |
| Wirth 2016 | −0.412 | 0.2447 | 11.2% | 0.66 [0.41, 1.07] |
| **Subtotal (95% CI)** | | | **100.0%** | **0.77 [0.63, 0.93]** |
| Heterogeneity: Tau² = 0.03; Chi² = 11.15, df = 4 (P = 0.02); I² = 64% | | | | |
| Test for overall effect: Z = 2.69 (P = 0.007) | | | | |
| **1.1.2 DASH diet** | | | | |
| Campos 2019 | −0.3628 | 0.2824 | 6.7% | 0.70 [0.40, 1.21] |
| Chang 2022 (DASH) | −0.0008 | 0.0204 | 23.9% | 1.00 [0.96, 1.04] |
| Del Gobbo 2015 | 0.0516 | 0.0916 | 19.0% | 1.05 [0.88, 1.26] |
| Goyal 2021 | −0.3141 | 0.1177 | 16.6% | 0.73 [0.58, 0.92] |
| Levitan 2009 (female) | −0.4662 | 0.1366 | 15.0% | 0.63 [0.48, 0.82] |
| Levitan 2009 (male) | −0.2463 | 0.0941 | 18.8% | 0.78 [0.65, 0.94] |
| **Subtotal (95% CI)** | | | **100.0%** | **0.83 [0.70, 0.98]** |
| Heterogeneity: Tau² = 0.03; Chi² = 25.52, df = 5 (P = 0.0001); I² = 80% | | | | |
| Test for overall effect: Z = 2.14 (P = 0.03) | | | | |

Test for subgroup differences: Chi² = 0.41, df = 1 (P = 0.52), I² = 0%

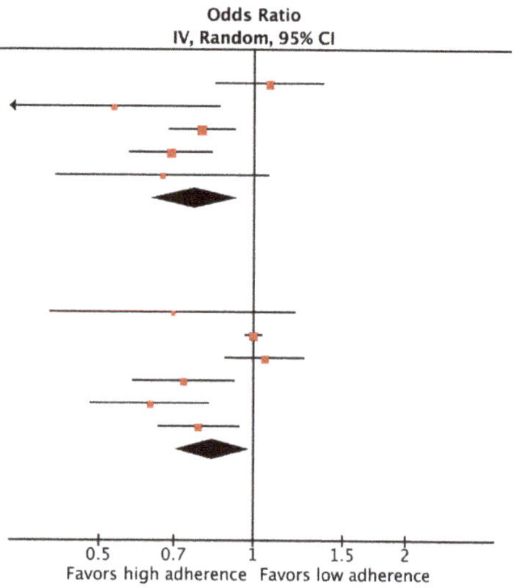


**Figure 2.** The forest plot of the effect of the Mediterranean diet and the DASH diet pattern on the risk of heart failure [15,16,18,19,26,29–33].

Similarly, in the pooled analysis employing a random effects model, it was revealed that there was a significant and inverse association between high adherence to the DASH diet pattern (compared to low adherence) and the risk of incident HF among patients without a previous diagnosis of HF (OR = 0.83, 95% CI: 0.70–0.98, $p = 0.03$) (Figure 2). Significant and substantial heterogeneity was detected within the studies evaluating the DASH diet in relation to the risk of incident HF risk ($Tau^2 = 0.03$, $Chi^2 = 25.52$, $I^2 = 80\%$, $p < 0.001$). Hence, in light of the noticeable heterogeneity, the analysis was conducted utilizing the random effects model. Analyses indicated no evidence of bias, as confirmed by Egger's test (Intercept = −2.28, t = −2.60, $p = 0.06$) and Begg and Mazumdar's rank correlation test (z = −1.69, $p = 0.09$). The visualization of the funnel plot is provided in Supplemental Figure S1.

### *3.5. Outcomes of the Meta-Analysis on Mortality in Patients with Heart Failure*

In the meta-analysis, which employed a fixed effects model, a noteworthy inverse association was observed between high adherence to the Mediterranean diet model (compared to low adherence) and all-cause mortality among patients with HF (OR = 0.88, 95% CI: 0.78–0.99, $p = 0.03$) (Figure 3). No significant heterogeneity was evident in the studies examining the relationship between the Mediterranean diet and all-cause mortality in patients with HF ($Tau^2 = 0.00$, $Chi^2 = 1.15$, $I^2 = 0.0\%$, $p = 0.56$). Furthermore, the analyses carried out did not reveal any substantial evidence of bias. This conclusion was supported by the results of Egger's test (Intercept = −2.62, t = −1.49, $p = 0.37$) and Begg and Mazumdar's rank correlation test (z = −1.57, $p = 0.11$). The visual examination of the funnel plot is presented in Supplemental Figure S2).

In a pooled analysis of two independent studies examining high adherence to the DASH diet model (compared to low adherence) and all-cause mortality in patients with HF, no significant association was found between the DASH diet and all-cause mortality among patients with HF (OR = 0.89, 95% CI: 0.75–1.05, $p = 0.15$) (Figure 3). It appears that no significant and substantial heterogeneity was observed within the studies assessing the DASH diet in relation to the all-cause mortality in patients with HF ($Tau^2 = 0.00$, $Chi^2 = 1.15$, $I^2 = 13\%$, $p = 0.28$). Since there were only two reports, bias analysis was not conducted.

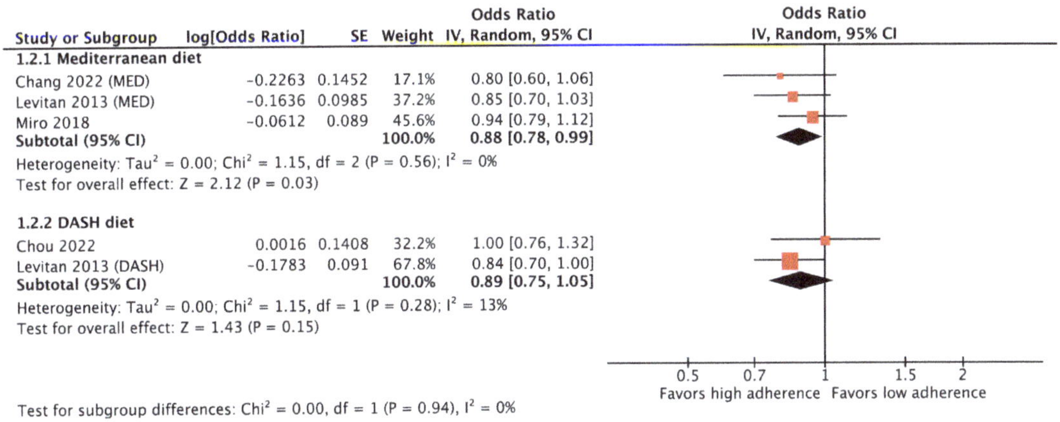


**Figure 3.** The forest plot of the effect of the Mediterranean diet and the DASH diet pattern on all-cause mortality in patients with heart failure [14,17,27,28].

### 3.6. Subgroup Analysis

We executed various subgroup analyses from eligible studies to address individual dietary components of the Mediterranean and DASH diet patterns in terms of incident HF risk among patients without previous diagnosis of HF and all-cause mortality among patients with HF. Consistently across all the analyzed data, it was observed that a high-quantile consumption of fruits and legumes was linked to a notably reduced risk of incident HF (Table 2). Moderate alcohol intake, particularly wine—a characteristic feature of the Mediterranean diet—also exhibited a protective effect against incident HF risk. Of note, consumption of legumes and fruits was linked to decreased incident HF risk as well. On the contrary, a high-quantile consumption of vegetables and fish did not exhibit a statistically significant association with incident HF risk. However, consumption of vegetables and less dairy consumption were significantly associated with reduced all-cause mortality among patients with HF (Table 3). Of note, low sodium did not have any significant impact on all-cause mortality risk among patients with HF.

**Table 2.** Subgroup analyses of dietary components and heart failure risk of eligible studies included in the systematic review and meta-analysis.

| Analysis | Analysis Model | Number of Reports ($n$) | Effect Size (OR) | 95% CI | $p$ Value | $I^2$ | $p$ Value |
|---|---|---|---|---|---|---|---|
| Fruits | Fixed | 4 | 0.92 | 0.85–0.99 | 0.03 | 0.00% | 0.76 |
| Legumes | Fixed | 4 | 0.93 | 0.86–0.99 | 0.04 | 0.01% | 0.48 |
| Moderate Alcohol | Fixed | 4 | 0.91 | 0.83–0.98 | 0.02 | 0.03% | 0.38 |
| Vegetables | Fixed | 4 | 0.97 | 0.85–1.08 | 0.61 | 60.48% | 0.07 |
| Fish | Fixed | 4 | 0.94 | 0.86–1.01 | 0.11 | 0.00% | 0.54 |
| Less Dairy | Fixed | 3 | 0.92 | 0.84–1.00 | 0.05 | 0.08% | 0.19 |
| Fiber | Fixed | 2 | 0.92 | 0.84–1.00 | 0.06 | 0.00% | 0.89 |

CI confidence interval, OR odds ratio.

### 3.7. Sensitivity Analysis

In the sensitivity analyses designed to test the stability of our findings, we employed a sequential exclusion method where each study was individually removed from the pooled analysis to observe the effect on the effect size (ES). The subsequent re-evaluation of the ES after each study's exclusion revealed minimal fluctuations, thereby affirming the robustness of our initial findings. The outcomes of these analyses are documented in Supplemental

Figures S3 and S4. The outcome suggests that our results are not disproportionately affected by any single study included in the meta-analysis.

**Table 3.** Subgroup analyses of dietary components and all-cause mortality of eligible studies included in the systematic review and meta-analysis.

| Analysis | Model | Number of Reports (*n*) | Effect Size (RR) | 95% CI | *p* Value | I² | *p* Value |
|---|---|---|---|---|---|---|---|
| Fruits | Fixed | 3 | 0.99 | 0.90–1.09 | 0.99 | 0.77% | 0.36 |
| Legumes | Fixed | 3 | 0.89 | 0.78–1.00 | 0.06 | 24.78% | 0.27 |
| Moderate Alcohol | Random | 2 | 1.07 | 0.78–1.36 | 0.62 | 75.28% | 0.04 |
| Vegetables | Fixed | 3 | 0.82 | 0.72–0.92 | 0.001 | 0.00% | 0.56 |
| Fish | Fixed | 2 | 1.01 | 0.86–1.16 | 0.87 | 0.00% | 0.69 |
| Less Diary | Fixed | 2 | 0.80 | 0.65–0.95 | 0.01 | 0.00% | 0.78 |
| Less sodium | Fixed | 2 | 1.09 | 0.94–1.25 | 0.25 | 0.00% | 0.77 |

CI confidence interval, RR risk ratio.

## 4. Discussion

The aim of this meta-analysis was to clarify the impact of high adherence to the Mediterranean and DASH diets on the incident HF risk and all-cause mortality among individuals with HF. A substantial body of data consisting of 16 reports of 14 studies with a total sample size of 424,502 participants was examined, confirming a beneficial connection between adherence to Mediterranean and DASH dietary patterns and a decreased risk of incident HF among individuals without a previous diagnosis of HF. Notably, high adherence to a Mediterranean diet was furthermore associated with a lower rate of overall mortality in patients with HF. However, there was insufficient evidence regarding the influence of the DASH diet on all-cause mortality among patients with HF.

According to the DASH diet [29,30], people should eat less red meat, fat, and sugar and more fruits, vegetables, grains, grain products, lean meats, fish, and poultry, low- or nonfat dairy products, nuts, seeds, and legumes. They should also limit their intake of sodium. This diet was first recommended for hypertension, though, our meta-analysis has indicated on top of the existing literature that the DASH diet prevents incident HF by 17%. The DASH diet may help prevent HF by lowering blood pressure and preventing coronary heart disease.

The molecular mechanisms underlying the protective effects of the Mediterranean and DASH diets involve complex interactions between dietary components and key cellular pathways. The Mediterranean diet, through its high content of polyphenols (e.g., oleuropein, hydroxytyrosol), modulates epigenetic regulators such as DNA methyltransferases and histone deacetylases, leading to alterations in gene expression that suppress inflammatory and oxidative stress responses [35]. These compounds also inhibit nuclear factor-κB (NF-κB) activation, a key driver of pro-inflammatory cytokine production, thereby attenuating chronic low-grade inflammation implicated in cardiovascular diseases and neurodegenerative disorders [36]. Furthermore, olive oil, a cornerstone of the Mediterranean diet, contains phenolic compounds like hydroxytyrosol, which inhibit inflammatory enzymes such as COX-2 and MMP-9 while suppressing PKCα and PKCβ1 pathways in monocytes, thereby offering vascular protection [36]. Similarly, the DASH diet's emphasis on potassium, magnesium, and bioactive antioxidants from fruits and vegetables reduces oxidative damage by neutralizing free radicals and enhancing glutathione synthesis, critical for maintaining cellular redox homeostasis [37]. Additionally, both diets influence metabolic pathways linked to lipid metabolism and vascular health. The Mediterranean diet's monounsaturated fatty acids (MUFAs) from olive oil and omega-3 fatty acids from fish suppress lipogenesis and improve endothelial function by enhancing nitric oxide bioavailability while reducing adhesion molecule expression, which mitigates atherosclerotic plaque development [38]. The DASH diet's low sodium content and high potassium-to-sodium ratio further contribute to blood pressure reduction by modulating renal sodium handling and reducing vascular resistance [37]. Both dietary patterns underscore the pivotal role of nutritional components in modulating inflammatory and oxidative pathways, thereby fostering systemic health and preventing chronic disease progression [38]. Collectively, these molecular and cellular effects highlight the synergistic action of dietary components in preventing metabolic and inflammatory diseases while promoting longevity and optimal health.

The protective effects of the Mediterranean and DASH diets on cardiovascular health are not merely confined to their well-known antihypertensive benefits. Both dietary patterns also impart additional cardiovascular advantages, such as enhancing diastolic function and ameliorating arterial stiffness [28,39]. Importantly, these diets could mitigate oxidative stress—a key antecedent to HF. The composition of these diets, abundant in fruits, vegetables, whole grains, and lean proteins, lends itself to these cardioprotective effects [29]. However, the inclusion of dairy products in the DASH diet remains a subject of ongoing scrutiny, as its role in HF is yet to be understood [30].

The Mediterranean diet is particularly lauded for its anti-inflammatory and antioxidant properties, contributing to its inverse relation with HF severity. Mechanistically, this diet may exert its beneficial effects through the suppression of proinflammatory markers like IL1β, IL1RN, TNF-α, ICAM1, hs-CRP, and IL-6 [16,31,34]. Furthermore, it is worth noting that certain nutrients within the Mediterranean diet, such as mono-unsaturated fatty acids, may have the capacity to inhibit detrimental metabolic shifts in cardiac function, thereby mitigating HF risk [33]. Both diets are also commendable for their low sodium content, a critical element in preventing incident HF. Moreover, there is emerging evidence to suggest that these diets, replete with antioxidants and micronutrients, could influence the gut microbiome in a manner that offers additional protection against HF [40].

Hence, both the Mediterranean and DASH diets appear to offer broad-spectrum cardiovascular benefits that extend beyond their well-established antihypertensive effects. These findings accentuate the utility of these dietary patterns in both the prevention and management of HF and beckon further rigorous research to validate their roles comprehensively. Of note, the Mediterranean diet appears to positively influence sleep-disordered breathing (SDB) and its downstream effects on diastolic function, mechanisms that are particularly relevant to HFpEF. Studies have demonstrated that adherence to the Mediterranean diet, particularly when combined with physical activity, significantly reduces the apnea–hypopnea index during REM sleep in patients with obstructive sleep apnea syndrome (OSAS). This improvement is largely attributed to reductions in central obesity and metabolic risk markers, which are key contributors to SDB pathophysiology [41]. Moreover, systemic inflammation, which is prevalent in SDB and HFpEF patients, has been directly associated with diastolic dysfunction. The Mediterranean diet's anti-inflammatory properties may mitigate these effects, improving diastolic performance in patients with both conditions [42]. Additionally, weight loss interventions based on the Mediterranean diet have shown significant reductions in oxidative stress and inflammatory markers when combined with CPAP therapy, suggesting a synergistic effect in alleviating SDB-related cardiovascular dysfunction [43]. Furthermore, the Mediterranean diet's ability to enhance endothelial function and reduce diastolic blood pressure may contribute to its cardioprotective effects, particularly in improving diastolic function in patients with HFpEF [44]. These findings highlight the potential of the Mediterranean diet as a non-pharmacological intervention to address the interplay between SDB, inflammation, and diastolic dysfunction, offering a promising strategy for managing HFpEF and related comorbidities.

The Mediterranean diet plays a significant role in managing obesity, a critical contributing factor to arrhythmia-induced HF, and its preventive and therapeutic potential is increasingly recognized [45,46]. Obesity is a well-established risk factor for atrial fibrillation, the most common arrhythmia leading to HF, due to its effects on left atrial enlargement, systemic inflammation, and oxidative stress [45]. The Mediterranean diet, characterized by high consumption of fruits, vegetables, whole grains, nuts, olive oil, and lean proteins, particularly fish, has demonstrated efficacy in addressing obesity through caloric balance, improved satiety, and metabolic regulation. Research indicates that adherence to the Mediterranean diet reduces body weight, waist circumference, and visceral adiposity, factors directly linked to atrial remodeling and arrhythmogenesis. For instance, weight loss facilitated by the Mediterranean diet is associated with reduced left atrial volume and improved atrial conduction, lowering AF risk and its progression to HF [41]. Furthermore, the diet's anti-inflammatory and antioxidant properties mitigate the systemic inflammatory burden and oxidative damage that exacerbate arrhythmogenesis and cardiac remodeling [43]. The Mediterranean diet also improves lipid profiles and glycemic control, reducing other obesity-related risk factors such as hypertension and diabetes, which further contribute to arrhythmia-induced cardiac dysfunction. By addressing both obesity and its downstream effects, the Mediterranean diet emerges as a holistic strategy for preventing and managing arrhythmia-induced HF, supporting its integration into comprehensive cardiac care. Future research should explore its role in specific patient subgroups to optimize its therapeutic potential further.

Epicardial adipose tissue (EAT) is a metabolically active fat depot closely associated with myocardial function, and its inflammation and expansion are critical contributors to cardiac dysfunction. The anti-inflammatory properties of the Mediterranean diet, driven by its high content of omega-3 fatty acids, polyphenols, and monounsaturated fats, reduce the pro-inflammatory cytokine profile of EAT, including TNF-$\alpha$ and IL-6, which are known to promote myocardial fibrosis and dysfunction [47]. Furthermore, the diet improves insulin sensitivity and lipid metabolism, addressing the impaired glucose and lipid handling observed in EAT of heart failure patients, which exacerbates cardiac stress [48]. Reductions in EAT volume associated with adherence to the Mediterranean diet decrease mechanical stress and inflammatory signaling in the myocardium, contributing to improved cardiac function and reduced risk of heart failure [49]. Additionally, the Mediterranean diet enhances the secretion of protective adipokines, such as adiponectin, which counteracts oxidative stress and inflammation, supporting myocardial health [50]. These findings underscore the therapeutic potential of the Mediterranean diet in targeting EAT as a modifiable risk factor, providing a promising avenue for managing heart failure pathophysiology, particularly in conditions like HFpEF. Therefore, it is suggested that this type of plant-based diet contributes significantly to its potential effect on HF and is consistent with our outcomes.

Of note, resveratrol, a polyphenolic compound found in grapes and red wine, exhibits cardioprotective properties that may hold significant therapeutic potential in the management of HF. Resveratrol's benefits stem from its ability to modulate multiple molecular pathways involved in oxidative stress, inflammation, and cardiac remodeling. Research has demonstrated that resveratrol enhances nitric oxide bioavailability and upregulates proteins such as endothelial nitric oxide synthase and inducible nitric oxide synthase, which contribute to improved myocardial function and reduced ischemic damage [51]. Additionally, resveratrol acts as a potent antioxidant, attenuating oxidative stress and inflammation through pathways like PI3K/Akt and AMPK, while also promoting autophagy to remove damaged cellular components [52]. In experimental models of HF, resveratrol has been shown to improve left ventricular function, reduce fibrosis, and prevent pathological cardiac hypertrophy by regulating stress signaling pathways and oxidative markers such as COX-2 and ROS [53]. Its ability to modulate inflammasome activation and mitochondrial function further underscores its protective role against myocardial injury and arrhythmias, as evidenced by reductions in atrial fibrillation susceptibility in HF models [54]. Collectively, these findings suggest that resveratrol's multifaceted cardioprotective mechanisms make it a promising candidate for dietary or pharmacological intervention in HF, particularly when integrated into broader lifestyle modifications. Further clinical studies are warranted to validate these effects and establish optimal dose strategies. Taken together, plant-based dietary patterns contain abundant resveratrol; thus, their potential benefits in heart failure are compatible with our study. It sheds light on the long-term effects in HF.

The high heterogeneity observed in analyses of the DASH diet warrants deeper exploration to identify potential sources of variability. Population differences, such as genetic predispositions, baseline dietary habits, and cultural food practices, likely contribute significantly to this heterogeneity. For example, studies show that the impact of the DASH diet on cardiometabolic markers varies across populations due to differences in baseline health status and dietary environments [55]. Furthermore, varying definitions and measures of dietary adherence, such as the use of self-reported food frequency questionnaires versus biomarkers, introduce inconsistencies that complicate the aggregation of findings [56]. Reliance on observational studies introduces potential confounding factors that may bias the results. Unmeasured lifestyle variables, such as physical activity levels, alcohol consumption, and smoking, or socioeconomic factors like education and income, could independently influence the observed benefits of the DASH diet. For instance, higher adherence to the DASH diet is often associated with greater health awareness and access to healthcare, which may independently reduce disease risk [57]. Addressing these confounders through stratified analyses or the inclusion of comprehensive demographic and lifestyle data can help improve the validity of future studies. By standardizing adherence metrics and employing diverse, representative samples in future randomized controlled trials, researchers can reduce heterogeneity and strengthen the evidence base. Moreover, integrating qualitative assessments to understand barriers to adherence can provide actionable insights for tailoring dietary interventions across different populations.

The limited representation of low- and middle-income countries (LMICs) in dietary intervention studies, including those examining the DASH and Mediterranean diets, presents a notable limitation. Dietary patterns, food availability, and socioeconomic factors in LMICs differ significantly from those in high-income countries, which could influence the generalizability of findings. For instance, the affordability and accessibility of foods emphasized in these diets, such as fresh produce and lean proteins, may pose significant challenges in LMICs, potentially reducing adherence and effectiveness [57]. Future research should prioritize studies in these settings to understand how socioeconomic and cultural factors modify the impact of such diets and explore locally appropriate adaptations. Moreover, variability in dietary adherence scoring methods across studies introduces clinical heterogeneity that complicates the synthesis of results. Adherence is often assessed using tools such as food frequency questionnaires or biomarkers, each with distinct limitations, including recall bias or variations in cutoff thresholds for adherence [56]. Standardizing scoring methods and employing more objective measures of adherence, such as food diaries or nutrient biomarkers, would improve the comparability and reliability of findings across diverse populations and study designs. Addressing these limitations will enhance the global applicability and clinical relevance of dietary intervention research.

This meta-analysis examining high and low adherence to the Mediterranean and DASH diets has several limitations that need to be addressed. One of the important limitations of the study is the use of cohort studies, which likely result in the relationship between diet and outcomes being affected by confounding factors. All studies are observational, and observational studies on diet are very prone to bias and confounders. Other limitations include significant disparities in the comparison groups, different methodologies employed to evaluate adherence, inherent biases in food intervention trials, and the majority of studies conducted in high-income countries. As a result, the generalizability of the findings to low- and middle-income countries, where dietary patterns and food options may significantly differ, may be affected. Especially, given the diversity in dietary assessment tools and methodologies used in nutritional research, it is reasonable to suppose that there might not be uniformity across studies in defining levels of adherence. This potential inconsistency can introduce significant clinical heterogeneity, complicating the interpretation of results and the comparison of outcomes across different investigations. This heterogeneity makes it challenging to draw firm conclusions about the effectiveness of these dietary patterns in preventing or managing specific health conditions, such as cardiovascular disease and HF. To address this issue, future research should aim for greater standardization in the assessment of diet adherence. The study also presents inconsistencies in findings regarding the relationship between alcohol intake and cardiovascular disease. These inconsistencies are attributed to the lack of comprehensive evaluation and inconsistent data reporting among the analyzed studies. The utilization of a simplistic binary scale to assess alcohol intake and the absence of gender-based adjustments for variables such as BMI and physical activity further complicate the interpretation of the results.

Another notable limitation is the scarcity of studies reporting on all-cause mortality outcomes for Mediterranean and DASH diets. Only three studies investigated the impact of the Mediterranean diet on all-cause mortality in HF patients, while only two studies examined the DASH diet. This lack of studies addressing this crucial clinical outcome may undermine the statistical power and precision of our estimates. Despite these limitations, the sensitivity analysis demonstrates the robustness of the overall results. No individual study exerted an abnormal influence on the outcomes, thereby lending credibility to the findings. However, these limitations underscore the necessity for more uniform and standardized reporting in future dietary intervention studies, particularly in terms of defining and quantifying dietary adherence. The inclusion of more studies in various contexts is imperative to enhance the generalizability of the findings.

## 5. Conclusions

The findings of this meta-analysis suggest that high adherence to the Mediterranean and DASH diets is associated with a considerable reduction in the incidence of HF compared to low adherence. High adherence to the Mediterranean diet has also been related to decreased all-cause mortality among patients with HF compared to low adherence. However, high DASH diet adherence did not yield a significant reduction in all-cause mortality among patients with HF. Of note, adherence to some components of both diets was more closely related to the lower risk, such as consumption of fruits, legumes, and moderate alcohol, which was linked to decreased incident HF, whereas only consumption of vegetables and less dairy persisted in decreasing mortality risk as a secondary prevention in patients with HF.

**Supplementary Materials:** The following supporting information can be downloaded at: https://www.mdpi.com/article/10.3390/life15010063/s1, Table S1. The PRISMA checklist. Table S2. Search strategy used for the systematic review in PubMed, Embase, EBSCO Academic Search Ultimate, ICTRP, and NIH clinical trials databases. Table S3. Quality assessment of selected observational studies included in meta-analysis (Newcastle–Ottawa Scale). Figure S1. The funnel plot of the effect of the Mediterranean diet and the DASH diet on the risk of heart failure is approximately symmetrical and, in accordance with the results of Egger's ($p = 0.65$) fades the possibility of potential publication bias. Figure S2. The funnel plot of the effect of the Mediterranean diet and the DASH diet on mortality is approximately symmetrical and, in accordance with the results of Egger's ($p = 0.06$) fades the possibility of potential publication bias. Figure S3. Sensitivity analysis of the effect of the Mediterranean diet on the risk of heart failure. Figure S4. Sensitivity analysis of the effect of the DASH diet on the risk of heart failure.

**Author Contributions:** Conceptualization, M.E.A. and M.B.Y.; methodology, M.E.A., M.E.K. and M.B.Y.; software, M.E.A. and M.B.Y.; validation, M.E.A., M.E.K. and M.B.Y.; formal analysis, M.E.A. and M.B.Y.; investigation, M.E.A., M.E.K. and M.B.Y.; resources, M.E.A., M.E.K. and M.B.Y.; data curation, M.E.A. and M.B.Y.; writing—original draft, M.E.A., M.E.K. and M.B.Y.; writing—review and editing, M.E.A., M.E.K. and M.B.Y.; visualization, M.E.A., M.E.K. and M.B.Y.; supervision, M.E.A. and M.B.Y.; project administration, M.E.A., M.E.K. and M.B.Y.; funding acquisition, M.B.Y. All authors have read and agreed to the published version of the manuscript.

**Funding:** This research received no external funding.

**Institutional Review Board Statement:** Ethical approval is not required for this study, and all techniques followed the Declaration of Helsinki.

**Informed Consent Statement:** Not applicable.

**Data Availability Statement:** The datasets used and/or analyzed in this study are available upon reasonable request from the corresponding author.

**Conflicts of Interest:** M.E.A. and M.E.K. declare that they have no conflicts of interest to be disclosed. M.B.Y. has received institutional research fees from Bayer Healthcare Pharmaceuticals, Amgen, Novartis, Dalcor Pharmaceuticals, Novo Nordisk, Astra Zeneca, and Boehringer Ingelheim.

## References

1. Groenewegen, A.; Rutten, F.H.; Mosterd, A.; Hoes, A.W. Epidemiology of Heart Failure. *Eur. J. Heart Fail.* **2020**, *22*, 1342–1356. [CrossRef] [PubMed]
2. Celik, A.; Ural, D.; Sahin, A.; Colluoglu, I.T.; Kanik, E.A.; Ata, N.; Arugaslan, E.; Demir, E.; Ayvali, M.O.; Ulgu, M.M.; et al. Trends in Heart Failure between 2016 and 2022 in Türkiye (TRends-HF): A Nationwide Retrospective Cohort Study of 85 Million Individuals across Entire Population of All Ages. *Lancet Reg. Health Eur.* **2023**, *33*, 100723. [CrossRef] [PubMed]
3. Heidenreich, P.A.; Albert, N.M.; Allen, L.A.; Bluemke, D.A.; Butler, J.; Fonarow, G.C.; Ikonomidis, J.S.; Khavjou, O.; Konstam, M.A.; Maddox, T.M.; et al. Forecasting the Impact of Heart Failure in the United States: A Policy Statement from the American Heart Association. *Circ. Heart Fail.* **2013**, *6*, 606–619. [CrossRef] [PubMed]
4. Huffman, M.D.; Berry, J.D.; Ning, H.; Dyer, A.R.; Garside, D.B.; Cai, X.; Daviglus, M.L.; Lloyd-Jones, D.M. Lifetime Risk for Heart Failure among White and Black Americans: Cardiovascular Lifetime Risk Pooling Project. *J. Am. Coll. Cardiol.* **2013**, *61*, 1510–1517. [CrossRef]
5. Ishikawa, Y.; Sattler, E.L.P. Nutrition as Treatment Modality in Heart Failure. *Curr. Atheroscler. Rep.* **2021**, *23*, 13. [CrossRef] [PubMed]
6. Perk, J.; De Backer, G.; Gohlke, H.; Graham, I.; Reiner, Z.; Verschuren, M.; Albus, C.; Benlian, P.; Boysen, G.; Cifkova, R.; et al. European Guidelines on Cardiovascular Disease Prevention in Clinical Practice (Version 2012). The Fifth Joint Task Force of the European Society of Cardiology and Other Societies on Cardiovascular Disease Prevention in Clinical Practice (Constituted by Representatives of Nine Societies and by Invited Experts). *Eur. Heart J.* **2012**, *33*, 1635–1701. [CrossRef] [PubMed]
7. Sanches Machado d'Almeida, K.; Ronchi Spillere, S.; Zuchinali, P.; Corrêa Souza, G. Mediterranean Diet and Other Dietary Patterns in Primary Prevention of Heart Failure and Changes in Cardiac Function Markers: A Systematic Review. *Nutrients* **2018**, *10*, 58. [CrossRef] [PubMed]
8. Anand, S.S.; Hawkes, C.; de Souza, R.J.; Mente, A.; Dehghan, M.; Nugent, R.; Zulyniak, M.A.; Weis, T.; Bernstein, A.M.; Krauss, R.M.; et al. Food Consumption and Its Impact on Cardiovascular Disease: Importance of Solutions Focused on the Globalized Food System: A Report From the Workshop Convened by the World Heart Federation. *J. Am. Coll. Cardiol.* **2015**, *66*, 1590–1614. [CrossRef]
9. Arayici, M.E.; Basbinar, Y.; Ellidokuz, H. High and Low Dietary Fiber Consumption and Cancer Risk: A Comprehensive Umbrella Review with Meta-Meta-Analysis Involving Meta-Analyses of Observational Epidemiological Studies. *Crit. Rev. Food Sci. Nutr.* **2023**, *63*, 1–14. [CrossRef]

10. Filippou, C.D.; Tsioufis, C.P.; Thomopoulos, C.G.; Mihas, C.C.; Dimitriadis, K.S.; Sotiropoulou, L.I.; Chrysochoou, C.A.; Nihoyannopoulos, P.I.; Tousoulis, D.M. Dietary Approaches to Stop Hypertension (DASH) Diet and Blood Pressure Reduction in Adults with and without Hypertension: A Systematic Review and Meta-Analysis of Randomized Controlled Trials. *Adv. Nutr.* **2020**, *11*, 1150–1160. [CrossRef] [PubMed]
11. Arayici, M.E.; Yucel, U.; Ocek, Z.A. Knowledge and Attitudes of Ege University Midwifery, Nutrition-Dietetic, and Nursing Students About Natural Functional Foods. *J. Basic Clin. Health Sci.* **2020**, *4*, 364–370. [CrossRef]
12. Arayici, M.E.; Mert-Ozupek, N.; Yalcin, F.; Basbinar, Y.; Ellidokuz, H. Soluble and Insoluble Dietary Fiber Consumption and Colorectal Cancer Risk: A Systematic Review and Meta-Analysis. *Nutr. Cancer* **2022**, *74*, 2412–2425. [CrossRef]
13. Kerley, C.P. Dietary Patterns and Components to Prevent and Treat Heart Failure: A Comprehensive Review of Human Studies. *Nutr. Res. Rev.* **2019**, *32*, 1–27. [CrossRef] [PubMed]
14. Levitan, E.B.; Lewis, C.E.; Tinker, L.F.; Eaton, C.B.; Ahmed, A.; Manson, J.E.; Snetselaar, L.G.; Martin, L.W.; Trevisan, M.; Howard, B.V.; et al. Mediterranean and DASH Diet Scores and Mortality in Women with Heart Failure: The Women's Health Initiative. *Circ. Heart Fail.* **2013**, *6*, 1116–1123. [CrossRef]
15. Wirth, J.; di Giuseppe, R.; Boeing, H.; Weikert, C. A Mediterranean-Style Diet, Its Components and the Risk of Heart Failure: A Prospective Population-Based Study in a Non-Mediterranean Country. *Eur. J. Clin. Nutr.* **2016**, *70*, 1015–1021. [CrossRef] [PubMed]
16. Tektonidis, T.G.; Åkesson, A.; Gigante, B.; Wolk, A.; Larsson, S.C. A Mediterranean Diet and Risk of Myocardial Infarction, Heart Failure and Stroke: A Population-Based Cohort Study. *Atherosclerosis* **2015**, *243*, 93–98. [CrossRef] [PubMed]
17. Miró, Ò.; Estruch, R.; Martín-Sánchez, F.J.; Gil, V.; Jacob, J.; Herrero-Puente, P.; Herrera Mateo, S.; Aguirre, A.; Andueza, J.A.; Llorens, P.; et al. Adherence to Mediterranean Diet and All-Cause Mortality After an Episode of Acute Heart Failure: Results of the MEDIT-AHF Study. *JACC Heart Fail.* **2018**, *6*, 52–62. [CrossRef]
18. Levitan, E.B.; Wolk, A.; Mittleman, M.A. Consistency with the DASH Diet and Incidence of Heart Failure. *Arch. Intern. Med.* **2009**, *169*, 851–857. [CrossRef] [PubMed]
19. Goyal, P.; Balkan, L.; Ringel, J.B.; Hummel, S.L.; Sterling, M.R.; Kim, S.; Arora, P.; Jackson, E.A.; Brown, T.M.; Shikany, J.M.; et al. The Dietary Approaches to Stop Hypertension (DASH) Diet Pattern and Incident Heart Failure. *J. Card. Fail.* **2021**, *27*, 512–521. [CrossRef]
20. Page, M.J.; McKenzie, J.E.; Bossuyt, P.M.; Boutron, I.; Hoffmann, T.C.; Mulrow, C.D.; Shamseer, L.; Tetzlaff, J.M.; Moher, D. Updating Guidance for Reporting Systematic Reviews: Development of the PRISMA 2020 Statement. *J. Clin. Epidemiol.* **2021**, *134*, 103–112. [CrossRef]
21. Deeks, J.J.; Dinnes, J.; D'Amico, R.; Sowden, A.J.; Sakarovitch, C.; Song, F.; Petticrew, M.; Altman, D.G.; International Stroke Trial Collaborative Group; European Carotid Surgery Trial Collaborative Group. Evaluating Non-Randomised Intervention Studies. *Health Technol. Assess.* **2003**, *7*, iii–x, 1–173. [CrossRef]
22. Viechtbauer, W. Conducting Meta-Analyses in R with the Metafor Package. *J. Stat. Softw.* **2010**, *36*, 1–48. [CrossRef]
23. Review Manager (RevMan) [Computer Program]. Version 5.4 (2020). The Cochrane Collaboration. Available online: https://revman.cochrane.org (accessed on 6 January 2025).
24. ProMeta-3 Professional Statistical Software for Conducting Meta-Analysis (2015). It Is Based on ProMeta 2.1 Deployed by Internovi in 2015. Available online: https://Idostatistics.Com/Prometa3/ (accessed on 6 January 2025).
25. Egger, M.; Davey Smith, G.; Schneider, M.; Minder, C. Bias in Meta-Analysis Detected by a Simple, Graphical Test. *BMJ* **1997**, *315*, 629–634. [CrossRef] [PubMed]
26. Del Gobbo, L.C.; Kalantarian, S.; Imamura, F.; Lemaitre, R.; Siscovick, D.S.; Psaty, B.M.; Mozaffarian, D. Contribution of Major Lifestyle Risk Factors for Incident Heart Failure in Older Adults: The Cardiovascular Health Study. *JACC Heart Fail.* **2015**, *3*, 520–528. [CrossRef]
27. Chou, T.-Y.; Liu, W.-J.; Lee, C.-L.; Wang, J.-S. Adherence to the Dietary Approaches to Stop Hypertension Diet and All-Cause Mortality in Patients with a History of Heart Failure. *Front. Nutr.* **2022**, *9*, 1015290. [CrossRef] [PubMed]
28. Chang, C.-Y.; Lee, C.-L.; Liu, W.-J.; Wang, J.-S. Association of Adherence to the Mediterranean Diet with All-Cause Mortality in Subjects with Heart Failure. *Nutrients* **2022**, *14*, 842. [CrossRef]
29. Campos, C.L.; Wood, A.; Burke, G.L.; Bahrami, H.; Bertoni, A.G. Dietary Approaches to Stop Hypertension Diet Concordance and Incident Heart Failure: The Multi-Ethnic Study of Atherosclerosis. *Am. J. Prev. Med.* **2019**, *56*, 819–826. [CrossRef]
30. Chang, R.S.; Xu, M.; Brown, S.H.; Cohen, S.S.; Yu, D.; Akwo, E.A.; Dixon, D.; Lipworth, L.; Gupta, D.K. Relation of the Dietary Approaches to Stop Hypertension Dietary Pattern to Heart Failure Risk and Socioeconomic Status (from the Southern Community Cohort Study). *Am. J. Cardiol.* **2022**, *169*, 71–77. [CrossRef] [PubMed]
31. Strengers, J.G.; den Ruijter, H.M.; Boer, J.M.A.; Asselbergs, F.W.; Verschuren, W.M.M.; van der Schouw, Y.T.; Sluijs, I. The Association of the Mediterranean Diet with Heart Failure Risk in a Dutch Population. *Nutr. Metab. Cardiovasc. Dis.* **2021**, *31*, 60–66. [CrossRef] [PubMed]

32. Tektonidis, T.G.; Åkesson, A.; Gigante, B.; Wolk, A.; Larsson, S.C. Adherence to a Mediterranean Diet Is Associated with Reduced Risk of Heart Failure in Men. *Eur. J. Heart Fail.* **2016**, *18*, 253–259. [CrossRef] [PubMed]
33. Levitan, E.B.; Wolk, A.; Mittleman, M.A. Relation of Consistency with the Dietary Approaches to Stop Hypertension Diet and Incidence of Heart Failure in Men Aged 45 to 79 Years. *Am. J. Cardiol.* **2009**, *104*, 1416–1420. [CrossRef] [PubMed]
34. Papadaki, A.; Martínez-González, M.Á.; Alonso-Gómez, A.; Rekondo, J.; Salas-Salvadó, J.; Corella, D.; Ros, E.; Fitó, M.; Estruch, R.; Lapetra, J.; et al. Mediterranean Diet and Risk of Heart Failure: Results from the PREDIMED Randomized Controlled Trial. *Eur. J. Heart Fail.* **2017**, *19*, 1179–1185. [CrossRef] [PubMed]
35. Kontogiorgis, C.A.; Bompou, E.-M.; Ntella, M.; Berghe, W.V. Natural Products from Mediterranean Diet: From Anti-Inflammatory Agents to Dietary Epigenetic Modulators. *Anti-Inflamm. Anti-Allergy Agents Med. Chem.* **2010**, *9*, 101–124. [CrossRef]
36. Scoditti, E.; Nestola, A.; Massaro, M.; Calabriso, N.; Storelli, C.; De Caterina, R.; Carluccio, M.A. Hydroxytyrosol Suppresses MMP-9 and COX-2 Activity and Expression in Activated Human Monocytes via PKCα and PKCβ1 Inhibition. *Atherosclerosis* **2014**, *232*, 17–24. [CrossRef]
37. Asemi, Z.; Samimi, M.; Tabassi, Z.; Sabihi, S.; Esmaillzadeh, A. A Randomized Controlled Clinical Trial Investigating the Effect of DASH Diet on Insulin Resistance, Inflammation, and Oxidative Stress in Gestational Diabetes. *Nutrition* **2013**, *29*, 619–624. [CrossRef] [PubMed]
38. Bonaccio, M.; Cerletti, C.; Iacoviello, L.; de Gaetano, G. Mediterranean Diet and Low-Grade Subclinical Inflammation: The Moli-Sani Study. *Endocr. Metab. Immune Disord. Drug Targets* **2015**, *15*, 18–24. [CrossRef]
39. Tuttolomondo, A.; Di Raimondo, D.; Casuccio, A.; Velardo, M.; Salamone, G.; Cataldi, M.; Corpora, F.; Restivo, V.; Pecoraro, R.; Della Corte, V.; et al. Mediterranean Diet Adherence and Congestive Heart Failure: Relationship with Clinical Severity and Ischemic Pathogenesis. *Nutrition* **2020**, *70*, 110584. [CrossRef] [PubMed]
40. Huedo-Medina, T.B.; Garcia, M.; Bihuniak, J.D.; Kenny, A.; Kerstetter, J. Methodologic Quality of Meta-Analyses and Systematic Reviews on the Mediterranean Diet and Cardiovascular Disease Outcomes: A Review. *Am. J. Clin. Nutr.* **2016**, *103*, 841–850. [CrossRef] [PubMed]
41. Papandreou, C.; Schiza, S.E.; Bouloukaki, I.; Hatzis, C.M.; Kafatos, A.G.; Siafakas, N.M.; Tzanakis, N.E. Effect of Mediterranean Diet versus Prudent Diet Combined with Physical Activity on OSAS: A Randomised Trial. *Eur. Respir. J.* **2012**, *39*, 1398–1404. [CrossRef] [PubMed]
42. Hegner, P.; Wester, M.; Tafelmeier, M.; Provaznik, Z.; Klatt, S.; Schmid, C.; Maier, L.S.; Arzt, M.; Wagner, S.; Lebek, S. Systemic Inflammation Predicts Diastolic Dysfunction in Patients with Sleep Disordered Breathing. *Eur. Respir. J.* **2024**, *63*, 2400579. [CrossRef] [PubMed]
43. Georgoulis, M.; Yiannakouris, N.; Tenta, R.; Fragopoulou, E.; Kechribari, I.; Lamprou, K.; Perraki, E.; Vagiakis, E.; Kontogianni, M.D. A Weight-Loss Mediterranean Diet/Lifestyle Intervention Ameliorates Inflammation and Oxidative Stress in Patients with Obstructive Sleep Apnea: Results of the "MIMOSA" Randomized Clinical Trial. *Eur. J. Nutr.* **2021**, *60*, 3799–3810. [CrossRef] [PubMed]
44. Rallidis, L.S.; Lekakis, J.; Kolomvotsou, A.; Zampelas, A.; Vamvakou, G.; Efstathiou, S.; Dimitriadis, G.; Raptis, S.A.; Kremastinos, D.T. Close Adherence to a Mediterranean Diet Improves Endothelial Function in Subjects with Abdominal Obesity. *Am. J. Clin. Nutr.* **2009**, *90*, 263–268. [CrossRef] [PubMed]
45. Franquesa, M.; Pujol-Busquets, G.; García-Fernández, E.; Rico, L.; Shamirian-Pulido, L.; Aguilar-Martínez, A.; Medina, F.X.; Serra-Majem, L.; Bach-Faig, A. Mediterranean Diet and Cardiodiabesity: A Systematic Review through Evidence-Based Answers to Key Clinical Questions. *Nutrients* **2019**, *11*, 655. [CrossRef]
46. Mattioli, A.V.; Palmiero, P.; Manfrini, O.; Puddu, P.E.; Nodari, S.; Dei Cas, A.; Mercuro, G.; Scrutinio, D.; Palermo, P.; Sciomer, S.; et al. Mediterranean Diet Impact on Cardiovascular Diseases: A Narrative Review. *J. Cardiovasc. Med.* **2017**, *18*, 925–935. [CrossRef] [PubMed]
47. Esposito, K.; Ciotola, M.; Giugliano, D. Mediterranean Diet, Endothelial Function and Vascular Inflammatory Markers. *Public Health Nutr.* **2006**, *9*, 1073–1076. [CrossRef]
48. Burgeiro, A.; Fuhrmann, A.; Cherian, S.; Espinoza, D.; Jarak, I.; Carvalho, R.A.; Loureiro, M.; Patrício, M.; Antunes, M.; Carvalho, E. Glucose Uptake and Lipid Metabolism Are Impaired in Epicardial Adipose Tissue from Heart Failure Patients with or without Diabetes. *Am. J. Physiol. Endocrinol. Metab.* **2016**, *310*, E550–E564. [CrossRef] [PubMed]
49. Ansaldo, A.M.; Montecucco, F.; Sahebkar, A.; Dallegri, F.; Carbone, F. Epicardial Adipose Tissue and Cardiovascular Diseases. *Int. J. Cardiol.* **2019**, *278*, 254–260. [CrossRef]
50. Patel, V.B.; Basu, R.; Oudit, G.Y. ACE2/Ang 1-7 Axis: A Critical Regulator of Epicardial Adipose Tissue Inflammation and Cardiac Dysfunction in Obesity. *Adipocyte* **2016**, *5*, 306–311. [CrossRef]
51. Das, S.; Alagappan, V.K.T.; Bagchi, D.; Sharma, H.S.; Maulik, N.; Das, D.K. Coordinated Induction of iNOS-VEGF-KDR-eNOS after Resveratrol Consumption: A Potential Mechanism for Resveratrol Preconditioning of the Heart. *Vascul Pharmacol.* **2005**, *42*, 281–289. [CrossRef]

52. Petrovski, G.; Gurusamy, N.; Das, D.K. Resveratrol in Cardiovascular Health and Disease. *Ann. N. Y. Acad. Sci.* **2011**, *1215*, 22–33. [CrossRef]
53. Riba, A.; Deres, L.; Sumegi, B.; Toth, K.; Szabados, E.; Halmosi, R. Cardioprotective Effect of Resveratrol in a Postinfarction Heart Failure Model. *Oxid. Med. Cell. Longev.* **2017**, *2017*, 6819281. [CrossRef]
54. Chong, E.; Chang, S.-L.; Hsiao, Y.-W.; Singhal, R.; Liu, S.-H.; Leha, T.; Lin, W.-Y.; Hsu, C.-P.; Chen, Y.-C.; Chen, Y.-J.; et al. Resveratrol, a Red Wine Antioxidant, Reduces Atrial Fibrillation Susceptibility in the Failing Heart by PI3K/AKT/eNOS Signaling Pathway Activation. *Heart Rhythm.* **2015**, *12*, 1046–1056. [CrossRef]
55. Barak, F.; Falahi, E.; Keshteli, A.H.; Yazdannik, A.; Esmaillzadeh, A. Adherence to the Dietary Approaches to Stop Hypertension (DASH) Diet in Relation to Obesity among Iranian Female Nurses. *Public Health Nutr.* **2015**, *18*, 705–712. [CrossRef]
56. Fung, T.T.; Chiuve, S.E.; McCullough, M.L.; Rexrode, K.M.; Logroscino, G.; Hu, F.B. Adherence to a DASH-Style Diet and Risk of Coronary Heart Disease and Stroke in Women. *Arch. Intern. Med.* **2008**, *168*, 713–720. [CrossRef] [PubMed]
57. Soltani, S.; Arablou, T.; Jayedi, A.; Salehi-Abargouei, A. Adherence to the Dietary Approaches to Stop Hypertension (DASH) Diet in Relation to All-Cause and Cause-Specific Mortality: A Systematic Review and Dose-Response Meta-Analysis of Prospective Cohort Studies. *Nutr. J.* **2020**, *19*, 37. [CrossRef] [PubMed]


**Disclaimer/Publisher's Note:** The statements, opinions and data contained in all publications are solely those of the individual author(s) and contributor(s) and not of MDPI and/or the editor(s). MDPI and/or the editor(s) disclaim responsibility for any injury to people or property resulting from any ideas, methods, instructions or products referred to in the content.

life

MDPI

Article

# Clinicopathological Studies on the Impact of Grape Seed Extract and L-Carnitine as Cardioprotective Agents Against Doxorubicin-Induced Toxicity in Rats

**Tahany Saleh Aldayel [1], Omnia E. Kilany [2], Heba Nageh Gad El-Hak [3], Heba M. A. Abdelrazek [4], Osama Abdallah [2] and Donia E. Omar [2,*]**

1 Department of Health Sciences, Clinical Nutrition, College of Health and Rehabilitation Sciences, Princess Nourah bint Abdulrahman University, Riyadh 11671, Saudi Arabia; TSALdayel@pnu.edu.sa
2 Department of Clinical Pathology, Faculty of Veterinary Medicine, Suez Canal University, Ismailia 41522, Egypt; omniakilany@vet.suez.edu.eg (O.E.K.); dr_oabdallah@hotmail.com (O.A.)
3 Depatrment of Zoology, Faculty of Sciences, Suez Canal University, Ismailia 41522, Egypt; heba_ahmed@science.suez.edu.eg
4 Department of Physiology, Faculty of Veterinary Medicine, Suez Canal University, Ismailia 41522, Egypt; heba_abdelrazek@vet.suez.edu.eg
* Correspondence: donia_essam@vet.suez.edu.eg; Tel.: +20-1000769246

**Abstract:** Doxorubicin (DOX) cancer therapy induces serious cardiotoxicity as a side effect. This study aimed to investigate the cardioprotective effects of grape seed extract (GSE) and L-Carnitine (L-CA) against DOX-induced cardiac toxicity in male rats. Six groups of male albino rats were used: G1 (control); G2 (GSE), given grape seed extract (100 mg/kg b.wt.) orally for 35 days; G3 (L-CA) (150 mg/kg b.wt.); Group 4 (DOX-induced cardiotoxicity), given DOX (10 mg/kg b.wt., i.p.) on the 28th day of the experiment; G5 (GSE + DOX), given GSE and DOX as previously mentioned; and G6 (L-CA + DOX), given L-CA and DOX as previously mentioned. Electrocardiographic evaluation, lipid profile, lipid peroxidation and antioxidants, serum cardiac markers, and inflammatory markers were estimated. Histopathological evaluation of cardiac tissue was also examined. Key findings showed that DOX induced ECG abnormalities lipid peroxidation, reduced antioxidants, and elevated cardiac and inflammatory markers. GSE and L-CA significantly ameliorated ECG abnormalities, reduced lipid peroxidation, improved antioxidant enzymes and serum cardiac markers, and reduced inflammation. These findings suggest that GSE and L-CA exhibit substantial cardioprotective effects in DOX-induced cardiotoxicity via their antioxidant and anti-inflammatory potentials.

**Keywords:** cardiotoxicity; doxorubicin; grape seed extract; L-Carnitine

## 1. Introduction

Cancer is one of the main causes of death all over the world [1]. Despite the undeniable successes of chemotherapy, two critical problems remain unresolved: resistance to anticancer drugs and their associated toxicity [2]. One of the most significant drawbacks of anticancer therapy is its cardiovascular side effects, which can sometimes require reducing the drug dosage to ineffective levels or even discontinuing the treatment, posing severe health risks [3]. Doxorubicin (DOX), a potent cytotoxic antibiotic, falls under the anthracycline class and is developed from the *Streptomyces peucetius* var. *caesius* mutant variant as a secondary metabolite [4]. DOX is highly effective against a wide range of cancers, including malignancies of hematological origin like non-Hodgkin's lymphomas, Hodgkin's disease, and pediatric leukemia, as well as solid tumors such as those in the bladder, breast, and lung [5]. Nevertheless, DOX's use is restricted due to its dramatic adverse effects, which include vomiting, hair loss, nausea, hematological suppression, and a unique cardiotoxicity [6].

The mechanism behind DOX-induced heart failure involves a significant increase in free radicals and a decline in myocardial endogenous antioxidant activities [7]. This imbalance renders cardiac tissues particularly vulnerable to oxidative damage owing to their diminished antioxidant enzyme levels. Furthermore, DOX has a strong affinity for the phospholipids in the heart cells' mitochondrial membranes, resulting in its deposition in cardiac tissues. This accumulation triggers damage to intracellular components and the myocardium, as well as their membranes [8].

Mitigating heart damage caused by DOX could be achieved through treatments aimed at reducing oxidative stress [9]. Hence, there has been an increasing interest in using natural antioxidants as a preventive measure against heart issues [10]. Numerous polyphenols possessing substances with cardioprotective and antioxidant properties have recently been recognized. They can prevent DOX-induced injury to myocardial function and structure in rats by lowering the production of free radicals, increasing mitochondrial function, and reducing apoptosis [7].

Grapes, known for their rich polyphenol content, including proanthocyanidins (PAs), anthocyanins, and resveratrol, offer a diverse array of biological benefits, including anti-inflammatory, antioxidant, antidiabetic, antitumor, and cardioprotective effects [11]. Preclinical experiments have demonstrated that PAs can protect against the harmful effects of DOX on cardiac tissue. This protective effect is linked to a reduction in blood markers for cardiac damage and oxidative stress in the myocardium of experimental animals [12].

Carnitine (3-hydroxy-4-N-trimethylaminobutyrate), a small water-soluble molecule similar to a vitamin, is found in nearly all mammalian species [13]. Its primary role is to transport long-chain fatty acids in active form from the cellular cytosol to the matrix of the mitochondria, where β-oxidation happens [14]. L-Carnitine (L-CA) has several antioxidant mechanisms, including the capacity to quench free radicals directly; chelate catalytic metals-promoters of reactive oxygen species (ROS), like Cu and Fe; keep the integrity of the mitochondria; hinder ROS generation; and prohibit ROS-generating enzymes like NADPH oxidases and xanthine oxidase with further generation of antioxidant enzymes [15]. Grapes are one of the most widely cultivated fruits worldwide, owing to their diverse applications, including fresh consumption and the production of wine, grape juice, jam, and raisins. However, the massive manufacture of grape products produces large masses of byproducts, such as grape pomace and grape seeds, which can pose environmental problems and represent a major waste of valuable resources. There has been a growing interest in using these byproducts due to their rich composition of polyphenols. These compounds are renowned for their diverse beneficial properties [11], including anti-inflammatory, antioxidant, antidiabetic, antitumor, and cardioprotective effects [11]. On the other hand, L-CA is widely used as a nutritional supplement and is available in several forms, such as glycine-propionyl L-CA and L-CA L-tartrate; it has gained popularity for its role in enhancing athletic performance and improving muscle recovery. Its recovery-enhancing effects are attributed to its ability to boost the activity of antioxidant enzymes [16], which can effectively mitigate exercise-induced muscle damage [17].

The present study was designed to investigate the potential cardioprotective influences of GSE and L-CA against DOX-induced cardiac damage in male rats. This aim was achieved through the detection of electrocardiographic changes, lipid profile, lipid peroxidation and antioxidants, serum cardiac markers, and inflammatory markers, which were estimated. Also, the histopathological evaluation of cardiac tissue was examined, as well as the cardiac fibrous tissue installation.

## 2. Materials and Methods

### 2.1. Animals

Sixty male albino rats (300–400 g) were housed in the Laboratory Animal House of the Faculty of Veterinary Medicine at Suez Canal University, Egypt. The rats were allocated randomly into six groups, with ten rats per group (five rats per cage). To allow acclimation, they were kept under standard conditions, including room temperature (24 ± 2 °C), a natural daylight cycle, and free access to a basal diet for one week. Throughout the 35-day experimental duration, the rats were maintained at a room temperature of 24 ± 2 °C and a 55 ± 5% relative humidity. The experimental procedures were authorized by the institutional review board of the Faculty of Veterinary Medicine, Suez Canal University (protocol No. 2022013).

### 2.2. Plant Material, L-Carnitine, and Doxorubicin

Grape seed extract was obtained from Shaanxi Jintai Biological Engineering Co., Ltd. (Xi'an, China) (CAS No.: 84929-27-1). L-Carnitine was sourced from MARTINEZ NIETO (Murcia, Spain)in the form of 2000 mg liquid L-Carnitine tartrate. Doxorubicin hydrochloride (Adriadox®) was purchased from RMPL Pharma LLP (Mumbai, Maharashtra, India) in a 50 mg vial.

### 2.3. Study Design

The experimental rats were allocated randomly into six groups (ten in each) as follows:

Group 1 (control) was considered as the normal control group. Five rats received oral CMC, and the other five rats received distal water via gavage for 35 days. All of them were injected with IP saline on the 28th day.

The Group 2 (GSE) rats were given 100 mg/kg b.wt. of 1% *w/v* CMC via gavage daily for 35 days. The dosage was determined according to Nassiri-Asl and Hosseinzadeh [18]. The Group 3 (L-CA) rats received 150 mg/kg b.wt. of 33.3% *v/v* via gavage twice weekly for 35 days, with the dosage according to Tousson, Hafez [19].

In Group 4 (DOX), the cardiotoxicity was provoked by an IP injection of 10 mg/kg b.wt. DOX on the 28th experimental day. The dosage used to induce cardiotoxicity followed the protocol of Adıyaman, Adıyaman [9].

The Group 5 (GSE + DOX) rats received 100 mg/kg b.wt. of 1% *w/v* CMC via gavage daily for 35 days, and on the 28th experimental day, the rats were injected IP with 10 mg/kg b.wt. DOX.

The Group 6 (L-CA + DOX) rats received 150 mg/kg b.wt. of 33.3% *v/v* via gavage twice per week for 35 days, and on the 28th experimental day, the rats were injected IP with 10 mg/kg b.wt. DOX.

### 2.4. Phytochemical Analysis of Grape Seed Extract

Phytochemical analysis was performed using an Agilent 1260 series. The separation was carried out using an Eclipse C18 column (4.6 mm × 250 mm i.d., 5 μm). The mobile phase consisted of water (A) and 0.05% trifluoroacetic acid in acetonitrile (B) at a flow rate of 0.9 mL/min. The mobile phase was programmed consecutively in a linear gradient as follows: 0 min (82% A); 0–5 min (80% A); 5–8 min (60% A); 8–12 min (60% A); 12–15 min (82% A); 15–16 min (82% A); and 16–20 (82% A). The multi-wavelength detector was monitored at 280 nm. The injection volume was 5 μL for each of the sample solutions. The column temperature was maintained at 40 °C. The quantification method was carried out using the following standards: catechin, gallic acid, caffeic acid, methyl gallate, pyro catechol, syringic acid, ellagic acid, chlorogenic acid, rutin, coumaric acid, vanillin, naringenin, ferulic acid, quercetin, daidzein, apigenin, cinnamic acid, kaempferol, and hesperetin.

### 2.5. Electrocardiography (ECG)

ECG recordings were taken for all the experimental groups. The experimental animals were fully anaesthetized through tetrahydrofuran (THF) inhalation. Electrodes of ECG were attached subcutaneously to the paws of the rats where they were positioned on their backs. The electrodes were connected to a Kaden Yasen™ ECG-903 device (Zhuhai City, Guangdong, China). The recorded ECG parameters included heart rate (HR), QT and QRS complex intervals, and ST segment amplitude. The later parameters were obtained as four readings/rats in all the groups. All the rats (5 rats/group) were subjected to ECG analyses on the 29th day and 35th day.

### 2.6. Blood and Sample Collection

Rats were sacrificed twice: on day 29 (24 h post–cardiotoxicity induction) and day 35 (experiment completed). Blood was drawn from the retro-orbital sinus under mild THF anesthesia after an overnight fast. The blood samples were processed for biochemical, antioxidant, and cytokines analyses. The rats were subsequently euthanized with an overdose of THF. The hearts were divided for histological analysis and stored at −80 °C for oxidant and antioxidant assays. Cardiac tissue homogenates were prepared using the Lowry protein assay described by Lu, Yiao [20].

### 2.7. Determination of Lipid Profile

Serum triglycerides (TG), total cholesterol (TC), and high-density lipoprotein cholesterol (HDL-C) were determined using Clinchem kits (Hungary) according to the manufacturer's protocols [21–23], respectively. Low-density lipoprotein cholesterol (LDL-C) (1)and very low-density lipoprotein cholesterol (VLDL-C) (2) were calculated via the equations described by Obasi and Ogugua [24]. (1) Serum LDL-C (mg/dL) = TC − HDL-C − TG/5. (2) Serum VLDL-C (mg/dL) = TG/5.

### 2.8. Cardiac Lipid Peroxidation and Antioxidants

Catalase (CAT), reduced glutathione (GSH), malondialdehyde (MDA), and total nitric oxide (TNO) were measured by kits from Cell Biolabs, Inc. (San Diego, CA, USA), following the manufacturer's protocols [25–27], respectively. The total oxidative capacity (TOC) and total antioxidative capacity (TAC) were evaluated using kits from Labor Diagnostika Nord GmbH & Co. KG (Nordhorn, Germany), adhering to the protocols provided by the manufacturer [28]. The procedures of the kits were carried out according to [29,30]. In addition, LOOH was assayed using the Cayman Chemical kits' protocol [25].

### 2.9. Determination of Serum Cardiac Marker

Creatine Kinase (CK-MB), lactate dehydrogenase (LDH), and aspartate aminotransferase (AST) activities in serum were measured using Clinchem kits (Budapest, Hungary) according to the manufacturer's protocols [31–33]. Serum cardiac troponin I (cTnI) and NT-proBNP were measured using ELISA kits from Kamiya Biomedical Company (Seattle, WA, USA) and Cusabio Technology LLC (Wuhan, China) in accordance with the manufacturer's guidelines [34,35].

### 2.10. Inflammatory Markers

The ELISA kits for measuring serum IL-1β, TNF-α (Kamiya Biomedical Company, Seattle, WA, USA), MPO, and NF-Kß were obtained from (Cusabio Technology LL-C, Wuhan, China). The assay procedures were followed as the kit manufacturer's protocol.

### 2.11. Histopathological Examination of the Heart Tissue

Samples of the heart tissues were put in 10% neutral buffered formalin for fixation, subjected to dehydration via passage of graded alcohol concentration, subjected to xylene clearing, and immersed in paraffin. Sections 5 microns in thickness were subjected to staining via Masson's trichrome (on day 35) and Hematoxylin and Eosin (H&E) (on day 29 and day 35) for light microscopic examination according to Bancroft and Cook [36]. Four random fields per slide were imaged to determine the percentage area of collagen fibers in the Masson's trichrome slides. A total of 3 slides/rats were examined.

### 2.12. Statistical Analysis

The data from the study were tested using the Shapiro–Wilk test, which revealed that all the data were normal except the ECG parameters and that the percentage area of collagen fibers was not found to be parametric. The Kruskal–Wallis H test was performed to determine the differences in the later parameters between the groups. Additionally, SPSS 29 employed a violin plot of the ECG data. The rest of the study data were analyzed via SPSS version 25. The results were expressed as mean ± SE. One-way ANOVA followed by Tukey's test was used for analysis, with $p < 0.05$ considered statistically significant.

## 3. Results

### *3.1. Phytochemical Analysis of Grape Seed Extract*

The phytochemical screening of the standard laboratory procedures revealed the presence of phenolic compounds (chlorogenic acid, catechin, gallic acid, methyl gallate, pyrocatechol, caffeic acid, syringic acid, coumaric acid, quercetin, and apigenin) (Table 1, Figure 1). The highest concentration among the active compounds was observed in catechin, with a content of 11,385.07 µg/g, while the lowest concentration was in apigenin, with a content of 12.91 µg/g.

**Table 1.** Phytochemical analysis of grape seed extract.

| Chemical Class | Compound | Wavelength (nm) | Retention Time (min) | Contents (µg/g) |
|---|---|---|---|---|
| Phenolic compounds | Gallic acid | 280 | 3.333 | 1623.68 |
| | Chlorogenic acid | 280 | 4.091 | 2925.33 |
| | Caffeic acid | 280 | 5.843 | 1990.29 |
| | Syringic acid | 280 | 6.479 | 121.76 |
| | Coumaric acid | 280 | 8.981 | 342.14 |
| | Pyro Catechol | 280 | 6.771 | 719.14 |
| Flavonoids | Quercetin | 280 | 12.700 | 110.31 |
| | Catechin | 280 | 4.539 | 11,385.07 |
| | Methyl Gallate | 280 | 5.357 | 1692.11 |
| | Apigenin | 280 | 14.538 | 12.91 |

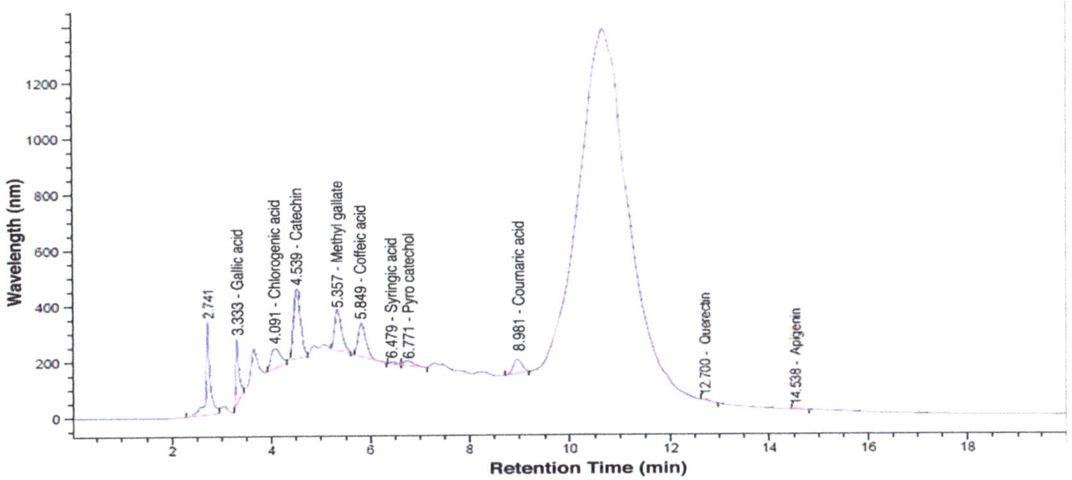


**Figure 1.** Phytochemical analysis of grape seed extract.

### *3.2. ECG*

As seen in (Figures 2 and 3), there were no statistical differences among the control, GSE, and L-CA groups in both the 29th and 35th days of the experiment. The DOX group exhibited a marked decrease in HR and a statistical elevation in the ST segment. On the 29th day, there were non-significant changes in the QT and QRS complex intervals, but by the 35th day, these intervals were significantly elongated in comparison to the control group. The groups pretreated with GSE and L-CA demonstrated a significant increase in HR and a significant decrement in ST segment amplitude in comparison to the DOX group on both days. However, there were no significant changes in the QT and QRS complex intervals on the 29th day. By the 35th day, the data revealed no significant change in the QRS complex, while a statistically significant shortening of the QT interval was noted in comparison to the DOX rats.

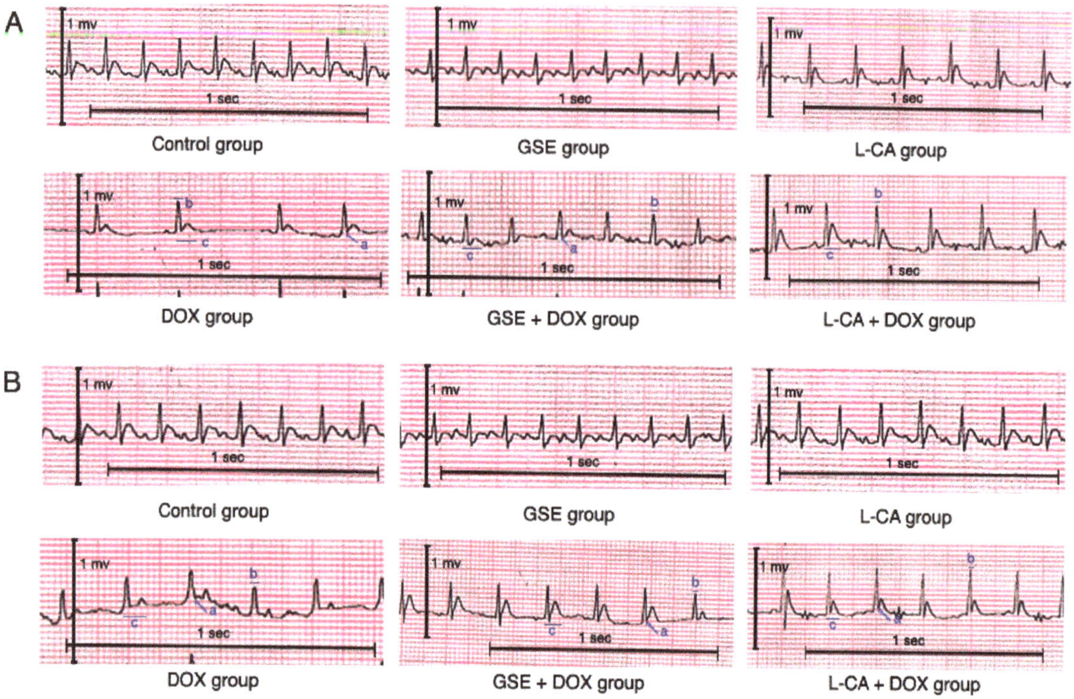


**Figure 2.** (**A**) Representative ECG on day 29 of the experiment. (**B**) Representative ECG on day 35 of the experiment. Group GSE: grape seed extract, Group L-CA: L-Carnitine; Group DOX: Doxorubicin, Group GSE + DOX: Grape seed extract with Doxorubicin, Group L-CA+ DOX: L-Carnitine with Doxorubicin. Labels a, b, and c denote the following ECG parameters: (a) ST-segment elevation, (b) QRS interval and (c) QT interval.

### 3.3. *Lipid Profile*

As mentioned in Table 2, the present results demonstrated non-significant variations in TG, TC, HDL-C, LDL-C, and VLDL-C levels in the groups that received GSE and L-CA in comparison to the control group on the 29th and 35th days of the experimental duration. In contrast, DOX injection resulted in a significant increase in TG, TC, LDL-C, and VLDL-C and a significant decline in HDL-C in comparison to the control rats on the 29th and 35th days. Pretreatment with GSE and L-CA led to significant improvements in these parameters compared to the DOX group, with a notable decrease in TG, TC, LDL-C, and VLDL-C and a statistical promotion in HDL-C. Moreover, the L-CA pretreated group showed a significant reduction in TC and LDL-C on the 29th and 35th days, along with improvements in TG and VLDL-C levels on day 35, compared to the rats pretreated with GSE.

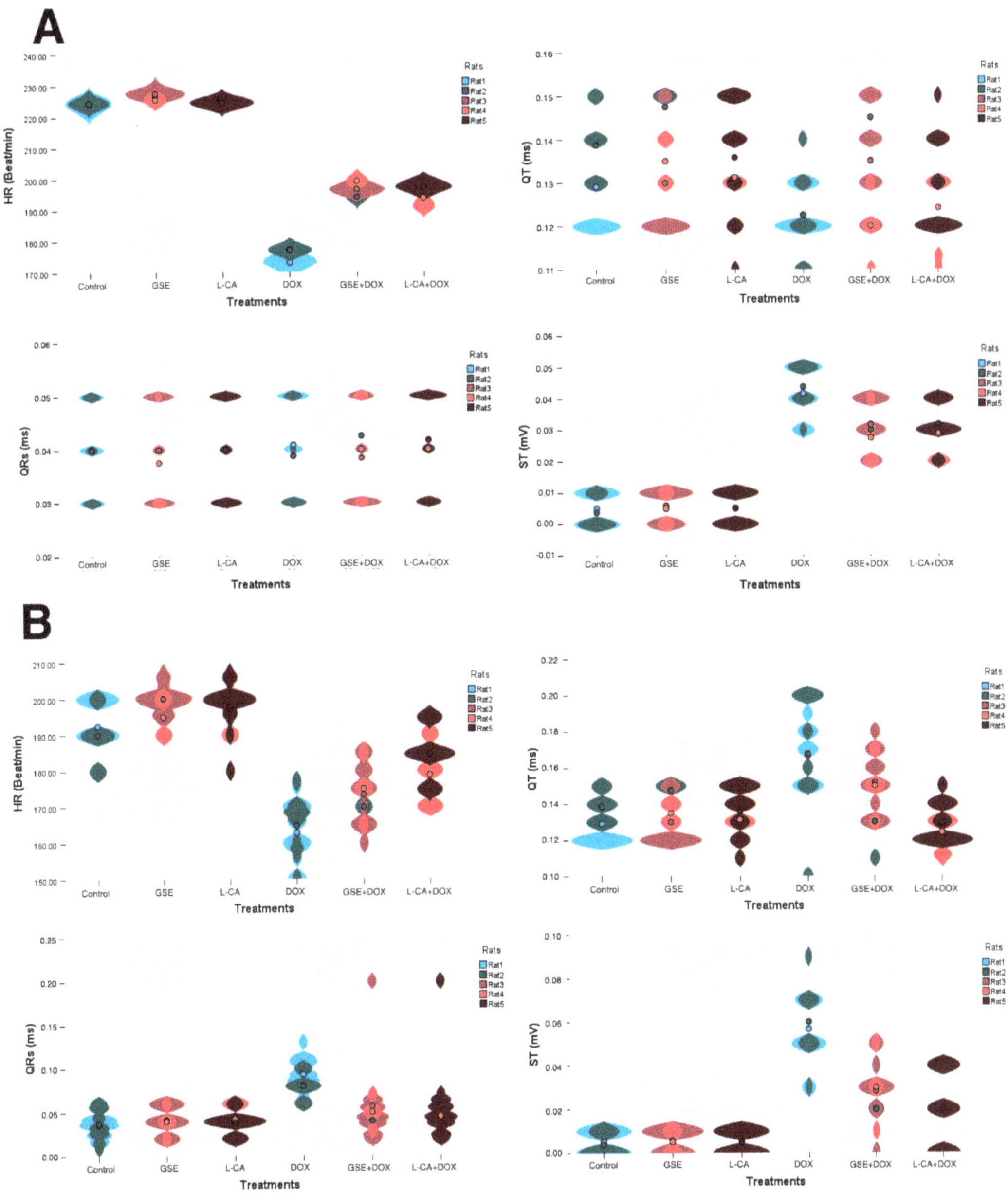


**Figure 3.** The impact of doxorubicin, grape seed extract, and L-carnitine on heart rate (HR), QRS complex, QT interval, and ST segment amplitude. (**A**) Representation of the changes in ECG on day 29 of the experiment ($n$ = 5). Data for each rat were obtained from 4 readings/rat. (**B**) Representation of the changes in ECG on day 35 of the experiment ($n$ = 5). Data for each rat were obtained from 4 readings/rat.

**Table 2.** The impact of doxorubicin, grape seed extract, and L-Carnitine on serum lipid profile on days 29 and 35 of the experiment.

| Treatment | | Triglycerides (mg/dL) | Total Cholesterol (mg/dL) | HDL-C (mg/dL) | LDL-C (mg/dL) | VLDL-C (mg/dL) |
|---|---|---|---|---|---|---|
| Control | Day 29 | $63.36^{c} \pm 0.62$ | $55.20^{d} \pm 0.55$ | $13.59^{a} \pm 0.35$ | $28.73^{d} \pm 1.05$ | $12.67^{c} \pm 0.12$ |
| | Day 35 | $64.26^{d} \pm 0.64$ | $55.65^{d} \pm 0.50$ | $14.29^{a} \pm 0.36$ | $28.50^{d} \pm 0.40$ | $12.85^{d} \pm 0.13$ |
| GSE | Day 29 | $62.68^{c} \pm 0.64$ | $55.30^{d} \pm 0.55$ | $14.32^{a} \pm 0.61$ | $28.17^{d} \pm 0.09$ | $12.54^{c} \pm 0.13$ |
| | Day 35 | $63.27^{d} \pm 0.64$ | $54.49^{d} \pm 0.64$ | $14.60^{a} \pm 0.64$ | $27.23^{d} \pm 0.20$ | $12.65^{d} \pm 0.13$ |
| L-CA | Day 29 | $62.39^{c} \pm 0.53$ | $55.60^{d} \pm 0.61$ | $14.63^{a} \pm 0.55$ | $26.23^{d} \pm 0.24$ | $12.48^{c} \pm 0.11$ |
| | Day 35 | $63.18^{d} \pm 1.01$ | $54.24^{d} \pm 0.49$ | $14.86^{a} \pm 0.55$ | $26.75^{d} \pm 0.90$ | $12.63^{d} \pm 0.09$ |
| DOX | Day 29 | $107.32^{a} \pm 0.61$ | $92.20^{a} \pm 0.55$ | $8.67^{c} \pm 0.68$ | $49.20^{a} \pm 1.24$ | $21.46^{a} \pm 0.12$ |
| | Day 35 | $100.87^{a} \pm 0.58$ | $84.40^{a} \pm 0.53$ | $9.70^{c} \pm 0.21$ | $44.64^{a} \pm 1.21$ | $20.17^{a} \pm 0.12$ |
| GSE + DOX | Day 29 | $94.44^{b} \pm 0.67$ | $86.52^{b} \pm 0.64$ | $9.37^{c} \pm 0.26$ | $46.17^{b} \pm 1.34$ | $18.89^{b} \pm 0.13$ |
| | Day 35 | $85.77^{b} \pm 0.77$ | $77.75^{b} \pm 0.52$ | $10.23^{bc} \pm 0.23$ | $41.25^{b} \pm 0.56$ | $17.15^{b} \pm 0.14$ |
| L-CA + DOX | Day 29 | $95.55^{b} \pm 0.67$ | $80.37^{c} \pm 0.64$ | $11.27^{b} \pm 0.37$ | $39.70^{c} \pm 1.31$ | $19.11^{b} \pm 0.13$ |
| | Day 35 | $83.26^{c} \pm 0.64$ | $68.33^{c} \pm 0.61$ | $11.30^{b} \pm 0.23$ | $33.02^{c} \pm 0.10$ | $16.65^{c} \pm 0.13$ |

Superscripts a, b, c, d within the same row are considered significant at $p < 0.05$. Group GSE: grape seed extract, Group L-CA: L-Carnitine; Group DOX: Doxorubicin; Group GSE + DOX: Grape seed extract with Doxorubicin, Group L-CA + DOX: L-Carnitine with Doxorubicin.

### 3.4. Cardiac Lipid Peroxidation and Antioxidants

As declared in Table 3, the present study revealed a non-significant alteration in lipid peroxidation and antioxidant levels in the experimental groups orally administered with GSE and L-CA when compared to the control group on both day 29 and day 35 of the experiment. In contrast, the group intoxicated with DOX displayed a significant decline in GSH, CAT, and TAC, along with a significant increase in TOC, MDA, TNO, and LOOH on both days compared to the control group.

**Table 3.** The impact of doxorubicin, grape seed extract, and L-Carnitine on lipid peroxidation and antioxidant enzymes in the heart tissue on days 29 and 35 of the experiment.

| Treatment | | GSH (μM/mg) | CAT (U/mg) | TAC (mmol/g) | TOC (mmol/g) | MDA (μM/mg) | TNO (μM/mg) | LOOH (nmol/mg) |
|---|---|---|---|---|---|---|---|---|
| Control | Day 29 | $13.44^{a} \pm 0.47$ | $50.59^{a} \pm 0.30$ | $1.77^{a} \pm 0.15$ | $0.39^{c} \pm 0.03$ | $11.12^{d} \pm 0.47$ | $36.24^{d} \pm 0.18$ | $1.12^{c} \pm 0.06$ |
| | Day 35 | $13.76^{a} \pm 0.64$ | $50.4^{a} \pm 0.55$ | $1.80^{a} \pm 0.06$ | $0.37^{d} \pm 0.01$ | $10.51^{d} \pm 0.29$ | $35.63^{d} \pm 0.32$ | $1.15^{d} \pm 0.09$ |
| GSE | Day 29 | $13.88^{a} \pm 0.52$ | $51.31^{a} \pm 0.38$ | $1.86^{a} \pm 0.19$ | $0.40^{c} \pm 0.02$ | $11.35^{d} \pm 0.60$ | $35.78^{d} \pm 0.15$ | 1.15 c $\pm$ 0.03 |
| | Day 35 | $13.80^{a} \pm 0.67$ | $50.6^{a} \pm 0.61$ | $1.81^{a} \pm 0.06$ | $0.37^{d} \pm 0.01$ | $10.32^{d} \pm 0.20$ | $35.63^{d} \pm 0.32$ | $1.15^{d} \pm 0.09$ |
| L-CA | Day 29 | $13.95^{a} \pm 0.52$ | $51.61^{a} \pm 0.31$ | $1.85^{a} \pm 0.03$ | $0.39^{c} \pm 0.02$ | $11.25^{d} \pm 0.65$ | $35.71^{d} \pm 0.21$ | $1.16^{c} \pm 0.04$ |
| | Day 35 | $14.59^{a} \pm 0.61$ | $52.4^{a} \pm 0.69$ | $1.82^{a} \pm 0.06$ | $0.35^{d} \pm 0.01$ | $10.11^{d} \pm 0.25$ | $35.61^{d} \pm 0.31$ | $1.15^{d} \pm 0.09$ |
| DOX | Day 29 | $7.05^{c} \pm 0.33$ | $26.08^{d} \pm 0.25$ | $0.72^{c} \pm 0.01$ | $0.72^{a} \pm 0.02$ | $33.89^{a} \pm 0.06$ | $69.75^{a} \pm 0.14$ | $3.16^{a} \pm 0.02$ |
| | Day 35 | $9.11^{c} \pm 0.15$ | $32.5^{d} \pm 0.62$ | $1.03^{d} \pm 0.01$ | $0.64^{a} \pm 0.01$ | $25.61^{a} \pm 0.31$ | $52.56^{a} \pm 0.30$ | $2.59^{a} \pm 0.15$ |
| GSE + DOX | Day 29 | $8.61^{b} \pm 0.35$ | $31.42^{c} \pm 0.30$ | $1.03^{b} \pm 0.01$ | $0.67^{ab} \pm 0.03$ | 28.55 b $\pm$ 0.83 | $58.24^{b} \pm 0.30$ | $3.18^{a} \pm 0.36$ |
| | Day 35 | $10.56^{b} \pm 0.12$ | $41.9^{c} \pm 0.58$ | $1.33^{c} \pm 0.01$ | $0.53^{b} \pm 0.01$ | $19.36^{b} \pm 0.20$ | $46.46^{b} \pm 0.29$ | $2.08^{b} \pm 0.10$ |
| L-CA + DOX | Day 29 | $9.49^{b} \pm 0.29$ | $36.33^{b} \pm 0.35$ | $1.28^{b} \pm 0.01$ | $0.61^{b} \pm 0.03$ | $25.36^{c} \pm 0.41$ | $52.43^{c} \pm 0.23$ | $2.43^{b} \pm 0.03$ |
| | Day 35 | $11.77^{b} \pm 0.15$ | $45.5^{b} \pm 0.61$ | $1.63^{b} \pm 0.01$ | $0.42^{c} \pm 0.01$ | $13.77^{c} \pm 0.15$ | $39.17^{c} \pm 0.29$ | $1.50^{c} \pm 0.12$ |

Superscripts a, b, c, d within the same row are considered significant at $p < 0.05$. Group GSE: grape seed extract, Group L-CA: L-Carnitine; Group DOX: Doxorubicin; Group GSE + DOX: Grape seed extract with Doxorubicin, Group L-CA + DOX: L-Carnitine with Doxorubicin.

Moreover, the groups pretreated with GSE and L-CA demonstrated significant enhancements in GSH, CAT, and TAC, as well as a statistical reduction in TOC, MDA, and TNO on both days compared to the DOX group. Specifically, the group pretreated with L-CA showed an improvement in CAT, MDA, TNO, and LOOH on the 29th and 35th days, along with a significant increase in TAC on day 35 of the experiment.

### 3.5. Cardiac Injury Markers

As demonstrated in Table 4, the activity of CK-MB, LDH, AST, cTnI, and NT-ProBNP showed non-significant variations in the groups treated with GSE and L-CA as compared with the control group on both the 29th and 35th days of the experimental duration. In contrast, DOX administration provoked a notable increase in serum cardiac markers compared to the control group on both days. However, significant diminution in these markers was consistently detected in the groups pretreated with GSE and L-CA compared to the DOX group, suggesting a protective effect against DOX-induced cardiac injury. Furthermore, L-CA pretreatment exhibited significant reductions in cardiac injury markers compared to the GSE-pretreated group on both days, indicating a potentially superior protective effect of L-CA.

**Table 4.** The impact of doxorubicin, grape seed extract, and L-Carnitine on serum cardiac injury markers on days 29 and 35 of the experiment.

| Treatment | | CK-MB (U/L) | LDH (U/L) | AST (U/L) | cTnI (ng/mL) | NT-ProBNP (pg/mL) |
|---|---|---|---|---|---|---|
| Control | Day 29 | $14.52^{c} \pm 0.87$ | $235.23^{d} \pm 2.90$ | $121.13^{d} \pm 2.31$ | $0.21^{d} \pm 0.01$ | $9.75^{d} \pm 0.03$ |
| | Day 35 | $15.10^{d} \pm 0.52$ | $238.30^{d} \pm 0.05$ | $123.47^{d} \pm 0.61$ | $0.21^{d} \pm 0.00$ | $9.50^{d} \pm 0.40$ |
| GSE | Day 29 | $12.60^{c} \pm 0.86$ | $233.20^{d} \pm 1.74$ | $121.60^{d} \pm 1.78$ | $0.21^{d} \pm 0.01$ | $9.74^{d} \pm 0.03$ |
| | Day 35 | $14.62^{d} \pm 0.61$ | $236.50^{d} \pm 0.55$ | $122.43^{d} \pm 0.58$ | $0.21^{d} \pm 0.01$ | $9.52^{d} \pm 0.48$ |
| L-CA | Day 29 | $14.13^{c} \pm 0.60$ | $232.77^{d} \pm 4.68$ | $120.90^{d} \pm 1.50$ | $0.21^{d} \pm 0.00$ | $9.78^{d} \pm 0.03$ |
| | Day 35 | $14.64^{d} \pm 0.55$ | $235.97^{d} \pm 1.59$ | $122.63^{d} \pm 1.26$ | $0.21^{d} \pm 0.00$ | $9.51^{d} \pm 0.36$ |
| DOX | Day 29 | $32.95^{a} \pm 1.16$ | $574.77^{a} \pm 2.90$ | $285.47^{a} \pm 2.49$ | $1.19^{a} \pm 0.03$ | $45.63^{a} \pm 2.88$ |
| | Day 35 | $26.73^{a} \pm 0.61$ | $506.57^{a} \pm 0.66$ | $232.67^{a} \pm 0.55$ | $0.88^{a} \pm 0.01$ | $37.60^{a} \pm 0.35$ |
| GSE + DOX | Day 29 | $26.19^{b} \pm 0.74$ | $510.60^{b} \pm 5.80$ | $235.57^{b} \pm 2.94$ | $0.93^{b} \pm 0.02$ | $39.15^{b} \pm 1.89$ |
| | Day 35 | $22.61^{b} \pm 0.64$ | $439.23^{b} \pm 0.66$ | $183.23^{b} \pm 0.47$ | $0.65^{b} \pm 0.01$ | $26.71^{b} \pm 0.60$ |
| L-CA + DOX | Day 29 | $23.74^{b} \pm 0.38$ | $479.70^{c} \pm 2.90$ | $220.40^{c} \pm 2.91$ | $0.71^{c} \pm 0.02$ | $32.32^{c} \pm 2.52$ |
| | Day 35 | $18.52^{c} \pm 0.58$ | $361.33^{c} \pm 0.55$ | $151.73^{c} \pm 0.66$ | $0.36^{c} \pm 0.01$ | $14.42^{c} \pm 0.44$ |

Superscripts a, b, c, d within the same row are considered significant at $p < 0.05$. Group GSE: grape seed extract, Group L-CA: L-Carnitine; Group DOX: Doxorubicin; Group GSE + DOX: Grape seed extract with Doxorubicin, Group L-CA + DOX: L-Carnitine with Doxorubicin.

### 3.6. Cardiac Inflammatory Markers

As demonstrated in Table 5, the levels of IL-1β, TNF-α, MPO, and NF-Kß showed non-significant variations in the groups treated with GSE and L-CA compared to the control group on both day 29 and day 35 of the experiment. However, the DOX-injected group exhibited a statistical increase in the levels of IL-1β, TNF-α, MPO, and NF-Kß in comparison to the control group at both time intervals. Additionally, the groups pretreated with GSE and L-CA displayed a significant decrease in these markers compared to the DOX group on the 29th and 35th days. Notably, the group pretreated with L-CA demonstrated a more significant decrease in IL-1β, TNF-α, MPO, and NF-Kß levels compared to the group pretreated with GSE on the 29th and 35th days.

**Table 5.** The impact of doxorubicin, grape seed extract, and L-Carnitine on cardiac inflammatory markers on days 29 and 35 of the experiment.

| Treatment | | IL-1β (pg/mg) | TNF-α (pg/mg) | MPO (ng/mg) | NF-Kß (pg/mg) |
|---|---|---|---|---|---|
| Control | Day 29 | $35.26^{d} \pm 0.06$ | $61.75^{d} \pm 0.39$ | $1.19^{d} \pm 0.03$ | $6.25^{d} \pm 0.03$ |
| | Day 35 | $35.31^{d} \pm 0.32$ | $61.04^{d} \pm 1.04$ | $1.22^{d} \pm 0.01$ | $6.30^{d} \pm 0.17$ |
| GSE | Day 29 | $35.34^{d} \pm 0.24$ | $62.12^{d} \pm 0.58$ | $1.19^{d} \pm 0.02$ | $6.22^{d} \pm 0.03$ |
| | Day 35 | $34.60^{d} \pm 0.32$ | $60.54^{d} \pm 0.29$ | $1.21^{d} \pm 0.00$ | $6.25^{d} \pm 0.14$ |

**Table 5.** *Cont.*

| Treatment | | IL-1β (pg/mg) | TNF-α (pg/mg) | MPO (ng/mg) | NF-Kß (pg/mg) |
|---|---|---|---|---|---|
| L-CA | Day 29 | $34.84^{d} \pm 0.23$ | $61.49^{d} \pm 0.29$ | $1.19^{d} \pm 0.02$ | $6.19^{d} \pm 0.03$ |
| | Day 35 | $34.51^{d} \pm 0.31$ | $60.07^{d} \pm 0.23$ | $1.20^{d} \pm 0.01$ | $6.16^{d} \pm 0.09$ |
| DOX | Day 29 | $119.47^{a} \pm 0.29$ | $194.54^{a} \pm 0.29$ | $3.85^{a} \pm 0.03$ | $17.76^{a} \pm 0.13$ |
| | Day 35 | $89.45^{a} \pm 0.30$ | $150.91^{a} \pm 0.52$ | $2.80^{a} \pm 0.15$ | $14.25^{a} \pm 0.43$ |
| GSE + DOX | Day 29 | $91.81^{b} \pm 0.23$ | $163.53^{b} \pm 0.29$ | $3.25^{b} \pm 0.03$ | $15.19^{b} \pm 0.04$ |
| | Day 35 | $73.36^{b} \pm 0.29$ | $117.40^{b} \pm 0.35$ | $2.27^{b} \pm 0.18$ | $12.16^{b} \pm 0.60$ |
| L-CA + DOX | Day 29 | $76.12^{c} \pm 0.07$ | $134.22^{c} \pm 0.12$ | $2.65^{c} \pm 0.03$ | $13.75^{c} \pm 0.03$ |
| | Day 35 | $53.55^{c} \pm 0.29$ | $78.41^{c} \pm 0.42$ | $1.81^{c} \pm 0.14$ | $8.53^{c} \pm 0.46$ |

Superscripts a, b, c, d within the same row are considered significant at $p < 0.05$. Group GSE: grape seed extract, Group L-CA: L-Carnitine; Group DOX: Doxorubicin; Group GSE + DOX: Grape seed extract with Doxorubicin, Group L-CA + DOX: L-Carnitine with Doxorubicin.

### 3.7. Histopathology on Cardiac Tissue Sections

Light microscopy of the rat cardiac sample tissue sections on the control, L-CA, and GSE groups on day 29 (Figure 4a–c) and day 35 (Figure 5a–c) of the experiment revealed normal cardiomyocytes and typical connective tissue on day 35 (Figure 6a–c). The cardiac wall consists of striated, branched cardiomyocytes containing intercalated disks and typically mononucleated nuclei.

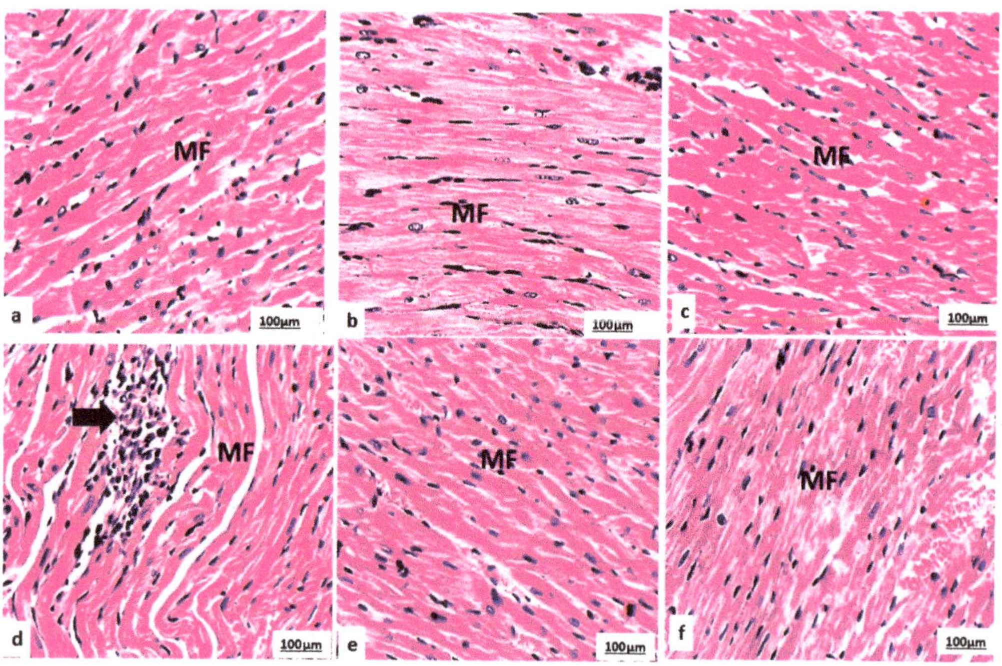


**Figure 4.** Photomicrographs of cardiac myocytes from the control, GSE, and L-CA groups (**a–c**) on day 29 of the experiment displayed normal cardiac myofibrillar structure (MF) with striations, branched appearance, central nucleus, and continuity with adjacent myofibrils. In contrast, the DOX group (**d**) revealed several abnormalities, including nuclear pyknosis and leukocyte infiltration (indicated by arrows). The DOX + GSE and DOX + L-CA groups (**e**,**f**) showed a restoration to normal cardiac myofibrillar structure (C) with clear striations. (H&E, 400×).

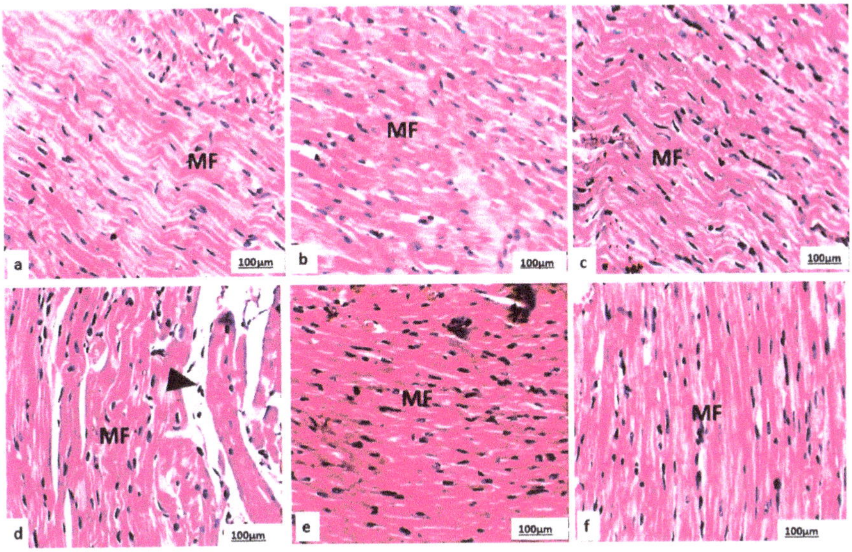


**Figure 5.** Photomicrographs of cardiac myocytes from the control, GSE, and L-CA groups (**a**–**c**) on day 35 of the experiment showed normal cardiac myofibrillar structure (MF) with striations, a branched appearance, a central nucleus, and continuity with adjacent myofibrils. In contrast, the DOX group (**d**) exhibited signs of myocardial infarction, including focal myolysis, non-visible nuclei, and darker, irregular necrotic contraction bands (indicated by arrowheads). The DOX + GSE and DOX + L-CA groups (**e**,**f**) displayed a return to normal cardiac myofibrillar structure (C) with clear striations. (H&E, 400×).

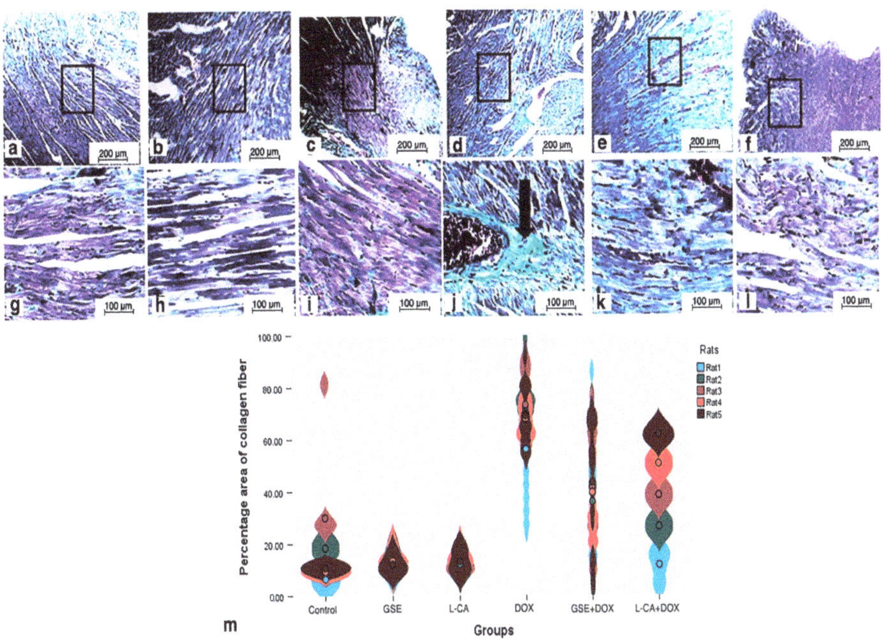


**Figure 6.** Photomicrographs of Masson-trichrome-stained cardiac myocytes of low and high magnification from the control (**a**,**g**), GSE (**b**,**h**), and L-CA groups (**c**,**i**) on day 35 of the experiment depicted normal cardiac myofibrillar structure with striations, a branched appearance, a central nucleus, and

continuity with adjacent myofibrils. In contrast, the DOX group (**d**,**j**) exhibited interstitial fibrosis, with an increase in the percentage area of collagen fiber (arrow). However, the GSE + DOX (**e**,**k**) and L-CA + DOX groups (**f**,**l**) displayed a restoration of normal cardiac myofibrillar structure with clear striations, accompanied by a decrease in the percentage area of collagen fiber. (100× & 400×). The mean percentage area of collagen fiber (**m**) was quantified across ($n$ = 5) rats/group. Each set of rat data was obtained from 12 measurements. Group GSE: grape seed extract; Group L-CA: L-Carnitine; Group DOX: Doxorubicin; Group GSE + DOX: Grape seed extract with Doxorubicin; Group L-CA + DOX: L-Carnitine with Doxorubicin.

Histopathological examination of the cardiac sample tissue sections on the DOX group on day 29 (Figure 4d) and day 35 (Figure 5d) revealed several abnormalities, including degeneration of the myofibrillar structure, myocardial atrophy, nuclear pyknosis, focal hemorrhage, edema, leukocyte infiltration, and interstitial fibrosis. There was an increased percentage area of collagen fibers on day 35, as evidenced by Masson trichrome staining (Figure 6d).

In contrast, the groups pretreated with L-CA or GSE on both day 29 (Figure 4e,f), and day 35 (Figure 5e,f) showed a marked reduction in the abnormalities observed in the DOX group. The heart tissue from these pretreated groups appeared to have normal myocardial muscle bundles with no interstitial fibrosis and a decreased percentage area of collagen fibers, as indicated by the Masson trichrome staining (Figure 6e,f).

## 4. Discussion

Doxorubicin is a highly effective chemotherapeutic agent extensively cast off in cancer treatment. However, its clinical use is significantly limited by its cardiotoxic side effects. DOX-induced cardiotoxicity is primarily linked to increased inflammation, oxidative stress, and apoptosis in cardiac tissue [37]. In the present study, we evaluated the possible alleviation of GSE and L-CA in DOX-induced cardiotoxicity.

Cardiotoxicity was confirmed by significant changes across multiple parameters, including ECG findings, serum biomarkers indicative of oxidative stress, cardiac injury, and histopathological analysis. Our results declared that DOX statistically reduced HR and caused alterations in ECG waves, including prolonged QRS duration and QT interval, as well as elevated ST segment amplitude. The reduction in HR was consistent with Prathumsap, Ongnok [38], who attributed the bradycardia to sinoatrial node dysfunction and disruptions in cardiac conduction caused by cell death and oxidative stress. However, Ammar, Said [39] found a contradictory result and reported an increase in HR shortly after DOX treatment, likely as a reflex to acute cardiomyopathy from a higher DOX dose (15 mg/kg, i.p.). The observed prolongation of the QRS duration and QT interval was in line with Sheibani, Nezamoleslami [40] and Sobhy, Ismail [41], suggesting that DOX-induced significant heart damage led to these abnormalities. Additionally, the elevated ST segment, a key marker of cardiomyocyte membrane damage, further confirmed the extent of cardiac injury. This was supported by the increased levels of cardiac enzymes, oxidative stress, and histopathological findings, all of which indicate underlying membrane damage and highlight the severity of DOX-induced cardiotoxicity.

The present study demonstrated that both GSE and L-CA exhibit cardioprotective effects against DOX-induced ECG abnormalities and help protect cell membranes from damage. Ammar, Said [39] suggested that GSE stabilizes cell membranes by limiting the interaction of lipid peroxyl radicals with nearby membrane polyunsaturated fatty acids, thus impeding the propagation phase of lipid peroxidation. Similarly, Mustafa, Hegazy [42] reported that L-CA's antioxidant properties reduce oxidative stress and promote membrane stabilization in cardiomyocytes. The active ingredients of GSE such as catechin may be incriminated in such effects, and ECG improvement as previously reported by Schön, Allegrini [43]. The protective effects of GSE were further supported by the decline in cardiac enzyme levels, improvements in oxidative status, and the restoration of both the functional and structural integrity of the myocardium.

In the DOX group, our study found significantly high levels of VLDL-C, TG, LDL-C, and TC with a significant decline in HDL-C. Similar findings were reported by Al-Sowayan [44] and Sobhy, Ismail [41]. According to Boghdady [45], DOX-induced hyperlipidemia is likely linked to nephrotic syndrome, which results from DOX-induced glomerulonephritis. The hyperlipidemia observed in our study is an important marker of DOX-induced metabolic disruption and correlates with cardiotoxicity.

The administration of GSE and L-CA, however, resulted in significant improvements in the lipid profile, indicating their ability to mitigate the adverse effects of DOX on the lipid metabolism. Previous studies declared the anti-hyperlipidemic influence of GSE phenolic constituents such as gallic acid [46], chlorogenic acid, caffeic acid [47], syringic acid [48], and coumaric acid [49]. Phenolic compounds are known to prevent TG absorption from the gut and stimulate lipoprotein lipase activity [50]. Moreover, flavonoids such as quercetin [51], catechin [52], apigenin [53], pyro catechol [54], and methyl gallate [55] possess ani-hyperlipidemic effects. L-CA, on the parallel side, was found to reduce DOX's harmful effects on lipid levels, as supported by Meky, Haggag [56]. L-CA could perform as a burner for body fat that encourages the lipids' metabolism and declines the blood LDL-C [57]. Additionally, Martín, Giráldez [58] suggested that L-CA decreases cholesterol levels by reducing acetyl coenzyme A, a precursor for cholesterol synthesis, as free carnitine binds with acetyl coenzyme A to form acetylcarnitine.

DOX-induced oxidative stress emerged as a key factor contributing to cardiac injury, as proved by raised levels of MDA and depletion of antioxidant enzymes. These findings align with Aziz, Abd El Fattah [59]. Birari, Wagh [60] attributed this effect to the quinone and hydroquinone groups within the DOX structure facilitating the formation of semiquinone radical intermediates. These intermediates intensify oxidative stress, leading to the depletion of the body's antioxidant reserves. Sheibani, Nezamoleslami [40] further supported this mechanism, highlighting that DOX cardiotoxicity results from an imbalance between ROS and antioxidant enzyme levels. The excessive ROS generated by DOX not only disrupts this balance but also causes significant cellular damage, leading to increased lipid peroxidation and MDA formation. Ogonowski, Mikusic [61] added that DOX cardiotoxicity can be amplified under metabolic perturbations or in other health ailments that comprise cardiovascular risk factors.

Our study revealed that both GSE and L-CA significantly improved the cardiac antioxidant defense system. This protective effect is consistent with their antioxidant properties. The greatest reduction was observed with L-CA treatment, followed by GSE, which suggests their potential role in mitigating DOX-induced cardiotoxicity by enhancing the heart's antioxidant defenses.

The protective effect of GSE is attributed to the rich composition of bioactive compounds, which includes a variety of phenolic ingredients, such as chlorogenic acid, caffeic acid, syringic acid, and gallic acid as well as flavonoids such as quercetin, catechin, and apigenin, as was demonstrated in our phytochemical analysis. These findings reflect the contribution of specific polyphenols and flavonoids in the antioxidant activity of GSE. GSE exerts its antioxidant effect by stabilizing cell membranes and facilitating electron transfer in oxidation-reduction reactions, thus neutralizing reactive species. GSE's ability to inhibit enzymes such as cyclooxygenase, lipoxygenase, and phospholipase A2, as well as its metal-chelating properties, further reduce oxidative damage [62]. The high catechin content identified in our phytochemical analysis exerts protective effects on vascular endothelial cells by inhibiting NADPH oxidase, an enzyme responsible for generating ROS [63]. Previous reports confirmed the antioxidative potential of the detected GSE's ingredients on cardiomyocytes; Xu, Yang [64] displayed that apigenin could reduce cardiomyocytes' oxidative stress parameters via modulating the SIRT1 pathway. Badavi, Sadeghi [65] demonstrated that gallic acid improved the antioxidant capacity of cardiomyocytes and enhanced the cell membrane integrity of rats' myocytes after ischemic perfusion. Chlorogenic acid was found to reduce the oxidative stress induced by myocardial injury in myocardial-infarction-induced Sprague Dawley male rats [66]. Another study, by Wang, Kaur [67], revealed that caffeic acid abridged the atherosclerogenic-diet-induced oxidative damage on cardiomyocytes via MDA reduction and free radicals' chelation in rats. Synergic acid can reduce oxidative stress cardiomyopathy in diabetic rats via its antioxidant potential [67]. Coumaric acid possesses antioxidant and anti-inflammatory influences on cardiac tissue that prevent its damage [68]. Methyl gallate was found to reverse DOX-induced MDA elevations and GSH depletion via its antioxidant potential in female rats [69]. Flavonoid constituents of GSE such as quercetin were previously found to diminish DOX-induced myocardial oxidative stress and injury in male rats [70]. Catechin is another GSE flavonoid that was proven to enhance antioxidant criteria in cardiomyocytes of SOD-knocked out mice [71].

In our research, the antioxidant properties of L-CA emerged as a significant protective factor against oxidative stress. This aligns with the verdicts of Sharma, Schmidt [72], who found that L-CA is a potent antioxidant and free radicals scavenger, protecting cells from oxidative stress and mitigating mitochondrial toxicity. This protective effect is achieved not only by neutralizing free radicals but also by promoting β-oxidation, which reduces the harmful impact of free fatty acids on cells. Furthermore, Meky, Haggag [56] found that L-CA reduces hydroxyl radical production, which is a key driver of oxidative damage, particularly during the Fenton reaction. This is achieved through the chelation of iron, a critical cofactor in hydroxyl radical formation.

Moreover, L-CA can inhibit NADPH oxidase, a source of superoxide anion in cardiomyocytes that protects cardiomyocytes against DOX-induced oxidative damage [73]. These mechanisms likely contribute to the overall cardioprotective effects of L-CA observed in our study. Sayed-Ahmed, Shaarawy [74] added that L-CA protects the heart against myocardial injury induced via DOX without changing DOX antitumor potentials by suppression of palmitate oxidation [74].

In our study, the DOX group had a statistical upsurge in cardiac injury biomarkers such as CK-MB, LDH, AST, cTnI, and NT-proBNP, all of which are released from damaged cardiomyocytes and serve as sensitive indicators of DOX-induced cardiotoxicity. This increase is likely attributable to the cardiac fiber lesions observed in the histopathological analysis. These outcomes were in agreement with Sobhy, Ismail [41] and Aziz, Abd El Fattah [59]. Bin Jardan, Ansari [8] demonstrated that DOX triggers the accumulation of free radicals within cardiac tissue, leading to oxidative damage to the myocardial walls. This damage compromises the integrity of myocardial cell membranes, causing the release of cardiac enzymes into the bloodstream. However, our findings of cTnI contradict those of Botelho, Lempek [75], whose results were negative for all the tested animals. Samples from the animals that got a single dosage after 7 days of DOX injury may have had reduced detection levels and thus were declared negative.

Serum biochemical analysis provided valuable insights into the cardioprotective potential of GSE and L-CA. Our findings demonstrated that both GSE and L-CA statistically abridged the elevated serum echelons of cardiac enzymes induced by DOX. Nazima, Manoharan [76] explained that GSE achieves this by stabilizing cellular membranes and donating hydrogen from its phenolic compounds to neutralize free radicals. Similarly, Mustafa, Hegazy [42] attributed that to the lessening of oxidative stress biomarkers and the restoration of cardiomyocyte membrane integrity. Several studies confirmed that the active constituents of GSE abridged serum cardiac injury biomarkers and inflammatory markers. Gallic acid induced significant reduction in LDH and CK-MB as a result of antioxidant potential against DOX administration in male rats [10]. Chlorogenic acid induced significant amelioration of CK-MB, LDH, and cTnI in an induced myocardial ischemic injury model of 57 BL/6 mice [77]. They added that chlorogenic acid possesses an anti-inflammatory effect against myocardial injury via suppressing NLRP3 inflammasome and Neat1. The study by Zare, Rakhshan [78] showed that apigenin significantly ameliorated LDH, CK-MB, cTnI, and AST in DOX-induced-cardiac-injury male rats due to antioxidant, anti-inflammatory, and antiapoptotic potentials. Oktar, Aydın [79] showed that administration of caffeic acid significantly reduced AST, LDH, MPO, and CK in the myocardial- injury rat model.

Synergic acid [80] and coumaric acid [81] induced antioxidant and anti-lipid peroxidation influence in myocardial-infarction-induced adult male rats that resulted in CK-MB, LDH, and AST reduction. Sharma, Parikh [82] demonstrated that quercetin ameliorated the DOX-induced cardiac toxicity, which statistically changed the cardiac biomarkers and improved myocardial histology. Ahmed, Satyam [69] demonstrated that methyl gallate reduced CK-MB, LDH, AST, MDA, and GSH levels in DOX-induced cardiotoxicity female Wistar rats with amelioration of DOX-induced ECG changes. Moreover, Aziz, Abd El Fattah [59] claimed the L-CA antioxidant potential for the reduction in cardiomyocytes damage and leakage of their enzymes into blood, whereas oxidative stress plays a central role in cardiomyocyte damage.

The significant upregulation of inflammatory markers, including IL-1β, TNF-α, MPO, and NF-Kß, in the DOX-treated group suggests an inflammatory response to oxidative damage. This aligns with the results of Aziz, Abd El Fattah [59]. Sadek, Mahmoud [83] explained that oxidative stress caused by DOX-induced cardiac injury results in endothelial cell damage, leading to leukocytes infiltration and the release of pro-inflammatory cytokines.

GSE and L-CA demonstrated protective effects by significantly reducing the levels of these markers in sera as matched with the DOX-intoxicated group. This suggests that both GSE and L-CA possess anti-inflammatory properties, but L-CA exhibited a more pronounced effect. The study's findings showed that, in comparison to the intoxicated group, pre-treatment with GSE and L-CA caused a substantial drop in the serum echelons of TNF-α, MPO, NF-Kß, and IL-1β. These findings align with Zhou, Li [11], who demonstrated that grape-derived compounds are highly effective in reducing inflammation by inhibiting pro-inflammatory cytokine release and regulating associated signaling pathways. Feringa, Laskey [84] also demonstrated that flavonoids in GSE inhibit the lipoxygenase pathways responsible for generating pro-inflammatory leukotrienes, and help balance cytokine patterns, thus offering anti-inflammatory effects. Regarding L-CA anti-inflammatory action, Fallah and Mahdavi [85] and Aziz, Abd El Fattah [59] suggested that L-CA's anti-inflammatory effects are primarily mediated by its ability to reduce ROS production, which in turn inhibits pro-inflammatory signaling, particularly the NF-Kß-mediated pathway.

The histopathological analysis provided visual confirmation of the biochemical and ECG findings, revealing significant structural damage in the DOX-treated hearts, including myofibrillar degeneration, myocardial atrophy, and infiltration of inflammatory cells. These results are in line with the oxidative stress-induced damage reported by Aziz, Abd El Fattah [59] and Sadek, Mahmoud [83]. Sheibani, Nezamoleslami [40] showed that there was a correlation between the increase in CK-MB in blood, a diagnostic marker with a high predictive value for myocardial damage, and substantial heart histopathology damage. The DOX-induced cardiomyocyte damage could be attributed to DOX triggering to catecholamine release, which promotes p53-release and macrophages-dependent mitochondrial apoptosis [86]. In addition, DOX accumulates in the mitochondria and extinguishes the mitochondrial electron chain, which provokes ROS production [7]. Moreover, DOX induces BAX production that leads to both apoptosis and necrosis of myocardial cells [87], therefore leaking their enzymes into circulation and causing histopathological damage.

The observed increase in collagen fiber deposition and interstitial fibrosis further supports the role of oxidative stress in promoting fibroblast proliferation. This aligns with Mustafa, Hegazy [42], who reported that cardiac stress promotes the proliferation of myofibroblasts, which are α-SMA positive and play a crucial part in the progression of fibrosis, causing the structural changes noticed in DOX-induced cardiac injury.

Pretreatment with GSE and L-CA resulted in marked histological improvements, with a significant reduction in myofibrillar damage, edema, and inflammation. Al-Sowayan [44] suggested that GSE's phenolic compounds, particularly catechins and proanthocyanidins, have been shown to enhance endogenous antioxidant defenses and prevent apoptosis, thus preserving cardiac tissue integrity. Moreover, GSE catechin and polyphenols were found to abridge DOX-induced cardiac damage by decreasing the cohort of ROS and the number of apoptotic cells, regulating the expression levels of the antiapoptotic protein Bcl-2 and the proapoptotic protein Bax α, impeding apoptotic signaling trails and averting DNA fragmentation [88]. Similarly, Tousson, Hafez [19] highlighted that L-CA and its derivatives are potent free radical scavengers, effectively reducing ROS production and protecting cells from oxidative stress. L-CA might provoke prostacyclin production, which is crucial for the anti-apoptotic effect that preserves cardiomyocytes against DOX damage [73]. This ability to preserve heart muscle structure and improve overall cardiac function further emphasizes the cardioprotective properties of both GSE and L-CA.

While GSE and L-CA mitigated DOX-induced myocardial damage, the degree of protection appeared to differ between the two. The group pretreated with L-CA showed a more marked reduction in collagen fiber deposition and fibrosis compared to the group pretreated with GSE. According to Mustafa, Hegazy [42], this superior effect of L-CA may be attributed to its capability to hinder the transformation of fibroblasts into myofibroblasts, thereby limiting collagen deposition and the progression of cardiac fibrosis.

These histopathological improvements align with the reductions in biochemical markers of oxidative stress and inflammation, suggesting that both GSE and L-CA effectively attenuate DOX-induced cardiotoxicity through a combination of antioxidant, anti-inflammatory, and membrane-stabilizing mechanisms.

## 5. Conclusions

Doxorubicin exerts cardiotoxic effects, as evidenced by ECG abnormalities, increasing oxidative stress, altered lipid profiles, elevated cardiac biomarkers, inflammation, and cardiac tissue damage. These impacts were effectively ameliorated via GSE and L-CA. Their cardioprotective effects were due to their antioxidant and anti-inflammatory possessions that improve cardiac biomarkers in sera.

**Author Contributions:** Conceptualization, O.E.K., D.E.O. and O.A.; methodology, D.E.O., H.M.A.A., H.N.G.E.-H. and O.A.; software, T.S.A., D.E.O., O.E.K., H.M.A.A. and H.N.G.E.-H.; validation, D.E.O., O.E.K., T.S.A. and O.A.; formal analysis, D.E.O.; investigation, T.S.A., D.E.O. and O.E.K.; resources, T.S.A., D.E.O., H.N.G.E.-H. and H.M.A.A.; data curation, T.S.A., D.E.O. and O.E.K.; writing—original draft preparation, D.E.O. and H.N.G.E.-H.; writing—review and editing, O.A., O.E.K., T.S.A. and H.M.A.A.; visualization, T.S.A.; supervision, O.A. and O.E.K.; project administration, T.S.A.; funding acquisition, D.E.O. and O.E.K. All authors have read and agreed to the published version of the manuscript.

**Funding:** This study was funded by the Princess Nourah bint Abdulrahman University Researchers Supporting Project, number PNURSP2024R74, Princess Nourah bint Abdulrahman University, Riyadh, Saudi Arabia.

**Institutional Review Board Statement:** The study was conducted in accordance with the Declaration of Helsinki, and approved by the Institutional Review Board of the Faculty of Veterinary Medicine, Suez Canal University (protocol code 2022013 approved on 22 August 2022).

**Informed Consent Statement:** Not applicable.

**Data Availability Statement:** The data presented in this study are available in the article.

**Acknowledgments:** The authors would like to acknowledge Princess Nourah bint Abdulrahman University Researchers Supporting Project for granting Project number (PNURSP2024R74), Princess Nourah bint Abdulrahman University, Riyadh, Saudi Arabia. And the statistical assistance done by Marwa A. Hassan, Department of Veterinary Public Health, Faculty of Veterinary Medicine, Suez Canal University.

**Conflicts of Interest:** The authors declare no conflicts of interest.

## References


1. Othman, S.N.N.; Lum, P.T.; Gan, S.H.; Mani, S.; Sekar, M. Protective Effect of Natural Products against Chemotherapy-Induced Cardiotoxicity: A Review. *Pharmacogn. J.* **2020**, *12*, 1180–1189. [CrossRef]
2. Koss-Mikołajczyk, I.; Todorovic, V.; Sobajic, S.; Mahajna, J.; Gerić, M.; Tur, J.A.; Bartoszek, A. Natural Products Counteracting Cardiotoxicity during Cancer Chemotherapy: The Special Case of Doxorubicin, a Comprehensive Review. *Int. J. Mol. Sci.* **2021**, *22*, 10037. [CrossRef]
3. Murabito, A.; Hirsch, E.; Ghigo, A. Mechanisms of anthracycline-induced cardiotoxicity: Is mitochondrial dysfunction the answer? *Front. Cardiovasc. Med.* **2020**, *7*, 35. [CrossRef]
4. Rawat, P.S.; Jaiswal, A.; Khurana, A.; Bhatti, J.S.; Navik, U. Doxorubicin-induced cardiotoxicity: An update on the molecular mechanism and novel therapeutic strategies for effective management. *Biomed. Pharmacother.* **2021**, *139*, 111708. [CrossRef] [PubMed]
5. Sheibani, M.; Azizi, Y.; Shayan, M.; Nezamoleslami, S.; Eslami, F.; Farjoo, M.H.; Dehpour, A.R. Doxorubicin-Induced Cardiotoxicity: An Overview on Pre-clinical Therapeutic Approaches. *Cardiovasc. Toxicol.* **2022**, *22*, 292–310. [CrossRef]
6. Ahmed, A.Z.; Mumbrekar, K.D.; Satyam, S.M.; Shetty, P.; D'souza, M.R.; Singh, V.K. Chia Seed Oil Ameliorates Doxorubicin-Induced Cardiotoxicity in Female Wistar Rats: An Electrocardiographic, Biochemical and Histopathological Approach. *Cardiovasc. Toxicol.* **2021**, *21*, 533–542. [CrossRef]
7. Sergazy, S.; Shulgau, Z.; Fedotovskikh, G.; Chulenbayeva, L.; Nurgozhina, A.; Nurgaziyev, M.; Krivyh, E.; Kamyshanskiy, Y.; Kushugulova, A.; Gulyayev, A.; et al. Cardioprotective effect of grape polyphenol extract against doxorubicin induced cardiotoxicity. *Sci. Rep.* **2020**, *10*, 14720. [CrossRef]
8. Bin Jardan, Y.A.; Ansari, M.A.; Raish, M.; Alkharfy, K.M.; Al-Jenoobi, F.I.; Haq, N.; Ahmad, A. Sinapic acid ameliorates oxidative stress, inflammation, and apoptosis in acute doxorubicin-induced cardiotoxicity via the NF-κB-mediated pathway. *BioMed Res. Int.* **2020**, *2020*, 3921796. [CrossRef] [PubMed]
9. Adıyaman, M.; Adıyaman, A.; Dağlı, A.F.; Karahan, M.Z.; Kaya, I.; Dağlı, M.N. Effects of grapeseed extract on doxorubicin-induced cardiotoxicity in rats. *Herz* **2021**, *46*, 103–108. [CrossRef]
10. Swamy, A.H.M.V.; Kulkarni, J. Cardioprotective effect of gallic acid against doxorubicin-induced myocardial toxicity in albino rats. *Indian J. Health Sci. Biomed. Res.* **2015**, *8*, 28. [CrossRef]
11. Zhou, D.-D.; Li, J.; Xiong, R.-G.; Saimaiti, A.; Huang, S.-Y.; Wu, S.-X.; Yang, Z.-J.; Shang, A.; Zhao, C.-N.; Gan, R.-Y.; et al. Bioactive Compounds, Health Benefits and Food Applications of Grape. *Foods* **2022**, *11*, 2755. [CrossRef] [PubMed]
12. Koneru, M.; Nalban, N.; Sahu, B.D.; Sistla, R. Natural products against drug-induced cardiotoxicity. In *Cardioprotective Natural Products: Promises and Hopes*; World Scientific: Singapore, 2018; pp. 121–147.
13. Bene, J.; Szabo, A.; Komlósi, K.; Melegh, B. Mass Spectrometric Analysis of L-Carnitine and its Esters: Potential Biomarkers of Disturbances in Carnitine Homeostasis. *Curr. Mol. Med.* **2020**, *20*, 336–354. [CrossRef]
14. Caballero-García, A.; Noriega-González, D.C.; Roche, E.; Drobnic, F.; Córdova, A. Effects of L-Carnitine Intake on Exercise-Induced Muscle Damage and Oxidative Stress: A Narrative Scoping Review. *Nutrients* **2023**, *15*, 2587. [CrossRef] [PubMed]
15. Abdel-Emam, R.A.; Ahmed, E.A. Ameliorative effect of L-carnitine on chronic lead-induced reproductive toxicity in male rats. *Veter. Med. Sci.* **2021**, *7*, 1426–1435. [CrossRef]
16. Mielgo-Ayuso, J.; Pietrantonio, L.; Viribay, A.; Calleja-González, J.; González-Bernal, J.; Fernández-Lázaro, D. Effect of acute and chronic oral l-Carnitine supplementation on exercise performance based on the exercise intensity: A systematic review. *Nutrients* **2021**, *13*, 4359. [CrossRef] [PubMed]
17. Sawicka, A.K.; Renzi, G.; Olek, R.A. The bright and the dark sides of L-carnitine supplementation: A systematic review. *J. Int. Soc. Sports Nutr.* **2020**, *17*, 49. [CrossRef]
18. Nassiri-Asl, M.; Hosseinzadeh, H. Review of the Pharmacological Effects of Vitis vinifera (Grape) and its Bioactive Constituents: An Update: Pharmacological Effects of Grape. *Phytother. Res.* **2016**, *30*, 1392–1403. [CrossRef]
19. Tousson, E.; Hafez, E.; Zaki, S.; Gad, A. The cardioprotective effects of L-carnitine on rat cardiac injury, apoptosis, and oxidative stress caused by amethopterin. *Environ. Sci. Pollut. Res.* **2016**, *23*, 20600–20608. [CrossRef] [PubMed]
20. Lu, T.-S.; Yiao, S.-Y.; Lim, K.; Jensen, R.V.; Hsiao, L.-L. Interpretation of biological and mechanical variations between the Lowry versus Bradford method for protein quantification. *N. Am. J. Med. Sci.* **2010**, *2*, 325–328. [PubMed]
21. Menezes, F.G.; Neves, A.C.; De Lima, D.F.; Lourenço, S.D.; Da Silva, L.C.; De Lima, K.M.G. Bioorganic concepts involved in the determination of glucose, cholesterol and triglycerides in plasma using the enzymatic colorimetric method. *Quím. Nova* **2015**, *38*, 588–594. [CrossRef]
22. Li, L.-H.; Dutkiewicz, E.P.; Huang, Y.-C.; Zhou, H.-B.; Hsu, C.-C. Analytical methods for cholesterol quantification. *J. Food Drug Anal.* **2019**, *27*, 375–386. [CrossRef] [PubMed]
23. Portela, R.D.P.; Neto, E.M.R.; Junior, F.J.G.; Ferreira, J.M.; Alves, R.d.S.; Carvalho, T.M.d.J.P.; Holanda, B.A.P. Comparative Analysis of Two Methodologies for Determination of HDL Cholesterol. *J. Young Pharm.* **2018**, *10*, 308. [CrossRef]
24. Obasi, D.C.; Ogugua, V.N. Effect of Ruzu Herbal Bitters on the Liver Function and Lipid Profile Parameters of Alloxan-Induced Diabetic Rats. *J. Clin. Exp. Hepatol.* **2024**, *14*, 100929. [CrossRef] [PubMed]
25. Katerji, M.; Filippova, M.; Duerksen-Hughes, P. Approaches and Methods to Measure Oxidative Stress in Clinical Samples: Research Applications in the Cancer Field. *Oxid. Med. Cell. Longev.* **2019**, *2019*, 1279250. [CrossRef]

26. Diniz, B.S.; Mendes-Silva, A.P.; Silva, L.B.; Bertola, L.; Vieira, M.C.; Ferreira, J.D.; Nicolau, M.; Bristot, G.; da Rosa, E.D.; Teixeira, A.L.; et al. Oxidative stress markers imbalance in late-life depression. *J. Psychiatr. Res.* **2018**, *102*, 29–33. [CrossRef] [PubMed]
27. Li, Y.; Tang, T.; Lee, H.; Song, K. Cold Atmospheric Pressure Plasma-Activated Medium Induces Selective Cell Death in Human Hepatocellular Carcinoma Cells Independently of Singlet Oxygen, Hydrogen Peroxide, Nitric Oxide and Nitrite/Nitrate. *Int. J. Mol. Sci.* **2021**, *22*, 5548. [CrossRef]
28. Rowicka, G.; Czaja-Bulsa, G.; Chełchowska, M.; Riahi, A.; Strucińska, M.; Weker, H.; Ambroszkiewicz, J. Oxidative and Antioxidative Status of Children with Celiac Disease Treated with a Gluten Free-Diet. *Oxidative Med. Cell. Longev.* **2018**, *2018*, 1324820. [CrossRef] [PubMed]
29. Cao, G.; Alessio, H.M.; Cutler, R.G. Oxygen-radical absorbance capacity assay for antioxidants. *Free Radic. Biol. Med.* **1993**, *14*, 303–311. [CrossRef] [PubMed]
30. Flohé, L.; Günzler, W.A. Assays of glutathione peroxidase. *Methods Enzymol.* **1984**, *105*, 114–121. [CrossRef] [PubMed]
31. Vanderthommen, M.; Chamayou, R.; Demoulin, C.; Crielaard, J.-M.; Croisier, J.-L. Protection against muscle damage induced by electrical stimulation: Efficiency of a preconditioning programme. *Clin. Physiol. Funct. Imaging* **2015**, *35*, 267–274. [CrossRef]
32. Tuncelli, G.; Tuncelli, I.C.; Dagsuyu, E.; Turkyilmaz, I.B.; Yanardag, R.; Erkan, N. The effect of different types of microplastic and acute cadmium exposure on the Mytilus galloprovincialis (Lamarck, 1819). *Sci. Total Environ.* **2024**, *936*, 173505. [CrossRef] [PubMed]
33. Alshehri, A.A.; Younes, N.M.; Kamel, R.; Shawir, S.M. Characterization and potential health benefits of millet flour and banana peel mixtures on rats fed with a high-fat diet. *Heliyon* **2024**, *10*, e39424. [CrossRef]
34. Abukhalil, M.H.; Althunibat, O.Y.; Aladaileh, S.H.; Al-Amarat, W.; Obeidat, H.M.; Al-Khawalde, A.A.-M.A.; Hussein, O.E.; Alfwuaires, M.A.; Algefare, A.I.; Alanazi, K.M.; et al. Galangin attenuates diabetic cardiomyopathy through modulating oxidative stress, inflammation and apoptosis in rats. *Biomed. Pharmacother.* **2021**, *138*, 111410. [CrossRef] [PubMed]
35. Giuliani, I.; Rieunier, F.; Larue, C.; Delagneau, J.-F.; Granier, C.; Pau, B.; Ferriere, M.; Saussine, M.; Cristol, J.-P.; Dupuy, A.-M.; et al. Assay for Measurement of Intact B-Type Natriuretic Peptide Prohormone in Blood. *Clin. Chem.* **2006**, *52*, 1054–1061. [CrossRef] [PubMed]
36. Bancroft, J.D.; Cook, H.C.; Stirling, R.W. *Manual of Histological Techniques and Their Diagnostic Application*; Churchill Livingstone: New York, NY, USA, 1994; p. 457.
37. Zhang, J.; Cui, L.; Han, X.; Zhang, Y.; Zhang, X.; Chu, X.; Zhang, F.; Zhang, Y.; Chu, L. Protective effects of tannic acid on acute doxorubicin-induced cardiotoxicity: Involvement of suppression in oxidative stress, inflammation, and apoptosis. *Biomed. Pharmacother.* **2017**, *93*, 1253–1260. [CrossRef]
38. Prathumsap, N.; Ongnok, B.; Khuanjing, T.; Arinno, A.; Maneechote, C.; Apaijai, N.; Chunchai, T.; Arunsak, B.; Kerdphoo, S.; Janjek, S.; et al. Vagus nerve stimulation exerts cardioprotection against doxorubicin-induced cardiotoxicity through inhibition of programmed cell death pathways. *Cell. Mol. Life Sci.* **2023**, *80*, 21. [CrossRef]
39. Ammar, E.-S.M.; Said, S.A.; El-Damarawy, S.L.; Suddek, G.M. Cardioprotective effect of grape-seed proanthocyanidins on doxorubicin-induced cardiac toxicity in rats. *Pharm. Biol.* **2013**, *51*, 339–344. [CrossRef] [PubMed]
40. Sheibani, M.; Nezamoleslami, S.; Faghir-Ghanesefat, H.; Emami, A.H.; Dehpour, A.R. Cardioprotective effects of dapsone against doxorubicin-induced cardiotoxicity in rats. *Cancer Chemother. Pharmacol.* **2020**, *85*, 563–571. [CrossRef] [PubMed]
41. Sobhy, M.H.; Ismail, A.; Abdel-Hamid, M.S.; Wagih, M.; Kamel, M. 2-Methoxyestradiol ameliorates doxorubicin-induced cardiotoxicity by regulating the expression of GLUT4 and CPT-1B in female rats. *Naunyn-Schmiedeberg's Arch. Pharmacol.* **2024**, *397*, 7129–7139. [CrossRef] [PubMed]
42. Mustafa, H.N.; Hegazy, G.A.; El Awdan, S.A.; AbdelBaset, M. Protective role of CoQ10 or L-carnitine on the integrity of the myocardium in doxorubicin induced toxicity. *Tissue Cell* **2017**, *49*, 410–426. [CrossRef]
43. Schön, C.; Allegrini, P.; Engelhart-Jentzsch, K.; Riva, A.; Petrangolini, G. Grape Seed Extract Positively Modulates Blood Pressure and Perceived Stress: A Randomized, Double-Blind, Placebo-Controlled Study in Healthy Volunteers. *Nutrients* **2021**, *13*, 654. [CrossRef] [PubMed]
44. Al-Sowayan, N.S. Antioxidant potential of grape seed extract and vitamin E in ameliorating doxorubicin-induced cardiotoxicity in rat. *Pensee* **2014**, *76*, 355–368.
45. Boghdady, N.A. Antioxidant and antiapoptotic effects of proanthocyanidin and ginkgo biloba extract against doxorubicin-induced cardiac injury in rats. *Cell Biochem. Funct.* **2013**, *31*, 344–351. [CrossRef]
46. Shaik, A.H.; Shaik, S.R.; Daddam, J.R.; Ali, D.; Manoharadas, S.; Arafah, M.W.; Kodidhela, L.D. Maslinic acid and gallic acid protective efficacy on lipids, lipoproteins and lipid metabolizing enzymes against isoproterenol administered cardiotoxicity: An in vivo and in silico molecular docking evidences. *J. King Saud Univ. Sci.* **2021**, *33*, 101230. [CrossRef]
47. Agunloye, O.M.; Oboh, G. High cholesterol diet promotes dysfunction of arginase and cholinergic enzymatic system in rats: Ameliorative role of caffeic and chlorogenic acids. *J. Complement. Integr. Med.* **2021**, *18*, 67–74. [CrossRef]
48. Somade, O.T.; Oyinloye, B.E.; Ajiboye, B.O.; Osukoya, O.A. Syringic acid through reduction of inflammation, oxidative injury, and downregulation of NF-κB-IL-6 pathway ameliorates HFD-induced pulmonary toxicity in male Wistar rats. *Comp. Clin. Pathol.* **2024**, 787–802.
49. Yuan, Z.; Lu, X.; Lei, F.; Sun, H.; Jiang, J.; Xing, D.; Du, L. Novel Effect of *p*-Coumaric Acid on Hepatic Lipolysis: Inhibition of Hepatic Lipid-Droplets. *Molecules* **2023**, *28*, 4641. [CrossRef] [PubMed]

50. Hasona, N.; Morsi, A. Grape Seed Extract Alleviates Dexamethasone-Induced Hyperlipidemia, Lipid Peroxidation, and Hematological Alteration in Rats. *Indian J. Clin. Biochem.* **2019**, *34*, 213–218. [CrossRef]
51. Rahmani, A.H.; Alsahli, M.A.; Khan, A.A.; Almatroodi, S.A. Quercetin, a Plant Flavonol Attenuates Diabetic Complications, Renal Tissue Damage, Renal Oxidative Stress and Inflammation in Streptozotocin-Induced Diabetic Rats. *Metabolites* **2023**, *13*, 130. [CrossRef] [PubMed]
52. Albedi, N.; Talib, R.H. The Influence of Catechin on Adiponectin and Insulin Resistance in Obese Rats. *Kufa J. Veter Med. Sci.* **2024**, *15*, 34–42. [CrossRef]
53. Aldayel, T.S. Apigenin attenuates high-fat diet-induced nephropathy in rats by hypoglycemic and hypolipidemic effects, and concomitant activation of the Nrf2/antioxidant axis. *J. Funct. Foods* **2022**, *99*, 105295. [CrossRef]
54. Ochalefu, D.O.; Adoga, G.I.; Luka, C.D.; Abu, A.H. Effects of Catechol containing fraction and other fractions of Nauclea latifolia aqueous root-bark extract on blood glucose, lipid profile and serum liver enzymes in streptozotocin–induced diabetic Wistar albino rats. *J. Stress Physiol. Biochem.* **2024**, *20*, 79–91.
55. Abdel-Hamed, A.R.; Mehanna, E.T.; Hazem, R.M.; Badr, J.M.; Abo-Elmatty, D.M.; Abdel-Kader, M.S.; Goda, M.S. *Plicosepalus acacia* Extract and Its Major Constituents, Methyl Gallate and Quercetin, Potentiate Therapeutic Angiogenesis in Diabetic Hind Limb Ischemia: HPTLC Quantification and LC-MS/MS Metabolic Profiling. *Antioxidants* **2021**, *10*, 1701. [CrossRef] [PubMed]
56. Meky, N.H.; Haggag, A.M.; Kamal, A.M.; Ahmed, Z.A. The Protective Effect of L-carnitine against Gamma Irradiation- Induced Cardiotoxicity in Male Albino Rats. *Egypt. Acad. J. Biol. Sci. C Physiol. Mol. Biol.* **2017**, *9*, 9–20. [CrossRef]
57. Huang, H.; Song, L.; Zhang, H.; Zhang, H.; Zhang, J.; Zhao, W. Influence of L-Carnitine Supplementation on Serum Lipid Profile in Hemodialysis Patients: A Systematic Review and Meta-Analysis. *Kidney Blood Press. Res.* **2014**, *38*, 31–41. [CrossRef] [PubMed]
58. Martín, A.; Giráldez, F.J.; Cremonesi, P.; Castiglioni, B.; Biscarini, F.; Ceciliani, F.; Santos, N.; Andrés, S. Dietary Administration of L-Carnitine During the Fattening Period of Early Feed Restricted Lambs Modifies Ruminal Fermentation but Does Not Improve Feed Efficiency. *Front. Physiol.* **2022**, *13*, 840065. [CrossRef]
59. Aziz, M.M.; Abd El Fattah, M.A.; Ahmed, K.A.; Sayed, H.M. Protective effects of olmesartan and l-carnitine on doxorubicin-induced cardiotoxicity in rats. *Can. J. Physiol. Pharmacol.* **2020**, *98*, 183–193. [CrossRef] [PubMed]
60. Birari, L.; Wagh, S.; Patil, K.R.; Mahajan, U.B.; Unger, B.; Belemkar, S.; Goyal, S.N.; Ojha, S.; Patil, C.R. Aloin alleviates doxorubicin-induced cardiotoxicity in rats by abrogating oxidative stress and pro-inflammatory cytokines. *Cancer Chemother. Pharmacol.* **2020**, *86*, 419–426. [CrossRef] [PubMed]
61. Ogonowski, N.; Mikusic, N.L.R.; Kouyoumdzian, N.M.; Choi, M.R.; Fellet, A.; Balaszczuk, A.M.; Celuch, S.M. Cardiotoxic Effects of the Antineoplastic Doxorubicin in a Model of Metabolic Syndrome: Oxidative Stress and Transporter Expression in the Heart. *J. Cardiovasc. Pharmacol.* **2021**, *78*, 784–791. [CrossRef]
62. Magrone, T.; Magrone, M.; Russo, M.A.; Jirillo, E. Recent Advances on the Anti-Inflammatory and Antioxidant Properties of Red Grape Polyphenols: In Vitro and In Vivo Studies. *Antioxidants* **2019**, *9*, 35. [CrossRef]
63. Sheng, Y.; Sun, Y.; Tang, Y.; Yu, Y.; Wang, J.; Zheng, F.; Li, Y.; Sun, Y. Catechins: Protective mechanism of antioxidant stress in atherosclerosis. *Front. Pharmacol.* **2023**, *14*, 1144878. [CrossRef]
64. Xu, K.; Yang, Y.; Lan, M.; Wang, J.; Liu, B.; Yan, M.; Wang, H.; Li, W.; Sun, S.; Zhu, K.; et al. Apigenin alleviates oxidative stress-induced myocardial injury by regulating SIRT1 signaling pathway. *Eur. J. Pharmacol.* **2023**, *944*, 175584. [CrossRef] [PubMed]
65. Badavi, M.; Sadeghi, N.; Dianat, M.; Samarbafzadeh, A. Effects of Gallic Acid and Cyclosporine A on Antioxidant Capacity and Cardiac Markers of Rat Isolated Heart After Ischemia/Reperfusion. *Iran. Red Crescent Med. J.* **2014**, *16*, e16424. [CrossRef] [PubMed]
66. Wang, D.; Tian, L.; Lv, H.; Pang, Z.; Li, D.; Yao, Z.; Wang, S. Chlorogenic acid prevents acute myocardial infarction in rats by reducing inflammatory damage and oxidative stress. *Biomed. Pharmacother.* **2020**, *132*, 110773. [CrossRef] [PubMed]
67. Wang, Y.; Kaur, G.; Kumar, M.; Kushwah, A.S.; Kabra, A.; Kainth, R. Caffeic Acid Prevents Vascular Oxidative Stress and Atherosclerosis against Atherosclerogenic Diet in Rats. *Evid. Based Complement. Altern. Med.* **2022**, *2022*, 8913926. [CrossRef] [PubMed]
68. Kheiry, M.; Dianat, M.; Badavi, M.; Mard, S.A.; Bayati, V. Does p-coumaric acid improve cardiac injury following LPS-induced lung inflammation through miRNA-146a activity? *Avicenna J. Phytomed.* **2020**, *10*, 50–57. [PubMed]
69. Ahmed, A.Z.; Satyam, S.M.; Shetty, P.; D'souza, M.R. Methyl Gallate Attenuates Doxorubicin-Induced Cardiotoxicity in Rats by Suppressing Oxidative Stress. *Scientifica* **2021**, *2021*, 6694340. [CrossRef] [PubMed]
70. Dulf, P.L.; Coadă, C.A.; Florea, A.; Moldovan, R.; Baldea, I.; Dulf, D.V.; Blendea, D.; Filip, A.G. Mitigating Doxorubicin-Induced Cardiotoxicity through Quercetin Intervention: An Experimental Study in Rats. *Antioxidants* **2024**, *13*, 1068. [CrossRef] [PubMed]
71. Oyama, J.-I.; Shiraki, A.; Nishikido, T.; Maeda, T.; Komoda, H.; Shimizu, T.; Makino, N.; Node, K. EGCG, a green tea catechin, attenuates the progression of heart failure induced by the heart/muscle-specific deletion of MnSOD in mice. *J. Cardiol.* **2017**, *69*, 417–427. [CrossRef]
72. Sharma, B.; Schmidt, L.; Nguyen, C.; Kiernan, S.; Dexter-Meldrum, J.; Kuschner, Z.; Ellis, S.; Bhatia, N.D.; Agriantonis, G.; Whittington, J.; et al. The Effect of L-Carnitine on Critical Illnesses Such as Traumatic Brain Injury (TBI), Acute Kidney Injury (AKI), and Hyperammonemia (HA). *Metabolites* **2024**, *14*, 363. [CrossRef]
73. Chao, H.-H.; Liu, J.-C.; Hong, H.-J.; Lin, J.-W.; Chen, C.-H.; Cheng, T.-H. L-carnitine reduces doxorubicin-induced apoptosis through a prostacyclin-mediated pathway in neonatal rat cardiomyocytes. *Int. J. Cardiol.* **2011**, *146*, 145–152. [CrossRef]

74. Sayed-Ahmed, M.M.; Shaarawy, S.; Shouman, S.A.; Osman, A.M. Reversal of doxorubicin-induced cardiac metabolic damage by L-carnitine. *Pharmacol. Res.* **1999**, *39*, 289–295. [CrossRef] [PubMed]
75. Botelho, A.F.M.; Lempek, M.R.; Branco, S.E.M.T.; Nogueira, M.M.; de Almeida, M.E.; Costa, A.G.; Freitas, T.G.; Rocha, M.C.R.C.; Moreira, M.V.L.; Barreto, T.O.; et al. Coenzyme Q10 Cardioprotective Effects Against Doxorubicin-Induced Cardiotoxicity in Wistar Rat. *Cardiovasc. Toxicol.* **2020**, *20*, 222–234. [CrossRef]
76. Nazima, B.; Manoharan; Miltonprabu, S. Oxidative stress induced by cadmium in the plasma, erythrocytes and lymphocytes of rats: Attenuation by grape seed proanthocyanidins. *Hum. Exp. Toxicol.* **2016**, *35*, 428–447. [CrossRef] [PubMed]
77. Chai, X.; Liang, Z.; Zhang, J.; Ding, J.; Zhang, Q.; Lv, S.; Deng, Y.; Zhang, R.; Lu, D. Chlorogenic acid protects against myocardial ischemia-reperfusion injury in mice by inhibiting Lnc Neat1/NLRP3 inflammasome-mediated pyroptosis. *Sci. Rep.* **2023**, *13*, 17803. [CrossRef]
78. Zare, M.F.R.; Rakhshan, K.; Aboutaleb, N.; Nikbakht, F.; Naderi, N.; Bakhshesh, M.; Azizi, Y. Apigenin attenuates doxorubicin induced cardiotoxicity via reducing oxidative stress and apoptosis in male rats. *Life Sci.* **2019**, *232*, 116623. [CrossRef] [PubMed]
79. Oktar, S.; Aydin, M.; Yonden, Z.; Alcin, E.; Ilhan, S.; Nacar, A. Effects of caffeic acid phenethyl ester on isoproterenol-induced myocardial infarction in rats. *Anadolu Kardiyol. Derg.* **2010**, *10*, 298–302. [CrossRef] [PubMed]
80. Shahzad, S.; Mateen, S.; Naeem, S.S.; Akhtar, K.; Rizvi, W.; Moin, S. Syringic acid protects from isoproterenol induced cardiotoxicity in rats. *Eur. J. Pharmacol.* **2019**, *849*, 135–145. [CrossRef]
81. Prince, P.S.M.; Roy, A.J. p-Coumaric acid attenuates apoptosis in isoproterenol-induced myocardial infarcted rats by inhibiting oxidative stress. *Int. J. Cardiol.* **2013**, *168*, 3259–3266. [CrossRef] [PubMed]
82. Sharma, A.; Parikh, M.; Shah, H.; Gandhi, T. Modulation of Nrf2 by quercetin in doxorubicin-treated rats. *Heliyon* **2020**, *6*, e03803. [CrossRef] [PubMed]
83. Sadek, K.M.; Mahmoud, S.F.E.; Zeweil, M.F.; Abouzed, T.K. Proanthocyanidin alleviates doxorubicin-induced cardiac injury by inhibiting NF-kB pathway and modulating oxidative stress, cell cycle, and fibrogenesis. *J. Biochem. Mol. Toxicol.* **2021**, *35*, e22716. [CrossRef] [PubMed]
84. Feringa, H.H.; Laskey, D.A.; Dickson, J.E.; Coleman, C.I. The Effect of Grape Seed Extract on Cardiovascular Risk Markers: A Meta-Analysis of Randomized Controlled Trials. *J. Am. Diet. Assoc.* **2011**, *111*, 1173–1181. [CrossRef] [PubMed]
85. Fallah, F.; Mahdavi, R. L-Carnitine and synbiotic co-supplementation: Beneficial effects on metabolic-endotoxemia, meta-inflammation, and oxidative-stress biomarkers in obese patients: A double blind, randomized, controlled clinical trial. *Food Funct.* **2023**, *14*, 2172–2187. [CrossRef] [PubMed]
86. Gambardella, J.; Santulli, G.; Fiordelisi, A.; Cerasuolo, F.A.; Wang, X.; Prevete, N.; Sommella, E.; Avvisato, R.; Buonaiuto, A.; Altobelli, G.G.; et al. Infiltrating macrophages amplify doxorubicin-induced cardiac damage: Role of catecholamines. *Cell. Mol. Life Sci.* **2023**, *80*, 323. [CrossRef] [PubMed]
87. Amgalan, D.; Garner, T.P.; Pekson, R.; Jia, X.F.; Yanamandala, M.; Paulino, V.; Liang, F.G.; Corbalan, J.J.; Lee, J.; Chen, Y.; et al. A small-molecule allosteric inhibitor of BAX protects against doxorubicin-induced cardiomyopathy. *Nat. Cancer* **2020**, *1*, 315–328. [CrossRef]
88. Demirkaya, E.; Avci, A.; Kesik, V.; Karslioglu, Y.; Oztas, E.; Kismet, E.; Gokcay, E.; Durak, I.; Koseoglu, V. Cardioprotective roles of aged garlic extract, grape seed proanthocyanidin, and hazelnut on doxorubicin-induced cardiotoxicity. *Can. J. Physiol. Pharmacol.* **2009**, *87*, 633–640. [CrossRef]


**Disclaimer/Publisher's Note:** The statements, opinions and data contained in all publications are solely those of the individual author(s) and contributor(s) and not of MDPI and/or the editor(s). MDPI and/or the editor(s) disclaim responsibility for any injury to people or property resulting from any ideas, methods, instructions or products referred to in the content.

*life*

MDPI

*Article*

# The Relationship Between the Kansas City Cardiomyopathy Questionnaire and Electrocardiographic Parameters in Predicting Outcomes After Cardiac Resynchronization Therapy

**Andrei-Mihnea Rosu [1,2], Luminita-Florentina Tomescu [3], Theodor-Georgian Badea [2,3], Emanuel-Stefan Radu [1], Andreea-Liana Rosu [4], Lavinia-Nicoleta Brezeanu [5], Maria-Daniela Tanasescu [6,*], Sebastian Isac [5,7], Teodora Isac [8], Oana-Andreea Popa [1] and Crina-Julieta Sinescu [9]**

1 Department of Cardiology, Prof. Dr. Agrippa Ionescu Emergency Hospital, Balotesti, 077015 Ilfov, Romania; andrei-mihnea.rosu@drd.umfcd.ro (A.-M.R.); radu.emanuel@dcti.ro (E.-S.R.); popa.oana@dcti.ro (O.-A.P.)
2 Doctoral School, Carol Davila University of Medicine and Pharmacy, 022328 Bucharest, Romania; theodor.badea@umfcd.ro
3 Department of Radiology, Prof. Dr. Agrippa Ionescu Emergency Hospital, Balotesti, 077015 Ilfov, Romania; luminita.tomescu@umfcd.ro
4 Department of Clinical Pharmacology, BBraun, 013714 Bucharest, Romania; andreea.rosu@bbraun.com
5 Department of Anesthesiology and Intensive Care I, Fundeni Clinical Institute, 022328 Bucharest, Romania; laviniajipa11@yahoo.com (L.-N.B.); sebastian.isac@umfcd.ro (S.I.)
6 Department of Semiology, Emergency University Hospital, Carol Davila University of Medicine and Pharmacy, 022328 Bucharest, Romania
7 Department of Physiology, Carol Davila University of Medicine and Pharmacy, 022328 Bucharest, Romania
8 Department of Internal Medicine, Fundeni Clinical Institute, 022328 Bucharest, Romania; teodora.isac@umfcd.ro
9 Department of Cardiology, Bagdasar-Arseni Emergency Hospital, Carol Davila University of Medicine and Pharmacy, 022328 Bucharest, Romania; crina.sinescu@umfcd.ro
* Correspondence: maria.tanasescu@umfcd.ro; Tel.: +40-74-504-2785

**Abstract:** Background: Cardiac resynchronization therapy (CRT) is an essential treatment for patients with symptomatic heart failure and ventricular conduction abnormalities. Low-ejection-fraction (EF) cardiomyopathy often involves a wide QRS complex displaying a left bundle branch block (LBBB) morphology and markedly delayed activation of the LV lateral wall. Following CRT, patients with heart failure and LBBB have better outcomes and quality-of-life improvements. Various electrocardiographic and clinical parameters are thought to be able to predict this improvement. The Kansas City Cardiomyopathy Questionnaire (KCCQ) is a reliable tool for measuring these patients' quality of life. Methods: This is an observational prospective study featuring over 69 individuals diagnosed with cardiac failure and dilatative cardiomyopathy with low-EF and major LBBB. This study analyzed the correlations between patient outcomes and demographic, clinical, and electrocardiographic parameters. Results: Following the analysis, we observed correlations between the QRS area, intraprocedural systolic blood pressure, Q-LV interval, the R-wave amplitude in the right precordial leads and the CRT outcomes indicated by the KCCQ score. Conclusions: The parameters found and their correlation with the KCCQ score show how CRT therapy impacts patients' quality of life, symptom burden, and functional status.

**Keywords:** Kansas City Cardiomyopathy Questionnaire; cardiac resynchronization therapy; electrocardiography; cardiac ischemia; left ventricular ejection fraction; dilatative cardiomyopathy

## 1. Introduction

Cardiac resynchronization therapy (CRT) is a fundamental treatment for patients with heart failure and ventricular conduction abnormalities [1]. Patients suitable for CRT typically exhibit cardiomyopathy along with an electrical substrate, such as delayed electrical activation within the left ventricular (LV) lateral wall [2]. Previous studies have shown that delayed activation of the LV lateral wall is more frequently observed in patients with a widened QRS complex and left bundle branch block (LBBB) [3]. These patients generally have better outcomes following CRT and experience a considerable improvement in their quality of life [4].

A critical aspect of CRT is distinguishing between "responders" and "non-responders", a division that has significant implications for patient outcomes and clinical decision-making. Responders are patients who demonstrate substantial improvements post-CRT, characterized by enhanced left ventricular function, reduced heart failure symptoms, and improved quality of life. These parameters are often measured by tools such as the KCCQ [5]. Conversely, non-responders, who can constitute 30–50% of the CRT patient population, fail to show meaningful clinical benefits despite undergoing the procedure. This variability underscores the need for more precise predictive markers and better patient selection criteria [6].

Numerous factors have been associated with CRT responses. Pre-implant characteristics such as baseline QRS duration, morphology (e.g., the presence of LBBB), and the extent of myocardial scar tissue are strong predictors of positive outcomes. Additionally, peri- and post-procedural factors, such as optimal lead placement and device programming, contribute to the effectiveness of CRT [6]. The identification of non-responders is equally important, as it can guide clinicians in the implementation of alternative strategies, such as more intensive monitoring or adjustments to the therapeutic approach. Understanding these predictors is essential for advancing individualized treatment plans, refining patient selection, and improving long-term CRT efficacy.

It is thought that various electrocardiographic [7] and clinical parameters [8] can be used to predict the quality-of-life improvement in patients undergoing therapy. The Kansas City Cardiomyopathy Questionnaire (KCCQ) is a reliable indicator used to quantify the quality of life in patients who have benefited from cardiac resynchronization [5,9]. It is widely regarded as the most comprehensive and extensively studied clinical tool for predicting overall well-being and clinical outcomes in real-world settings [1]. Research suggests that the KCCQ may be more precise in assessing the outcomes of patients with cardiomyopathy and reduced ejection fraction than the New York Heart Association (NYHA) functional class [10,11]. However, guidelines still do not offer individualized predictions of prognosis, and key markers, including the significance of QRS area reduction, are not fully understood. The KCCQ, while reliable, has limitations due to its reliance on self-reported data, which can introduce biases if patients underreport or overreport symptoms, and its correlation with specific clinical and electrocardiographic parameters post-CRT is still underexplored. Further research is needed to identify prognostic markers of patient response and their correlation with the KCCQ. This study aimed to assess improvements in patients' hemodynamic status and well-being, as measured by the total KCCQ score [2,8–10,12].

It also aimed to identify correlations between post-procedure outcomes and demographic, clinical, and electrocardiographic parameters, including systolic blood pressure, ECG morphology, QRS duration, QRS area, and comorbidities.

While the QRS duration has been extensively studied as a predictor of results after CRT, other factors, such as QRS morphology patterns [13], QRS area [14], and intraprocedural increases in blood pressure [15], are emerging areas of research [13].

A reduction in QRS area after CRT has been linked to improved survival, but current guidelines lack individual prognosis predictions, highlighting the need for further study [14]. Systolic blood pressure (SBP) may also be an important predictor of favorable CRT outcomes: some studies suggest that a rapid SBP increase immediately after CRT is more prevalent in responders compared to non-responders [15].

This study explored whether a decrease in QRS area and duration after CRT could indicate improvements in the electrical substrate and long-term response, along with potential correlations with increased systolic blood pressure. This insight could help to reduce hospitalization time and enhance post-operative follow-up efficiency for CRT patients [15].

## 2. Materials and Methods

### 2.1. Ethical Approval

The research was conducted in the Department of Cardiology of the Prof. Dr. Agrippa Ionescu Emergency Clinical Hospital in Balotesti, Ilfov, Romania, from 2017 to 2022 as a unicenter observational prospective study. Approval for the study protocol was obtained from the Ethics Committee of the Carol Davila University of Medicine and Pharmacy, Bucharest, Romania (15037/05.06.2017). Planning, data collection, and reporting involving human subjects were conducted following the principles outlined in the Declaration of Helsinki. Written informed consent was obtained from all participants in the study, following General Data Protection Regulation (GDPR) requirements.

### 2.2. Study Design

This prospective observational study included 69 individuals diagnosed with cardiac failure and dilatative cardiomyopathy with low ejection fraction (EF) and major LBBB who underwent CRT device implantation at the Agrippa Ionescu Hospital in Balotesti, Ilfov, Romania, between 2017 and 2022. Baseline data were collected from the hospital's patient information system and details regarding heart failure etiology, comorbidities, and medication were gathered from patients' histories and other medical records. The KCCQ was evaluated by conducting anamnesis on the patients.

Patients were considered eligible for the implantation of a CRT device based on specific criteria such as symptomatic heart failure with LBBB QRS morphology, a baseline QRS duration over 130 milliseconds, and an EF below 35% despite optimal medical treatment for at least 6 months [6]. The etiology of heart failure was categorized as ischemic if evidence of myocardial infarction, coronary artery disease, or coronary artery bypass grafting (CABG) was documented in the medical records.

The exclusion criteria were as follows: individuals with unipolar or bipolar pacemakers or those eligible for device replacement; patients with psychiatric disorders impeding their attendance at follow-up appointments; those patients unable to demonstrate satisfactory adherence to medical therapy; and individuals with recent infections or deemed to be at a significantly elevated risk of device-related infections.

For this study, both baseline 12-lead ECG and a paced 12-lead ECG were available post-implantation and at follow-up intervals of 6 months, 9 months, and 12 months after implantation. Patient selection, device implantation, and follow-up procedures were performed according to the local protocols at the time of enrollment. At the beginning of the study, these protocols were in accordance with the 2016 ESC [16] guidelines for the diagnosis and treatment of acute and chronic heart failure and were later updated to the newer 2021 version [6]. The analyzed outcome was the evolution of the total score on the KCCQ. This determined at the pre-procedure stage and at three post-procedure time points, namely, 6, 9, and 12 months.

### 2.3. CRT Device Implantation Procedure

CRT device implantation was performed under sterile conditions in the cardiac catheterization laboratory. Patients were placed in a supine position, and local anesthesia or conscious sedation was administered. Venous access was achieved, typically via the subclavian or cephalic vein, followed by the insertion of leads into the right atrium, right ventricle, and coronary sinus to achieve left ventricular pacing. Lead positioning was guided using fluoroscopy to ensure optimal placement in the right atrial appendage, in the right ventricular apex or septum, and the posterolateral or lateral vein of the coronary sinus to achieve left ventricular pacing.

Pacing thresholds, lead impedance, and sensing were measured to confirm proper function before the leads were secured. The device was then connected and implanted subcutaneously using a pre-formed pocket in the pectoral region. Post-implantation, device programming was optimized to achieve effective biventricular pacing and synchrony, with follow-up visits scheduled to assess device performance and patient response.

### 2.4. KCCQ—The Main Outcome Variable

The KCCQ consists of 23 questions that evaluate various aspects of health, including physical and social function, symptoms, knowledge, self-efficacy, and overall quality of life. Scores on the KCCQ range from 0 to 100 points, with higher values indicating better health status [17]. Changes in KCCQ scores span from a 5-point gain, indicating a small benefit, to a 10-point gain, signifying a moderate benefit, and up to a 22-point gain, indicating a large improvement. These changes reflect the indirect effects of therapy. Conversely, decreases of 5, 17, or 25 points represent small, moderate, or large deteriorations in quality of life, respectively [5].

There is a need to create a system in order to standardize the results of this test and implement a threshold to differentiate clinically significant changes. Some studies have considered a 5-point change to be small, but clinically important, while a 10- to 20-point variation would be a large change [5]. Kosiborod et al. stated that 5 points are usually significant. A 5-point increase correlates with a 10% reduction in cardiovascular risk, while a 5-point decrease in the KCCQ score would see risk increase by 10% [18]. It is also important to determine which score value should be taken into account. A study conducted at the University of Missouri [19] demonstrated that, considering the previous value, the current value, and the difference between them, the current value holds the highest prognostic significance.

### 2.5. Electrocardiographic Data

The study time points for ECG analysis were at the 6-, 9-, and 12-month follow-up visits. Electrocardiographic data were acquired by scanning the baseline ECG paper and the ECGs recorded after CRT device implantation at every follow-up using a multifunctional scanner. The freeware software IC-Measure version 3.0.0.521 [20] was used to measure ECGs. Calibration was performed for each ECG using the software's microscope and caliper settings, with the calipers placed on the large squares of the ECG and set to a value of 5 mm (Figure 1). While the use of paper ECGs introduces potential variability in measurements, several steps were taken to minimize user-dependent variability and ensure measurement accuracy. All measurements were conducted by well-trained physicians experienced in ECG interpretation, and a standardized protocol was used to ensure consistency. The same calibration procedure was applied to all ECGs, using IC-Measure's calibration tool to maintain uniformity across measurements. The calipers were consistently placed on the large squares of the ECG grid, and a strict protocol was followed when marking the beginning and end of the QRS complex. To further reduce variability, each measurement was double-checked by an independent observer, and discrepancies were resolved by a third observer.

Although digitizing ECG data could improve precision, these standardization techniques were employed to reduce the impact of user dependence and ensure the accuracy and reproducibility of the results.

The next step involved accurately measuring the QRS complex in each of the 12 ECG leads provided by the ECGs. All measurements were conducted by well-trained physicians. Since each millimeter on the horizontal axis corresponds to 40 milliseconds (0.04 s) and each millimeter on the vertical axis corresponds to 0.1 millivolts, the QRS complex measurements were converted to millivolt-seconds.

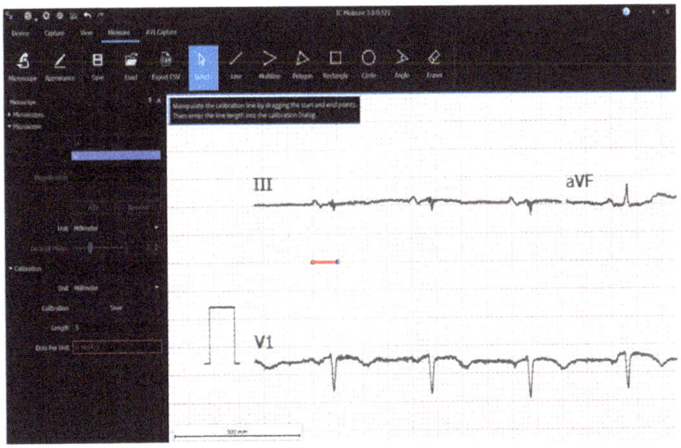


**Figure 1.** The calibration of the measurement tool using software-provided calipers.

### 2.6. Monitoring the Intraprocedural Systolic Blood Pressure

During each cardiac resynchronization procedure, arterial blood was continuously monitored using a radially or femorally placed catheter to assess any changes following the initiation of biventricular pacing. This monitoring was prompted by the expectation that correcting myocardial asynchrony would improve cardiac output as a sign of improvement. Some authors indicated a 5 mmHg threshold in their studies [15].

### 2.7. Statistical Analysis

Data analysis was performed in Python 3.7.4. For database processing, including the selection of variables, crosstabulation, division into patient groups, the extraction of descriptive statistics, etc., the pandas library was used [21]. Graphs were plotted using the matplotlib [22] and seaborn libraries [23].

For categorical variables, differences in distribution between two or more groups were assessed by constructing contingency tables and performing chi-square tests (SciPy library [24]). Student's *t* tests (SciPy) were used to compare numerical variables between two different groups. If more than two groups were compared, analysis was performed via one-way ANOVA, followed by analysis using Tukey's honestly significant difference test (Tukey's HSD), to correct for the number of comparisons.

To identify independent clinical factors predicting responses to the resynchronization therapy, multinomial logistic regression analysis was performed using the stats models package [25].

The Pearson correlation coefficient for each pair of variables was calculated using SciPy. A matrix of the results was then constructed, and the columns and rows were grouped by the unweighted pair group method with arithmetic mean (UPGMA) to identify related parameters.

To evaluate the prognostic value of the numerical parameters derived from EKG measurements before or after the resynchronization therapy, a linear logistic regression model was used. The results were visualized via Receiver Operating Characteristic (ROC) curves using the sklearn package [26]. Sensitivity and specificity were calculated for every possible threshold value and the threshold with the highest Youden J index was reported, along with its corresponding sensitivity and specificity values. In all statistical analyses, a significance threshold of $p = 0.05$ was used.

## 3. Results

### *3.1. KCCQ Score Evolution*

A progressive improvement in patients' quality of life after CRT was observed, as indicated by the median KCCQ scores at different time points. Initially, patients presented with a lower baseline quality of life, reflected by a median KCCQ score of approximately 35 at admission. By the 6-month mark, there was a notable increase to around 50, highlighting a significant early improvement in response to the therapy. This improvement continued to be evident at 9 and 12 months, where the median scores stabilized around 55, demonstrating the sustained benefit of CRT on functional capacity and symptom relief over time (Figure 2). Although individual variations in outcomes were captured by the interquartile ranges, the overall cohort consistently showed positive results, with only a few exceptions standing out as outliers.

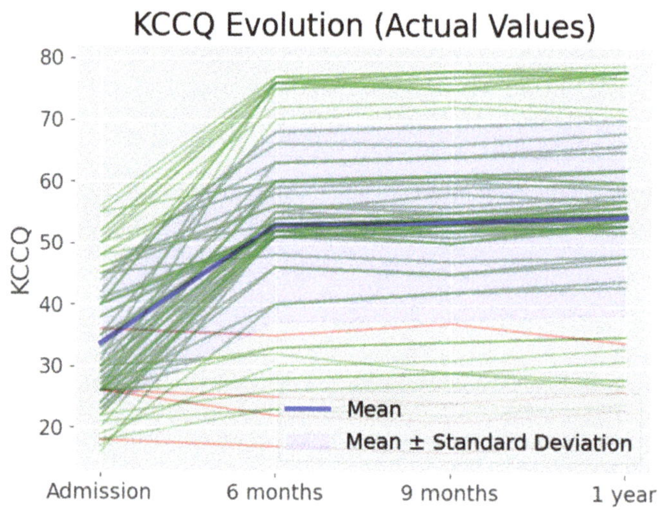


**Figure 2.** KCCQ scores at admission and a 6 months, 9 months, and 12 months following CRT. The graph shows the actual values of KCCQ, indicating a significant improvement in patient quality of life after therapy, with sustained benefits observed through the 12-month follow-up.

The distribution of KCCQ scores was assessed across four time points: at admission (baseline) and at 6 months, 9 months, and 1 year post-CRT. A significant improvement in KCCQ scores was observed following CRT, as reflected by the shift in the median scores over time. The median KCCQ score at baseline was approximately 40. This increased substantially by the 6-month follow-up to around 55, and remained consistent at both 9 months and 1 year (Figure 3). This is shown in Table S1 from the Supplementary File S1.

The statistical significance of these changes is denoted by the asterisks (**), indicating that there were significant differences ($p < 0.01$) between baseline scores and scores at each subsequent time point (6 months, 9 months, and 1 year), as assessed by ANOVA.

The interquartile ranges (IQRs) for each time point reflect the spread of data, which increases slightly in the later follow-ups. Additionally, a few outliers are visible, particularly at the 1-year mark, showing patients whose KCCQ scores did not improve as much or even worsened.

The overall trend suggests that CRT results in a sustained improvement in patient-reported outcomes, as reflected in the KCCQ score, with significant improvements observed as early as 6 months post-procedure and maintained through the 1-year follow-up.

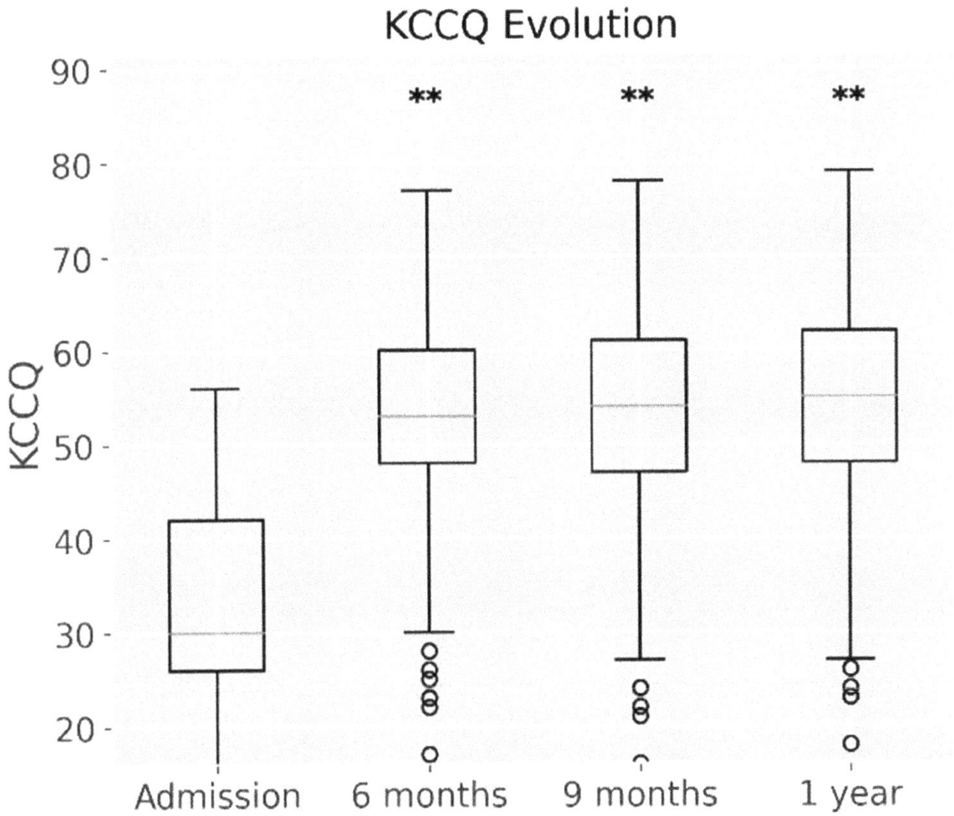


**Figure 3.** Boxplot showing the distribution of KCCQ scores at admission and at 6 months, 9 months, and 1 year following CRT. The boxes represent the interquartile range (IQR), with the median value indicated by the horizontal line. Asterisks (**) denote statistically significant differences ($p < 0.01$) compared to the baseline, as determined by the ANOVA test (** $p < 0.01$).

The distribution of changes in KCCQ scores (delta KCCQ), calculated as the difference between the 12-month and baseline scores, was found to reflect the overall improvement in quality-of-life following CRT. The mean improvement in KCCQ score across the study population was 20.8 points, with a standard deviation of 12.4 points indicating variability in patient responses. While most patients experienced a positive shift in their quality of life, the range of improvements varied from modest to more substantial gains, demonstrating the broad spectrum of outcomes obtained following CRT (Figure 4).

The following histogram shows the continuous distribution of KCCQ score improvements when patients were not divided into distinct responder and non-responder subgroups. Most patients exhibited an improvement of around 10 to 30 points, with a small proportion achieving gains exceeding 40 points. Based on this distribution, a delta KCCQ score greater than the median improvement of 23 points was considered a marker of a good response to CRT.

This analysis highlights the variability in patient outcomes, but overall suggests that CRT leads to significant improvements in quality of life for the majority of patients, with larger improvements being indicative of a more favorable therapeutic response.

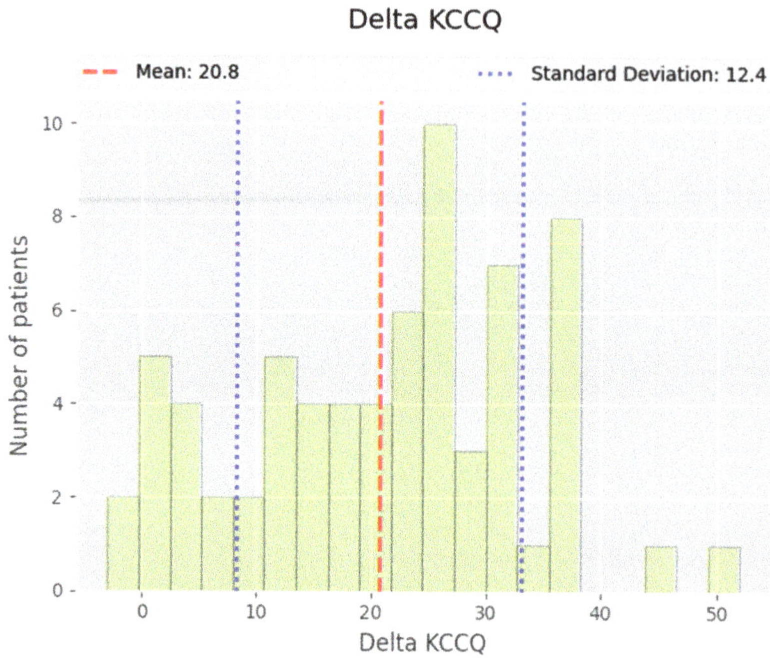


**Figure 4.** Histogram showing the post-implant evolution of the KCCQ parameters. Delta KCCQ represents KCCQ values at 12 months compared to KCCQ values at baseline. The study's population had a mean improvement in KCCQ of 20.8 points, with a standard deviation of 12.4 points. As no distinct populations were clearly differentiated on the histogram, a value over the median (23 points) was regarded as a good response to therapy.

### *3.2. Correlation Between the KCCQ Score and Clinical Parameters*

A comparison of demographic, clinical, and paraclinical characteristics between patients with KCCQ scores above or below the median value after CRT revealed several key differences (Table 1).

The age and sex distribution showed that the mean age of the entire cohort was 67.94 ± 9.57 years. Patients with KCCQ scores below the median tended to be slightly older (69.76 ± 8.33 years) than those with scores above the median (66.17 ± 10.44 years). While males made up the majority of the cohort (84.06%), the group with higher KCCQ scores had a larger proportion of females (22.86%) compared to the below-median group (8.82%).

In terms of heart failure severity, patients classified as NYHA Class III at admission were more frequently found in the group with KCCQ scores above the median (71.43%) than in the below-median group (58.82%). This suggests that individuals with more severe symptoms at admission may derive greater improvements in quality of life from CRT.

Regarding the living environment, there was a similar distribution of patients from urban (59.42%) and rural (40.58%) areas in both groups, indicating that living environment had no notable impact on KCCQ outcomes.

Comorbidities such as ischemia, atrial fibrillation, and diabetes mellitus were similarly distributed between the two groups. Ischemia was slightly more common in the under-median KCCQ group (44.12%) than in the over-median group (34.29%), while atrial fibrillation and diabetes mellitus showed no significant differences, with prevalence rates of 47.83% and 44.93%, respectively, across the cohort.

**Table 1.** A Comparison of clinical, demographic, and paraclinical parameters between patients with KCCQ scores above and below the median. The table highlights variables such as age, sex, NYHA class, comorbidities, and key laboratory values, offering insight into the characteristics associated with improved outcomes following CRT.

| | All | KCCQ Under Median | KCCQ over Median |
|---|---|---|---|
| Number | 69 | 34 | 35 |
| Age (mean ± stdev) | 67.94 ± 9.57 | 69.76 ± 8.33 | 66.17 ± 10.44 |
| Sex | | | |
| F | 11 (15.94%) | 3 (8.82%) | 8 (22.86%) |
| M | 58 (84.06%) | 31 (91.18%) | 27 (77.14%) |
| NYHA Class at Admission | | | |
| II | 24 (34.78%) | 14 (41.18%) | 10 (28.57%) |
| III | 45 (65.22%) | 20 (58.82%) | 25 (71.43%) |
| Living Environment | | | |
| Urban | 41 (59.42%) | 20 (58.82%) | 21 (60.00%) |
| Rural | 28 (40.58%) | 14 (41.18%) | 14 (40.00%) |
| Ischemia | 27 (39.13%) | 15 (44.12%) | 12 (34.29%) |
| Atrial Fibrillation | 33 (47.83%) | 18 (52.94%) | 15 (42.86%) |
| Diabetes Mellitus | 31 (44.93%) | 16 (47.06%) | 15 (42.86%) |
| Paraclinical | | | |
| Hemoglobin (mean ± stdev) | 13.46 ± 1.41 | 13.38 ± 1.53 | 13.54 ± 1.30 |
| Creatinine (mean ± stdev) | 1.13 ± 0.49 | 1.14 ± 0.38 | 1.13 ± 0.58 |
| Nt-Pro BNP (mean ± stdev) | 3303.26 ± 1911.92 | 3229.50 ± 1711.35 | 3374.91 ± 2111.29 |

Paraclinical parameters, including hemoglobin and creatinine levels, were comparable between the groups, suggesting no major differences in baseline anemia or renal function. Nt-Pro BNP levels, markers of heart failure severity, were slightly higher in the over-median KCCQ group (3374.91 ± 2111.29 pg/mL) compared to the under-median group (3229.50 ± 1711.35 pg/mL), though both groups had elevated levels, reflecting the overall severity of heart failure in the cohort.

In summary, patients with higher KCCQ scores were generally younger, were more likely to be female, and were more likely to present with more severe heart failure symptoms (NYHA Class III). Other factors, such as comorbidities and paraclinical markers, were not significantly different between the groups.

Further on, using the *t*-test, we compared the key clinical and electrocardiographic parameters of patients with stable outcomes and those classified as responsive in terms of KCCQ score improvement. The *t*-test results are presented in Table 2. The supplemental section (Supplementary File S2—Figures S1–S3) contains the visual representations of the *t*-tests performed for all the parameters and the ROC curves for the four parameters with the highest prognosis values.

**Table 2.** The *t*-test results comparing the clinical parameters of stable and responsive patients based on KCCQ score improvement after CRT. Significant parameters included Q-LV, immediate post-implant systolic BP increase, QRS area difference, and QRS area before CRT. The asterisks (*) in the "*p* Value Summary" column indicate the level of statistical significance. Parameters marked with "n.s." (not significant) have *p*-values greater than 0.05, indicating no statistical significance. A single asterisk (*) corresponds to a *p*-value between 0.01 and 0.05. Two asterisks (**) represent *p*-values between 0.001 and 0.01. Three asterisks (***) denote *p*-values between 0.0001 and 0.001, showing high statistical significance, while four asterisks (****) indicate *p*-values of 0.0001 or less, reflecting extremely significant results.

| Parameter | Mean Stable | Std Stable | Mean Responsive | Std Responsive | *T* Statistic | *p* Value | *p* Value Summary |
|---|---|---|---|---|---|---|---|
| Q-LV (ms) | 90.03 | 20.04 | 109.49 | 5.96 | −5.4323 | <0.0001 | **** |
| Immediate post-implantsystolic BP increase (mmHg) | 5.94 | 3.42 | 9.49 | 1.17 | −5.7259 | <0.0001 | **** |
| QRS area difference | 7.33 | 34.5 | 56.88 | 26.2 | −6.7038 | <0.0001 | **** |
| QRS area before (microV*s) | 105.18 | 46.55 | 148.01 | 61.47 | −3.2689 | 0.0017 | ** |
| R-wave amplitude in V1/V2 after (mm) | 1.27 | 1.32 | 1.82 | 1.06 | −1.9103 | 0.0606 | n.s. |
| R-wave amplitude in aVR after (mm) | 1.57 | 1.99 | 2.38 | 2.24 | −1.5959 | 0.1153 | n.s. |
| QRS duration after (ms) | 143.78 | 23.55 | 135.24 | 20.84 | 1.5931 | 0.116 | n.s. |
| Age | 69.76 | 8.33 | 66.17 | 10.44 | 1.5822 | 0.1185 | n.s. |
| QS wave duration in lead I after (ms) | 120.21 | 35.33 | 108.29 | 32.39 | 1.4594 | 0.1492 | n.s. |
| LVEDV (mL) | 241.62 | 64.34 | 263.09 | 68.86 | −1.3386 | 0.1852 | n.s. |
| QRS duration difference | 29.92 | 31.34 | 37.68 | 16.58 | −1.2794 | 0.2067 | n.s. |
| QS wave duration in lead aVL after (ms) | 94.84 | 40.76 | 84.01 | 32.2 | 1.2225 | 0.2261 | n.s. |
| PR interval before | 211.83 | 40.36 | 197.06 | 38.95 | 1.1271 | 0.2677 | n.s. |
| (S1 + R6) − (S6 + R1) after | 3 | 2.61 | 3.66 | 2.8 | −1.0035 | 0.3192 | n.s. |
| R6/S6 ratio after | 1.19 | 1.82 | 0.85 | 0.89 | 0.9682 | 0.3378 | n.s. |
| QRS area after (microV*s) | 97.85 | 53.98 | 91.13 | 45.47 | 0.5582 | 0.5787 | n.s. |
| Hemoglobin (Hgb) | 13.38 | 1.53 | 13.54 | 1.3 | −0.4696 | 0.6402 | n.s. |
| Percentage of biventricular pacing (%) | 98.76 | 0.85 | 98.69 | 1.11 | 0.3326 | 0.7405 | n.s. |
| Nt-Pro BNP | 3229.5 | 1711.35 | 3374.91 | 2111.29 | −0.3147 | 0.754 | n.s. |
| Creatinine | 1.14 | 0.38 | 1.13 | 0.58 | 0.1582 | 0.8749 | n.s. |
| QRS duration before (ms) | 173.7 | 30.84 | 172.92 | 19.01 | 0.126 | 0.9002 | n.s. |
| PR interval after | 100 | 0 | 100 | 0 | | | n.s. |

Significant differences were observed in the following parameters (also see the supplementary section for the visual representation of the *T* tests performed for each of the significant parameters—Supplementary File S2—Figure S1):

- Q-LV (ms): patients in the responsive group had significantly higher Q-LV intervals (109.49 ms) compared to the stable group (90.03 ms), with a $p$-value < 0.0001.
- Immediate post-implant dystolic BP increase (mmHg): a higher increase in systolic blood pressure immediately post-implantation was associated with a positive response (mean = 9.49 mmHg, $p < 0.0001$).

- QRS area before CRT (microV*s): responsive patients also had significantly higher baseline QRS areas ($p = 0.0017$).
- QRS area difference (microV*s): this parameter was significantly larger in the responsive group (mean = 56.88), indicating that a greater difference in QRS area before and after CRT strongly correlates with improved outcomes ($p < 0.0001$).

Non-significant parameters: Most other parameters, such as R-wave amplitude, age, LVEDV, and QRS duration after CRT, do not show significant differences between the stable and responsive groups, as indicated by the non-significant $p$-values (n.s.). These parameters did not appear to have a strong correlation with changes in KCCQ scores.

The predictive value of various EKG parameters for KCCQ score improvement following CRT was evaluated, identifying the optimal thresholds for each parameter, their corresponding Youden index, and their sensitivity and specificity in predicting a positive response (Table 3).

- The QRS area difference had the highest Youden index (0.678), with a threshold of 25.86 microV*s, indicating that this parameter is the most effective predictor of KCCQ improvement. It displayed a high sensitivity of 94.29% and specificity of 73.53%, meaning it can reliably identify patients who will experience significant improvements in quality of life after CRT.
- Q-LV (ms), with a threshold of 105 ms, showed a Youden index of 0.592, providing a sensitivity of 85.71% and specificity of 73.53%. This suggests that it is also a strong predictor of patient outcomes.
- Immediate post-implant systolic blood pressure increase (mmHg) had the highest sensitivity (97.14%) but relatively lower specificity (55.88%), with a Youden index of 0.53. This indicates that although this parameter can identify most patients who will benefit from CRT, it has a high rate of false positives.
- Parameters such as QRS duration after CRT, PR interval after CRT, and QS wave duration in lead aVL after CRT had lower Youden indices and either low sensitivity or specificity, suggesting they are less effective at predicting changes in KCCQ scores.

The sensitivity and specificity of each parameter reflect their ability to accurately predict a positive response to CRT. A higher sensitivity indicates a parameter's ability to correctly identify those patients who will experience a significant improvement in their KCCQ score. Conversely, a higher specificity indicates the ability to correctly identify those patients who may not experience a large improvement.

Overall, the results show that parameters such as QRS area difference, Q-LV, and immediate post-implant systolic BP increase are the most reliable predictors of KCCQ score improvement, helping clinicians to better identify which patients are likely to benefit most from CRT. The ROC curves for the most reliable predictors of KCCQ score improvements are included in the supplementary section to visually demonstrate the predictive accuracy of these EKG parameters in identifying patients likely to experience significant improvements in KCCQ scores following CRT (Supplementary File S2—Figure S3).

A forest plot was used to visually represent the results of a multinomial logistic regression analysis, which examined the predictive power of several clinical and demographic variables in determining a positive response to CRT, measured by the KCCQ improvement at 12 months. This is shown in Figure 5. Multinomial logistic regression can estimate the probability of a patient responding to CRT based on the values of various clinical or demographic parameters. As different patients may have overlapping or distinct patterns in terms of these parameters, this analysis models the role each one plays in determining the outcome, basically showing how the outcome changes when there is a one-unit increase in a predictor while the other variables remain constant. The analysis yields a list of odds ratios (ORs), representing the ability of each parameter to increase (for values higher than 1) or decrease (for values less than 1) the odds of responding to CRT. Forest plots are particularly useful for visualizing multinomial logistic regression results, as they provide a clear and concise summary of the OR for each variable, along with their 95% confidence intervals (CI), allowing for the easy comparison of the relative strengths of the predictors. In this plot, the odds ratio for each variable was displayed on a logarithmic scale, with the dashed vertical line representing an OR of 1.0, which indicated that there was no effect. Values to the right of this line suggest an increased likelihood of a positive response, while values to the left indicate a reduced likelihood. Confidence intervals that did not cross the line of no effect were considered to be statistically significant predictors of outcome.

**Table 3.** The predictive value of EKG parameters for KCCQ score improvement following CRT. The table shows the optimal thresholds, Youden index, sensitivity, and specificity for each parameter in predicting significant improvements in quality of life.

| Parameter | Threshold | Youden_j | Sensitivity (%) | Specificity (%) |
|---|---|---|---|---|
| QRS area difference | 25.86 | 0.678 | 94.29 | 73.53 |
| Q-LV (ms) | 105 | 0.592 | 85.71 | 73.53 |
| Immediate post-implant systolic BP increase (mmHg) | 8 | 0.53 | 97.14 | 55.88 |
| R-wave amplitude in V1/V2 after (mm) | 0.77 | 0.386 | 85.71 | 52.94 |
| QRS area before (microV*s) | 127 | 0.365 | 60 | 76.47 |
| R-wave amplitude in aVR after (mm) | 0.8 | 0.36 | 77.14 | 58.82 |
| QRS duration after (ms) | 130.4 | 0.279 | 51.43 | 76.47 |
| QRS duration difference | 28 | 0.271 | 80 | 47.06 |
| PR interval before | 223 | 0.271 | 80 | 47.06 |
| QS wave duration in lead I after (ms) | 112 | 0.248 | 57.14 | 67.65 |
| (S1 + R6) − (S6 + R1) after | 2.29 | 0.245 | 65.71 | 58.82 |
| LVEDV (mL) | 270 | 0.222 | 45.71 | 76.47 |
| QRS area after (microV*s) | 43.46 | 0.198 | 25.71 | 94.12 |
| QS wave duration in lead aVL after (ms) | 124 | 0.179 | 91.43 | 26.47 |
| R6/S6 ratio after | 2 | 0.148 | 97.14 | 17.65 |
| Percentage of biventricular pacing (%) | 100 | 0.139 | 28.57 | 85.29 |
| QRS duration before (ms) | 203.2 | 0.089 | 97.14 | 11.76 |
| PR interval after | 100 | 0 | 100 | 0 |

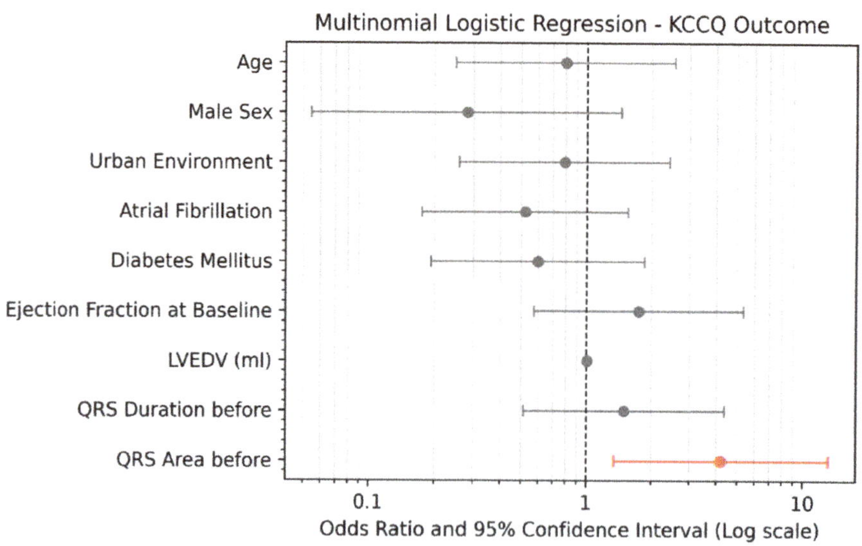


**Figure 5.** A forest plot showing the odds ratio for the response to therapy in terms of KCCQ improvement at 12 months. Patients with a QRS area above the median (106.91 microV*s) were 4.26 times more likely to respond to resynchronization therapy, as measured by the KCCQ, compared with patients with lower QRS area values.

The interactions between various clinical and electrocardiographic parameters and their relationship with outcomes such as KCCQ score improvement revealed several significant correlations. The strength and direction of these correlations were evident, with key parameters showing strong associations with one another.

Notably, QRS duration difference, QRS area difference, and delta KCCQ demonstrated significant correlations with other clinical variables. For example, QRS duration before and after CRT was strongly linked to multiple factors, highlighting its importance in predicting patient outcomes post-CRT. These findings emphasized how changes in electrical activity, particularly in QRS area difference and delta KCCQ, were closely tied to improvements in clinical outcomes following CRT.

In contrast, some variables showed weaker or non-significant correlations, suggesting they were less reliable in terms of predicting improvements in KCCQ scores. This differentiation allows clinicians to focus on the parameters that offer the most meaningful insights into patient response to CRT. By identifying these relationships, the analysis provided a clearer understanding of how specific clinical and electrocardiographic factors contributed to improving the post-therapy quality of life (Figure 6).

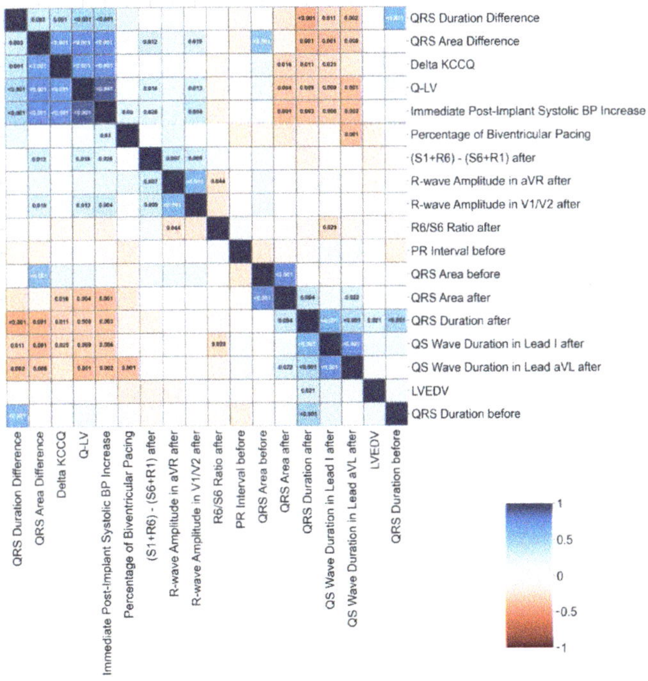


**Figure 6.** Correlation matrix showing the outcome measurements at baseline and at 12 months, and highlighting their differences (value at 12 months—value at baseline, denoted as a delta parameter). The graph color codes the strength of correlation (Pearson R value), with positive correlations in blue and negative correlations in red (see the color bar in the upper-left corner). Statistically significant correlations are indicated by the *p* value noted in the corresponding cell.

The logistic regression analysis identified several predictors of a positive response to CRT, as measured by KCCQ improvement at 12 months (Figure 5). Among the parameters, QRS area before CRT emerged as the strongest predictor, with an odds ratio of 4.26 (95% CI: [insert CI]). Patients with a QRS area above the median (106.91 microV*s) were more than four times as likely to experience significant improvements in their KCCQ scores compared to those with a lower QRS area, indicating a strong association with better outcomes.

Other parameters, such as the baseline ejection fraction, LVEDV, and QRS duration before CRT, showed weaker predictive power, with odds ratios closer to 1 and confidence intervals crossing the line of no effect, suggesting that there was no significant association with KCCQ improvement.

Clinical variables, including age, male sex, urban environment, atrial fibrillation, and diabetes mellitus, were not found to be strong predictors of responses to CRT. Their odds ratios were close to 1, with wide confidence intervals. This indicated that these variables had no substantial association with improvements in post-therapy quality of life.

Overall, the analysis underscored the relative importance of different variables, with the QRS area standing out as the most significant factor associated with enhanced patient outcomes following CRT.

## 4. Discussion

In this study, the KCCQ scale was used to assess the effectiveness of therapy in specific patient groups. By evaluating symptom severity, physical limitations, and social impact, the KCCQ proves to be a robust framework for evaluating health status outcomes and serves as a valuable indicator of improvements in quality of life. This score incorporates patient's perceptions of how symptoms affect their daily activities, offering clinicians insights into their clinical status. Moreover, KCCQ score reflects the dynamic evolution of health status over time, helping to monitor patients and identify changes that may require clinical action. Considering these aspects, the KCCQ score is an essential tool in ongoing monitoring and clinical management efforts, particularly in the context of multidisciplinary healthcare teams and the expanding reach of tele-medicine networks [5].

In comparison to traditional evaluation methods such as the New York Heart Association (NYHA) classification, the KCCQ offers certain advantages. The NYHA classification primarily focuses on the physical limitations observed by the physician, which can introduce variability depending on how the physician interprets the patient's condition. The KCCQ, on the other hand, provides a more nuanced, patient-reported measure of health status, allowing for a continuous and detailed assessment of how the patient perceives their own symptoms and limitations. Studies, such as Greene et al. [10], have shown that the KCCQ has superior prognostic value compared to the NYHA in predicting outcomes such as mortality and hospitalization. While a 5-point improvement in KCCQ scores is associated with reduced risk, the NYHA classification lacks this level of sensitivity to subtle yet clinically important changes in patient condition.

The KCCQ's ability to capture patient-centered data and offer more precise insights into health status changes makes it particularly valuable in guiding treatment decisions and evaluating the effectiveness of interventions like cardiac resynchronization therapy (CRT). By using the KCCQ alongside or even as an alternative to NYHA, clinicians may be better equipped to identify meaningful changes in patient well-being and optimize care accordingly.

The Q-LV interval, which represents the time delay between the onset of QRS and the activation of the left ventricle, plays a critical role in the effectiveness of CRT. A longer Q-LV after CRT has been shown to be associated with better synchronization and improved hemodynamics. This study shows that patients with a longer post-CRT Q-LV interval experienced greater improvements in their KCCQ scores, reflecting enhanced quality of life and symptom relief. This connection highlights the importance of achieving optimal electrical resynchronization in order to maximize the therapeutic benefits of CRT. The correlation between a longer Q-LV and higher KCCQ scores supports the notion that electrical remodeling, driven by CRT, is directly linked to improvements in functional capacity and overall patient well-being. These findings suggest that Q-LV could be a key factor in predicting the long-term success of CRT, especially in terms of patient-reported outcomes like KCCQ.

The present study also assessed the systolic blood pressure variation during the procedure and the QRS area to correlate them with the outcome. The immediate post-implant systolic blood pressure (BP) variation has emerged as a valuable predictor of CRT success. In this study, patients who experienced a greater increase in systolic BP immediately after CRT implantation also showed significant improvements in their KCCQ scores. This suggests that a larger systolic BP response may reflect better acute hemodynamic responses to CRT, which translate into improved functional capacity and quality of life, as captured by the KCCQ. The increase in systolic BP likely reflects enhanced cardiac output and more efficient ventricular contraction, both of which are key goals of CRT. These findings highlight the utility of monitoring systolic BP variation as a non-invasive, easily obtainable marker that correlates with positive patient outcomes, particularly in terms of subjective improvements in symptoms and overall well-being. As such, early post-implant BP variation could serve as a practical indicator of CRT effectiveness, aiding clinicians in identifying patients who are likely to experience significant benefits in terms of quality of life.

Furthermore, the study observed that variations in electrocardiographic parameters, such as the QRS complex area, following CRT are linked to changes in the KCCQ score. The QRS area, which is derived from vectorcardiography (VCG), has been recognized in recent studies as a potentially superior indicator compared to the QRS duration and morphology in predicting outcomes following CRT [27]. It has been suggested that a larger QRS area correlates closely with the delayed activation of the LV lateral wall, regardless of QRS morphology, and inversely correlates with myocardial scar size. Moreover, substantial evidence demonstrates that there is a robust association between QRS area and both clinical outcomes and echocardiographic response. These findings suggest that the QRS area reflects the electrical substrate suitable for CRT treatment and could serve as a criterion for identifying heart failure patients who would benefit from CRT [28]. Our results demonstrate the association of ΔQRS area with an increase in the KCCQ score following CRT, supporting the hypothesis that changes in the QRS area reflect alterations in the electrical substrate. Therefore, seeking a greater reduction in the QRS area after CRT may offer additional benefits to patients.

The R-wave amplitude in V1/V2 after CRT implantation provides insight into the electrical changes in the heart following therapy. In this study, higher R-wave amplitudes in these leads were associated with greater improvements in KCCQ scores. The R-wave amplitude reflects the depolarization of the ventricles, and an increase in this parameter post-implantation may indicate enhanced electrical activation and the synchronization of the heart's conduction system. This improved ventricular activation, particularly in the right ventricle and interventricular septum, could contribute to improved cardiac output and symptom relief. The correlation between the higher R-wave amplitude in V1/V2 and better KCCQ outcomes suggests that electrical remodeling in the early phases post-CRT is linked to improvements in patient-reported quality of life. Therefore, the R-wave amplitude in V1/V2 could serve as a useful marker for assessing the success of CRT in achieving electrical and symptomatic improvements.

It is very important to remember that several critical factors can influence the response to CRT, including technical and procedural elements such as the selection of the coronary sinus (CS) ventricular branch for left ventricular (LV) lead placement and the type of contrast media used during the procedure. The proper selection of the CS branch is crucial, as lead positioning impacts the electrical activation and mechanical synchronization of the left ventricle, thereby influencing overall therapeutic success. Research has shown that suboptimal lead placement can diminish CRT effectiveness and contribute to non-responder rates [29].

Additionally, the use of contrast media during CRT implantation poses another question. Contrast-induced nephropathy (CIN) has been identified as a potential risk that could impair the recovery of cardiac function, even in patients initially classified as responders. Certain studies underscore the importance of mitigating CIN to ensure maximal improvement in ejection fraction and overall patient outcomes. This highlights the need for careful patient management and the selection of low-risk contrast agents when performing CRT to optimize response rates and long-term benefits [30].

In recent years, there has been growing interest in physiological pacing, such as His bundle or left bundle branch area pacing, as an alternative or complement to traditional CRT for non-responders. These pacing techniques aim to restore the natural electrical activation of the heart by targeting the His–Purkinje system, potentially improving outcomes in patients who do not benefit from conventional CRT. Further research is ongoing to determine whether these physiological pacing strategies can reduce the percentage of non-responders and improve long-term clinical outcomes [12]. While the primary objective of this study was to explore the correlation between the KCCQ score and specific electrocardiographic parameters following cardiac resynchronization therapy (CRT), we acknowledge the potential interest in understanding the relationship between the KCCQ score and ejection fraction (EF). Although this correlation was not within the main scope of our research, we conducted supplementary analysis to provide additional insights. The statistical figures from this analysis are included in the supplementary section (Supplementary File S3) for readers interested in the broader implications of CRT outcomes. This supplemental analysis offers context and enhances the study's value. However, it should be interpreted as exploratory rather than definitive due to the primary focus on other clinical and electrocardiographic markers.

## 5. Study Limitations

There are several challenges in this research that should be noted. In the literature, both baseline and post-CRT implantation ECG data have been obtained from digitally stored information. However, some healthcare facilities lack access to digitally stored ECGs. For this study, all the correlations were established via measurements performed on paper ECGs and on post-CRT outcomes. Digitizing the entire process could save valuable time. Although the software used for the current measurements (i.e., IC Measure [20]) is very accurate, it is important to note that the current method is still user-dependent. Additionally, the numerous observations and measurements required to verify the response to CRT constitute a significant challenge. Optimization occurs hours or days after implantation, and interventions that require cardiac remodeling, such as CRT, affect the patient's overall health status. The QRS duration may remain unchanged, even after 6 months. All the factors that affect measurements and timing should be taken into consideration when evaluating the KCCQ score.

One limitation could be the small number of patients enrolled in the study over a 6-year timeline. While the results of our study provide valuable insights into the relationship between electrocardiographic parameters and KCCQ scores following cardiac resynchronization therapy (CRT), we acknowledge that the relatively small sample size limits the generalizability of our findings. The study cohort of 69 patients, although statistically significant for the purposes of this research, may not fully represent the broader population of heart failure patients undergoing CRT. Therefore, future research should aim to include larger, more diverse populations to validate these initial findings. Larger sample sizes could help to confirm the correlations observed in this study, refine the predictive models for CRT outcomes, and ensure that the findings are applicable across different patient demographics and clinical settings.

Another limitation of this study is the use of the KCCQ as the primary tool for assessing patient-reported outcomes. While the KCCQ is valuable for evaluating early improvements in quality of life and symptom burden, it may not be sensitive enough to capture the ongoing LV remodeling that can continue for up to 12 months or longer following CRT. To address this limitation, future studies should consider incorporating additional tools or conducting longitudinal follow-up using more sensitive measures, such as echocardiographic evaluations. The inclusion of other patient-reported outcomes and objective clinical metrics could provide a more comprehensive understanding of CRT's long-term effects on patients' health status.

Another potential bias is the reliance on self-reported Kansas City Cardiomyopathy Questionnaire (KCCQ) scores, which may introduce subjectivity into the results. Patients' perceptions of their symptoms and overall health can be influenced by a range of factors, including their emotional state, cognitive biases, and understanding of the questions. This subjectivity could result in variability in KCCQ scores that may not accurately reflect objective changes in clinical status. To mitigate this, KCCQ results were carefully interpreted alongside clinical measurements, such as systolic blood pressure and QRS area, ensuring that the subjective patient-reported outcomes aligned with objective data. While self-reported tools are valuable for assessing the patient's quality of life, future studies might consider supplementing KCCQ data with other standardized measures to reduce potential biases.

Another impediment that the study faced was related to patient education and willingness to complete the form, as it is not yet that widespread. Personalized healthcare and tailored treatment are in their infancy in many parts of the world. A possible solution to encourage the daily use of the KCCQ score would be to create a platform that patients can access individually before each visit, allowing them to familiarize themselves with it at their own pace.

## 6. Conclusions

In summary, this study highlights the value of using multiple clinical and electrocardiographic parameters, such as the Q-LV interval, systolic blood pressure variation, QRS area, and R-wave amplitude in V1/V2, as important predictors of CRT success. The strong correlation of these parameters with improvements in KCCQ scores underscores the importance of comprehensive patient evaluation to optimize CRT outcomes.

In particular, QRS area and systolic blood pressure emerged as key markers that can significantly influence both pre-operative planning and post-operative monitoring. Incorporating QRS area assessments into clinical practice may offer a more refined approach to selecting CRT candidates and tracking early therapeutic success. Similarly, monitoring systolic blood pressure changes immediately after CRT implantation provides a practical and minimally invasive measure of acute hemodynamic response, helping clinicians to quickly assess CRT efficacy.

By integrating these markers into routine clinical practice, clinicians can better identify patients who are most likely to benefit from CRT, ultimately enhancing quality of life and long-term patient care. Moving forward and understanding these correlations will guide personalized treatment strategies, optimize patient selection for interventions, and ultimately improve outcomes for individuals with cardiovascular disease.

**Supplementary Materials:** The following supporting information can be downloaded at: https://www.mdpi.com/article/10.3390/life14121564/s1, Table S1: Table showing significant KCCQ score improvements from baseline to later time points, with no significant differences between subsequent time points. Figure S1: Visual representation of the T tests performed for each of the significant parameters. Figure S2: Non-Significant Parameters. Figure S3: The ROC curves for the most reliable predictors of KCCQ score improvements. Figures S4 and S5: Charts comparing EF and KCCQ: The first shows group outcomes while the second highlights a strong correlation between Delta EF and Delta KCCQ.

**Author Contributions:** Conceptualization, A.-M.R., L.-F.T., T.-G.B. and E.-S.R.; methodology, A.-L.R., L.-N.B. and M.-D.T.; software S.I., T.I. and C.-J.S.; validation C.-J.S. and O.-A.P.; formal analysis A.-M.R., T.-G.B. and A.-L.R.; investigation S.I. and T.I.; resources, L.-F.T., E.-S.R. and L.-N.B.; data curation S.I., C.-J.S. and O.-A.P.; writing—original draft preparation, A.-M.R., O.-A.P. and L.-F.T.; writing—review and editing, S.I. and T.I.; visualization, T.-G.B. and E.-S.R.; supervision, A.-L.R.,

L.-N.B. and C.-J.S.; project administration A.-M.R.; funding acquisition A.-M.R. and O.-A.P. All authors have read and agreed to the published version of the manuscript.

**Funding:** Publication of this paper was supported by the University of Medicine and Pharmacy Carol Davila, through the institutional program "Publish not Perish".

**Institutional Review Board Statement:** The study was conducted in accordance with the Declaration of Helsinki, and approved by the Ethics Committee of Carol Davila University of Medicine and Pharmacy (15037/05.06.2017).

**Informed Consent Statement:** Written informed consent has been obtained from the patients to publish this paper.

**Data Availability Statement:** Data are contained within the article.

**Conflicts of Interest:** Andreea-Liana Rosu is employed by the company BBraun, but they were not part in our study. The authors declare no conflicts of interest.

## References

1. Nakai, T.; Ikeya, Y.; Kogawa, R.; Okumura, Y. Cardiac resynchronization therapy: Current status and near-future prospects. *J. Cardiol.* **2022**, *79*, 352–357. [CrossRef] [PubMed]
2. Kronborg, M.B.; Frausing, M.H.J.P.; Svendsen, J.H.; Johansen, J.B.; Riahi, S.; Haarbo, J.; Poulsen, S.H.; Eiskjær, H.; Køber, L.; Øvrehus, K.; et al. Does targeted positioning of the left ventricular pacing lead towards the latest local electrical activation in cardiac resynchronization therapy reduce the incidence of death or hospitalization for heart failure? *Am. Heart J.* **2023**, *263*, 112–122. [CrossRef] [PubMed]
3. van Stipdonk, A.M.W.; Rad, M.M.; Luermans, J.G.L.M.; Crijns, H.J.; Prinzen, F.W.; Vernooy, K. Identifying delayed left ventricular lateral wall activation in patients with non-specific intraventricular conduction delay using coronary venous electroanatomical mapping. *Neth. Heart J.* **2016**, *24*, 58–65. [CrossRef] [PubMed]
4. Strik, M.; Regoli, F.; Auricchio, A.; Prinzen, F. Electrical and mechanical ventricular activation during left bundle branch block and resynchronization. *J. Cardiovasc. Transl. Res.* **2012**, *5*, 117–126. [CrossRef]
5. Spertus, J.A.; Jones, P.G.; Sandhu, A.T.; Arnold, S.V. Interpreting the Kansas City Cardiomyopathy Questionnaire in Clinical Trials and Clinical Care: JACC State-of-the-Art Review. *J. Am. Coll. Cardiol.* **2020**, *76*, 2379–2390. [CrossRef]
6. Glikson, M.; Nielsen, J.C.; Kronborg, M.B.; Michowitz, Y.; Auricchio, A.; Barbash, I.M.; Barr, C.S.; Boriani, G.; Braunschweig, F.; Brignole, M.; et al. 2021 ESC Guidelines on cardiac pacing and cardiac resynchronization therapy: Developed by the Task Force on cardiac pacing and cardiac resynchronization therapy of the European Society of Cardiology (ESC) With the special contribution of the European Heart Rhythm Association (EHRA). *Eur. Heart J.* **2021**, *42*, 3427–3520. [CrossRef]
7. Végh, E.M.; Kandala, J.; Januszkiewicz, L.; Ren, J.; Miller, A.; Orencole, M.; Blendea, D.; Merkely, B.; Gellér, L.; Singh, J.P.; et al. A new simplified electrocardiographic score predicts clinical outcome in patients treated with CRT. *EP Europace* **2018**, *20*, 492–500. [CrossRef]
8. Lecoq, G.; Leclercq, C.; Leray, E.; Crocq, C.; Alonso, C.; Place, C.D.; Mabo, P.; Daubert, C. Clinical and electrocardiographic predictors of a positive response to cardiac resynchronization therapy in advanced heart failure. *Eur. Heart J.* **2005**, *26*, 1094–1100. [CrossRef]
9. Stogios, N.; Fezza, G.; Wong, J.V.; Ross, H.J.; Farkouh, M.E.; Nolan, R.P. Current challenges for using the Kansas City Cardiomyopathy Questionnaire to obtain a standardized patient-reported health status outcome. *Eur. J. Heart Fail.* **2021**, *23*, 205–207. [CrossRef]
10. Greene, S.J.; Butler, J.; Spertus, J.A.; Hellkamp, A.S.; Vaduganathan, M.; DeVore, A.D.; Albert, N.M.; Duffy, C.I.; Patterson, J.H.; Thomas, L.; et al. Comparison of New York Heart Association Class and Patient-Reported Outcomes for Heart Failure with Reduced Ejection Fraction. *JAMA Cardiol.* **2021**, *6*, 522–531. [CrossRef]
11. Sherrod, C.F.; Spertus, J.A.; Gosch, K.L.; Wang, A.; Elliott, P.M.; Lakdawala, N.K.; Reaney, M.; Zhong, Y.; Lam, J.; Wyrwich, K.W.; et al. The Kansas City Cardiomyopathy Questionnaire in Relation to New York Heart Association Class. *J. Card. Fail.* **2024**. In Press. [CrossRef] [PubMed]
12. Scheetz, S.D.; Upadhyay, G.A. Physiologic Pacing Targeting the His Bundle and Left Bundle Branch: A Review of the Literature. *Curr. Cardiol. Rep.* **2022**, *24*, 959–978. [CrossRef] [PubMed]
13. Oka, S.; Ueda, N.; Ishibashi, K.; Noda, T.; Miyazaki, Y.; Wakamiya, A.; Shimamoto, K.; Nakajima, K.; Kamakura, T.; Wada, M.; et al. Significance of effective cardiac resynchronization therapy pacing for clinical responses: An analysis based on the effective cardiac resynchronization therapy algorithm. *Heart Rhythm.* **2023**, *20*, 1289–1296. [CrossRef] [PubMed]
14. Marinko, S.; Platonov, P.G.; Carlson, J.; Borgquist, R. Baseline QRS Area and Reduction in QRS Area Are Associated with Lower Mortality and Risk of Heart Failure Hospitalization after Cardiac Resynchronization Therapy. *Cardiology* **2022**, *147*, 298–306. [CrossRef]

15. Tanaka, Y.; Tada, H.; Yamashita, E.; Sato, C.; Irie, T.; Hori, Y.; Goto, K.; Iwamoto, J.; Manni, H.; Yokokawa, M.; et al. Change in blood pressure just after initiation of cardiac resynchronization therapy predicts long-term clinical outcome in patients with advanced heart failure. *Circ. J.* **2009**, *73*, 288–294. [CrossRef]
16. Ponikowski, P.; Voors, A.A.; Anker, S.D.; Bueno, H.; Cleland, J.G.F.; Coats, A.J.S.; Falk, V.; González-Juanatey, J.R.; Harjola, V.-P.; Jankowska, E.A.; et al. 2016 ESC Guidelines for the diagnosis and treatment of acute and chronic heart failure. *Eur. Heart J.* **2016**, *37*, 2129–2200. [CrossRef]
17. Huo, X.; Pu, B.; Wang, W.; Peng, Y.; Li, J.; Lei, L.; Zhang, L.; Li, J. New York Heart Association Class and Kansas City Cardiomyopathy Questionnaire in Acute Heart Failure Key Points Question How is clinician-assigned New York Heart Association (NYHA) classification concordant with patient-reported Kansas City Cardiomyopathy + Supplemental content. *JAMA Netw. Open* **2023**, *6*, e2339458. [CrossRef]
18. Kosiborod, M.; Soto, G.E.; Jones, P.G.; Krumholz, H.M.; Weintraub, W.S.; Deedwania, P.; Spertus, J.A. Identifying heart failure patients at high risk for near-term cardiovascular events with serial health status assessments. *Circulation* **2007**, *115*, 1975–1981. [CrossRef]
19. Pokharel, Y.; Khariton, Y.; Tang, Y.; Nassif, M.E.; Chan, P.S.; Arnold, S.V.; Jones, P.G.; Spertus, J.A. Association of Serial Kansas City Cardiomyopathy Questionnaire Assessments With Death and Hospitalization in Patients With Heart Failure With Preserved and Reduced Ejection Fraction. *JAMA Cardiol.* **2017**, *2*, 1315–1321. [CrossRef]
20. The Imaging Source Europe GmbH. *IC Measure*; The Imaging Source Europe GmbH: Bremen, Germany, 2024; Available online: https://www.theimagingsource.com/en-us/product/software/icmeasure (accessed on 22 September 2024).
21. McKinney, W. Data Structures for Statistical Computing in Python. In Proceedings of the 9th Python in Science Conference, Austin, TX, USA, 28 June–3 July 2010; Volume 445, pp. 51–56.
22. Hunter, J.D. Matplotlib: A 2D Graphics Environment. *Comput. Sci. Eng.* **2007**, *9*, 90–95. [CrossRef]
23. Waskom, M. Seaborn: Statistical data visualization. *J. Open Source Softw.* **2021**, *6*, 3021. [CrossRef]
24. Virtanen, P.; Gommers, R.; Oliphant, T.E.; Haberland, M.; Reddy, T.; Cournapeau, D.; Burovski, E.; Peterson, P.; Weckesser, W.; Bright, J.; et al. SciPy 1.0: Fundamental Algorithms for Scientific Computing in Python. *Nat. Methods* **2020**, *17*, 261–272. [CrossRef] [PubMed]
25. Seabold, S.; Perktold, J. Statsmodels: Econometric and Statistical Modeling with Python. In Proceedings of the 9th Python in Science Conference, Austin, TX, USA, 28 June–3 July 2010; pp. 92–96.
26. Pedregosa, F.; Varoquaux, G.; Gramfort, A.; Michel, V.; Thirion, B.; Grisel, O.; Blondel, M.; Prettenhofer, P.; Weiss, R.; Dubourg, V.; et al. Scikit-learn: Machine Learning in Python. *J. Mach. Learn. Res.* **2011**, *12*, 2825–2830.
27. Eerenberg, F.; Luermans, J.; Lumens, J.; Nguyên, U.C.; Vernooy, K.; van Stipdonk, A. Exploring QRS Area beyond Patient Selection in CRT—Can It Guide Left Ventricular Lead Placement? *J. Cardiovasc. Dev. Dis.* **2024**, *11*, 18. [CrossRef] [PubMed]
28. Tokavanich, N.; Prasitlumkum, N.; Mongkonsritragoon, W.; Trongtorsak, A.; Cheungpasitporn, W.; Chokesuwattanaskul, R. QRS area as a predictor of cardiac resynchronization therapy response: A systematic review and meta-analysis. *Pacing Clin. Electrophysiol.* **2022**, *45*, 393–400. [CrossRef]
29. Butter, C.; Georgi, C.; Stockburger, M. Optimal CRT Implantation—Where and How To Place the Left-Ventricular Lead? *Curr. Heart Fail. Rep.* **2021**, *18*, 329–344. [CrossRef]
30. Teresa, S.; Giuseppe, A.; Valerio, P.; Livio, I.; Cristina, C.; Elisabeta, K.; Rosaria, C.; Fabio, G.A.; Vincenzo, M.F.; Aniello, V.; et al. Contrast-induced nephropathy after cardiac resynchronization therapy implant impairs the recovery of ejection fraction in responders. *ESC Heart Fail.* **2019**, *6*, 1266–1273.


**Disclaimer/Publisher's Note:** The statements, opinions and data contained in all publications are solely those of the individual author(s) and contributor(s) and not of MDPI and/or the editor(s). MDPI and/or the editor(s) disclaim responsibility for any injury to people or property resulting from any ideas, methods, instructions or products referred to in the content.

life

MDPI

*Article*

# Lipid Accumulation Product and Cardiometabolic Index as Effective Tools for the Identification of Athletes at Risk for Metabolic Syndrome

**Giuseppe Di Gioia [1,2], Armando Ferrera [1,3], Mihail Celeski [4], Raffaella Mistrulli [3], Erika Lemme [1], Federica Mango [1], Maria Rosaria Squeo [1] and Antonio Pelliccia [1,*]**

1 Institute of Medicine and Sport Science, National Italian Olympic Committee, Largo Piero Gabrielli, 1, 00197 Rome, Italy; dottgiuseppedigioia@gmail.com (G.D.G.); armando.ferrera95@gmail.com (A.F.); erikalemme@msn.com (E.L.); federicamango.md@gmail.com (F.M.); mariarosaria.squeo@coni.it (M.R.S.)

2 Department of Movement, Human and Health Sciences, University of Rome "Foro Italico", Piazza Lauro de Bosis, 15, 00135 Rome, Italy

3 Clinical and Molecular Medicine Department, Sapienza University of Rome, 00198 Rome, Italy; raffaella.mistrulli@uniroma1.it

4 Department of Cardiovascular Sciences, Fondazione Policlinico Universitario Campus Bio-Medico, Via Alvaro del Portillo, 200, 00128 Rome, Italy; mihail.celeski@unicampus.it

* Correspondence: ant.pelliccia@gmail.com

**Abstract:** Introduction: Metabolic syndrome (MS) is a growing global public health concern that is associated with increased risk for cardiovascular events, even in athletes. The lipid accumulation product (LAP) index and cardiometabolic index (CMI) have been shown to be efficient markers of MS in the general population; its applicability in athletes has not been discussed yet. We aimed to assess the role of LAP and CMI in predicting MS in athletes. Methods: We retrospectively enrolled 793 Olympic athletes practicing different sporting disciplines (power, skill, endurance, and mixed), classified arbitrarily into no risk (NR), low risk (LR), high risk (HR), or MS if they had 0, 1, 2, or 3 criteria for MS, respectively. Evaluations included a calculation of the LAP index, CMI, anthropometric measurements, and clinical and laboratorial variables. Results: Among our population, only 0.8% reached the criteria for MS, 9.1% were at HR for MS, 37.8% were defined as LR, and 52.3% had NR. Significant differences in anthropometric parameters and the principal components of MS criteria (blood pressure, lipidic profile, glycemia) were reported predominantly in HR athletes and those with MS ($p < 0.0001$). LAP and CMI presented linearly increasing values from individuals with NR to those with MS ($p < 0.0001$). In addition, HR and MS athletes were classified as "likely MS" (9.8%) and LR and NR athletes as "unlikely MS" (90.2%). After adjusting for potential confounders, LAP $\geq$ 34.66 and CMI $\geq$ 0.776 emerged as independent predictors for MS in the overall cohort (Hazar Ratio (HR) 7.22 [3.75–13.89], $p < 0.0001$, and HR 5.37 [2.96–9.73], $p < 0.0001$, respectively). The ROC curve revealed that these cut-offs in the general population predict MS with an area under the curve (AUC) of 0.80 and 0.79, respectively, for LAP and CMI. However, gender-related cut-offs seem to be more precise in predicting MS (LAP $\geq$ 38.79 for male, LAP $\geq$ 14.16 for female, and CMI $\geq$ 0.881 for male and $\geq$0.965 for female). Conclusion: The ROC curve analyses of LAP and CMI showed good diagnostic accuracy in predicting MS among athletes, despite the low prevalence of MS in our sample. Thus, these indexes may be used to promote screening for primary prevention and early detection of athletes at risk for MS to establish an early prevention strategy. Larger prospective studies are necessary to validate their benefit in the general population.

**Keywords:** metabolic syndrome; athletes; Olympics; lipid accumulation product; cardiometabolic index; cardiovascular disease

## 1. Introduction

Metabolic syndrome (MS) is a rising worldwide health issue. It is a pluri-pathological state defined by the co-occurrence of multiple cardiovascular risk factors, including high blood pressure, insulin resistance, abdominal obesity, and lipid metabolism disorders (high triglycerides, low high-density lipoprotein (HDL)-cholesterol) [1]. Additionally, it is linked to higher rates of morbidity, death, and healthcare costs [2,3].

There are numerous MS prediction models that have been put forward. Research has shown that variables such as age, sex, $\gamma$-glutamyl transpeptidase (GGT), uric acid, waist circumference (WC), blood pressure, triglyceride level, and HDL can predict MS [4]. Furthermore, anthropometric measures like body mass index (BMI), WC, and waist-to-height ratio (WhtR) are often used as early markers of MS. Nevertheless, these metrics are unable to differentiate between subcutaneous fat and visceral obesity, and do not show an optimal predictive value [5,6]. So, more sophisticated metrics known as the cardiometabolic index (CMI) and lipid accumulation product (LAP) were suggested as better predictors of MS [7,8].

LAP is determined by the following equation for women: (WC [cm] − 58) × (triglycerides (TG) [mmol/L]); and for men: [WC (cm) − 65] × TG (mmol/L) [9]. As it includes two of the five components, it is a reliable predictor of MS. In individuals of different ethnicities (i.e., Afro-Caribbean), regardless of weight, LAP has been proposed to be an early marker of metabolic dysfunction and appears to have more clinical usefulness than BMI in predicting metabolic diseases, including MS and type 2 diabetes mellitus (T2DM) [7]. Moreover, LAP is linked to non-alcoholic fatty liver disease (NAFLD) and arterial stiffness and is thought to be a therapeutically valuable diagnostic tool for estimating insulin resistance and cardiometabolic risk [10,11]. On the other hand, CMI has been created as an additional and more refined biomarker because it accounts for blood lipids and obesity. It is specifically determined by multiplying the triglyceride/high-density lipoprotein ratio by the WhtR. In order to determine a possible risk of metabolic abnormalities, such as the existence of MS and/or T2DM, this parameter takes into account both the accumulation of abdominal fat and the presence of dyslipidemia. While these two indicators have been extensively studied and validated in the general population, data on athletes remain scarce. Consequently, there is a gap in the literature regarding the potential role of LAP and CMI in athletes and their accuracy in predicting MS in healthy subjects. Therefore, the aim of our study was to determine, in a large cohort of Olympic athletes, the prevalence of MS and its risk factors and the likelihood and accuracy of LAP and CMI of predicting athletes at high-risk for MS.

## 2. Materials and Methods

The Institute of Sports Medicine and Science in Rome is the division of the Italian Olympic Committee responsible for the medical evaluation of the elite athletes selected for participation in the Olympic Games. In our study, we included a cohort of 793 Olympic athletes evaluated during pre-participation screening for the 2012–2022 Olympic Games. Body height and weight were obtained in each subject, and body mass index (BMI) was calculated as weight (kg)/height (m)$^2$. The WC was measured at the narrowest part between the lower border of the rib cage and the top of iliac crest to 0.1 cm with a tape measure while exhaling, with their feet set from 25 to 30 cm apart to distribute weight.

Body composition and fat mass percentage measurement was made with a Bioelectric Impedance Analysis (BIA 101 Quantum, Akern, Florence, Italy), with constant sinusoidal current, at an intensity of between 50 kHz and 400 μA. A blood test sample was collected, and the following biochemical indices were analyzed: total cholesterol, low-density lipoprotein cholesterol (LDL), HDL-cholesterol, triglycerides, and glycemia. Blood samples were collected in the institute of Sports Medicine and Science laboratory early in the morning and after at least 10 h fasting, and were analyzed on the same day. All of the blood tests were collected and analyzed in the same laboratory. Blood pressure was recorded in the sitting position before exercise testing, as recommended by the European Society of Cardiology guidelines [12].

MS was defined as meeting 3 or more of the 5 diagnostic criteria for MS that are defined according to the Adult Treatment Panel III (ATP III) report of the National Cholesterol Education Program (NCEP) [13]: fasting blood glucose $\geq$ 100 mg/dL or taking diabetes medications; TG $\geq$ 150 mg/dL; HDL-C < 40 mg/dL for men or <50 mg/dL for women; systolic blood pressure $\geq$ 130 mmHg or diastolic blood pressure $\geq$ 85 mmHg; and WC $\geq$ 90 cm for men or $\geq$80 cm for women [8,14].

Athletes who had 2 of the 5 diagnostic criteria and were arbitrarily defined as "high risk" for MS, while who had 1 of the 5 diagnostic criteria were defined as "low risk". Those who had no criteria were subsequently defined as having "no risk".

The LAP was calculated as follows for men: (WC $-$ 65) $\times$ TG; for women: (WC $-$ 58) $\times$ TG [8]. The cardiometabolic index (CMI) was calculated as the product of the triglycerides to high-density lipoprotein cholesterol (TG/HDL-C) and WHtR to predict cardiometabolic risk (CMR) in adults [15].

Athletes were engaged in a wide spectrum of sport disciplines, classified into four groups, as previously described [16]:

(1) Skill (technical disciplines): archery, golf, shooting, figure skating, sailing, curling, diving, and equestrian sports.
(2) Power (strength disciplines): weightlifting, Greco-Roman wrestling, judo, javelin, bobsleigh, skeleton, snowboard, swimming (<800 mt), alpine skiing, athletics (sprinting, shot put, and discus), and luge.
(3) Mixed discipline (alternate dynamic and strength components): soccer, volleyball, basketball, tennis, fencing, water polo, rhythmic gymnastics, taekwondo, badminton, beach volleyball, and softball.
(4) Endurance (primarily dynamic components): cycling, rowing, canoeing, triathlon, long-distance running, long-distance swimming (>800 mt), cross-country skiing, pentathlon, biathlon, speed skating, and Nordic combined.

CV risk factors were defined as follows:

(1) Family history for cardiovascular disease: Fatal or non-fatal CV events or/and established diagnosis of CV disease in first-degree male relatives aged under 55 years, or female relatives aged under 65 years [12], or evidence of carotid/peripheral atherosclerotic disease in first-degree relatives.
(2) Cigarette smoking: Defined as regular smokers of at least one cigarette per day.
(3) Overweight: BMI over 25; obesity: BMI over 30.

Each athlete of our cohort underwent a comprehensive pre-participation screening, including echocardiography, baseline ECG, and a stress test, which ruled out any significant cardiovascular diseases. This standardized screening ensures a healthy baseline within our cohort, allowing us to focus on relevant metabolic and performance metrics without the confounding effects of pre-existing cardiovascular conditions.

All of the athletes in our cohort trained more than 10 h per week.

The study design of the present investigation was evaluated and approved by the Review Board of the Institute of Medicine and Sports Science. All of the athletes included in this study were fully informed of the types and nature of the evaluation and signed a consent form, according to the Italian Law and Institute's policy. All of the clinical data collected from the study population are stored in an institutional database. The work described was performed in accordance with The Code of Ethics of the World Medical Association (Declaration of Helsinki).

*Statistical Analysis*

Categorical variables were expressed as frequencies and percentages, and were compared using Fisher's exact test or a Chi-square test, as appropriate. Normality criteria were checked for any continuous variables, which were presented as mean and standard deviation (SD) and compared using Student's *t*-test for independent data if they were normally distributed. Pearson's correlation coefficient was used for the correlation analysis. The comparative analysis between athletes with different numbers of criteria for MS was performed using the Dunn test and Pairwise comparison method. The tables show the pooled *p*-value [of the comparison test with the 4 categories: MS (with MS), HR (high risk), LR (low risk), and NR (no risk)]. If pooled $p < 0.05$, a pairwise test was performed. All pairwise tests were considered significant if $p < 0.05$. To confirm the ability of LAP and CMI to accurately discriminate the "likely MS" phenotypes, an area under the curve (AUC) was obtained using a receiver operating characteristic curve (ROC curve). The optimal cut-off value, sensitivity, specificity, and Youden Index of the LAP and CMI were obtained through the ROC curve. Moreover, the odds ratio and 95% confidence interval were obtained through logistic regression after adjusting for age, sex, fat mass, TC, LDL, and BMI. Statistical analysis was performed with STATA Statistics for Windows (SE, version 17) software.

## 3. Results

We enrolled 793 Olympic athletes, 433 males (54.6%), mean age 24.8 ± 5 years, mean body weight 73.6 ± 14.7 kg, and mean BMI 23.2 ± 3.1 kg/m$^2$. Athletes were divided according to sporting disciplines as follows: skill (90, 11.3%), power (246, 31%), mixed discipline (340, 42.9%), and endurance (117, 14.7%). Most of the athletes were Caucasians (755, 95.2%). In total, 62 athletes (7.8%) were smokers, 142 (17.9%) had familiarity with cardiovascular disease, and 82 (10.3%) had familiarity with dyslipidemia.

The main differences between athletes with an increasing number of criteria for MS are listed in Table 1. In total, 6 athletes (0.8%) reached the criteria for MS (at least three criteria over 5), 72 athletes (9.1%) had two criteria and were defined as "high risk" for MS, 300 athletes has one criteria (37.8%) defined as "low risk", and 415 athletes (52.3%) had no criteria and were subsequently defined as "no risk". LAP presented progressively increasing values starting from 11.3 ± 7.8 in those at no risk, 37.1 ± 26.6 in those at low risk, 54.7 ± 45.4 for athletes at high risk, and 109.4 ± 57.6 in athletes with MS ($p < 0.0001$). The same numerical behavior was observed for CMI, with 0.45 ± 0.22 for those at no risk, 0.76 ± 0.46 for those with low risk, 1.21 ± 0.87 for those with high risk, and 4.23 ± 4.42 for those with MS ($p < 0.0001$).

**Table 1.** Differences in main clinical and anthropometric parameters, blood test results, and indexes between athletes with different numbers of criteria for metabolic syndrome.

| *N* = 793 | MS | High Risk | Low Risk | No Risk | *p* Pooled | *p* Pairwise |
|---|---|---|---|---|---|---|
| | Three criteria | Two criteria | One criteria | No criteria | | |
| *N*, (%) | 6 (0.8) | 72 (9.1) | 300 (37.8) | 415 (52.3) | | |
| LAP | 109.4 ± 57.6 | 54.7 ± 45.4 | 37.1 ± 26.6 | 11.3 ± 7.8 | <0.0001 | MS vs. HR, $p = 0.007$; MS vs. LR, $p < 0.0001$; MS vs. NR, $p < 0.0001$; HR vs. LR, $p < 0.0001$; HR vs. NR, $p < 0.0001$; LR vs. NR, $p < 0.0001$ |
| CMI | 4.23 ± 4.42 | 1.21 ± 0.87 | 0.76 ± 0.46 | 0.45 ± 0.22 | <0.0001 | MS vs. HR, $p < 0.0001$; MS vs. LR, $p < 0.0001$; MS vs. NR, $p < 0.0001$; HR vs. LR, $p < 0.0001$; HR vs. NR, $p < 0.0001$; LR vs. NR, $p < 0.0001$ |
| Male, *n* (%) | 6 (100) | 53 (73.6) | 147 (49) | 227 (54.7) | 0.0002 | MS vs. LR, $p = 0.013$; MS vs. NR, $p = 0.026$; HR vs. LR, $p = 0.0002$; HR vs. NR, $p = 0.002$; LR vs. NR, $p = 0.132$; MS vs. HR, $p = 0.151$. |
| Age, years | 26.7 ± 4.7 | 25.4 ± 6 | 24.4 ± 5 | 24.9 ± 4.8 | 0.303 | - |
| Weight, kg | 106.5 ± 20.6 | 81.9 ± 16.9 | 72.7 ± 13.8 | 72.3 ± 13.8 | <0.0001 | MS vs. HR, $p = 0.001$; MS vs. LR, $p < 0.0001$; MS vs. NR, $p < 0.0001$; HR vs. LR, $p < 0.0001$; HR vs. NR, $p < 0.0001$; LR vs. NR, $p = 0.696$. |

**Table 1.** *Cont.*

| N = 793 | MS | High Risk | Low Risk | No Risk | p Pooled | p Pairwise |
|---|---|---|---|---|---|---|
| BMI, kg/m$^2$ | 29.3 ± 5.4 | 25.2 ± 4.1 | 23.2 ± 2.9 | 22.7 ± 2.6 | <0.0001 | MS vs. HR, $p = 0.027$; MS vs. LR, $p < 0.0001$; MS vs. NR, $p < 0.0001$; HR vs. LR, $p < 0.0001$; HR vs. NR, $p < 0.0001$; LR vs. NR, $p = 0.006$ |
| BMI > 25 kg/m$^2$ | 5 (83.3) | 29 (40.3) | 76 (25.3) | 75 (18.1) | <0.0001 | MS vs. HR, $p = 0.041$; MS vs. LR, $p = 0.001$; MS vs. NR, $p < 0.0001$; HR vs. LR, $p < 0.0001$; HR vs. NR, $p < 0.0001$; LR vs. NR, $p = 0.018$. |
| BSA | 2.35 ± 0.26 | 2 ± 0.24 | 1.87 ± 0.23 | 1.87 ± 0.24 | <0.0001 | MS vs. HR, $p = 0.001$; MS vs. LR, $p < 0.0001$; MS vs. NR, $p < 0.0001$; HR vs. LR, $p < 0.0001$; HR vs. NR, $p < 0.0001$; LR vs. NR, $p = 0.945$. |
| Fat mass, % | 17.1 ± 7.8 | 16.5 ± 8.1 | 16.6 ± 7.2 | 14.4 ± 6.2 | 0.0004 | HR vs. NR, $p = 0.018$; LR vs. NR, $p < 0.0001$; MS vs. HR, $p = 0.877$; MS vs. LR, $p = 0.866$; MS vs. NR, $p = 0.300$; HR vs. LR, $p = 0.973$; |
| WC, cm | 121.7 ± 22 | 111.6 ± 23.9 | 105.4 ± 24.3 | 77.5 ± 9.8 | <0.0001 | MS vs. NR, $p < 0.0001$; HR vs. NR, $p < 0.0001$; LR vs. NR, $p < 0.0001$; MS vs. HR, $p = 0.326$; MS vs. LR, $p = 0.107$; HR vs. LR, $p = 0.056$. |
| Afro-Caribbean, *n* (%) | 0 (0) | 0 (0) | 13 (4.3) | 25 (6) | 0.142 | - |
| Smokers, *n* (%) | 1 (16.7) | 12 (16.7) | 26 (8.7) | 23 (5.5) | 0.006 | HR vs. LR, $p = 0.037$; HR vs. NR, $p = 0.0005$; MS vs. HR, $p = 0.976$; MS vs. LR, $p = 0.500$; MS vs. NR, $p = 0.245$; LR vs. NR, $p = 0.099$. |
| Family history for CVD, *n* (%) | 0 (0) | 11 (15.3) | 47 (15.7) | 84 (20.2) | 0.258 | - |
| Training hours/week | 23 ± 2.3 | 22.3 ± 9 | 22.3 ± 9.3 | 24 ± 10.2 | 0.310 | - |
| TC, mg/dL | 184.8 ± 24 | 172.3 ± 8.1 | 175.7 ± 27.4 | 161 ± 27.7 | <0.0001 | MS vs. NR, $p = 0.036$; HR vs. NR, $p = 0.001$; LR vs. NR, $p < 0.0001$; MS vs. HR, $p = 0.209$; MS vs. LR, $p = 0.421$; HR vs. LR, $p = 0.320$; |
| LDL, mg/dL | 97 ± 35 | 98.5 ± 21.9 | 97.8 ± 22.4 | 84.3 ± 22.7 | <0.0001 | HR vs. NR, $p < 0.0001$; LR vs. NR, $p < 0.0001$; MS vs. HR, $p = 0.877$; MS vs. LR, $p = 0.931$; MS vs. NR, $p = 0.180$; HR vs. LR, $p = 0.804$; |
| HDL, mg/dL | 42 ± 15 | 54 ± 13 | 63 ± 15 | 64.7 ± 14 | <0.0001 | MS vs. HR, $p = 0.037$; MS vs. LR, $p = 0.0006$; MS vs. NR, $p < 0.0001$; HR vs. LR, $p < 0.0001$; HR vs. NR, $p < 0.0001$; LR vs. NR, $p = 0.245$. |
| TG, mg/dL | 228.8 ± 184 | 94.5 ± 50.1 | 74.3 ± 35.7 | 62.9 ± 22.1 | <0.0001 | MS vs. HR, $p < 0.0001$; MS vs. LR, $p < 0.0001$; MS vs. NR, $p < 0.0001$; HR vs. LR, $p < 0.0001$; HR vs. NR, $p < 0.0001$; LR vs. NR, $p < 0.0001$ |
| SBP, mmHg | 129.2 ± 6.1 | 121.7 ± 10.9 | 110.2 ± 11.5 | 108.7 ± 9.9 | <0.0001 | MS vs. LR, $p < 0.0001$; MS vs. NR, $p < 0.0001$; HR vs. LR, $p < 0.0001$; HR vs. NR, $p < 0.0001$; LR vs. NR, $p = 0.064$; MS vs. HR, $p = 0.104$. |
| DBP, mmHg | 81.7 ± 6.2 | 74.9 ± 8 | 68.8 ± 7.6 | 67.3 ± 7.1 | <0.0001 | MS vs. LR, $p < 0.0001$; MS vs. NR, $p < 0.0001$; HR vs. LR, $p < 0.0001$; HR vs. NR, $p < 0.0001$; LR vs. NR, $p = 0.005$; MS vs. HR, $p = 0.052$; |
| Glycemia, mg/dL | 104.3 ± 21.5 | 95.6 ± 7.1 | 90.8 ± 8.9 | 88.3 ± 5.5 | <0.0001 | MS vs. HR, $p = 0.027$; MS vs. LR, $p = 0.0005$; MS vs. NR, $p < 0.0001$; HR vs. LR, $p < 0.0001$; HR vs. NR, $p < 0.0001$; LR vs. NR, $p < 0.0001$. |

**Table 1.** *Cont.*

| $N$ = 793 | MS | High Risk | Low Risk | No Risk | $p$ Pooled | $p$ Pairwise |
|---|---|---|---|---|---|---|
| WC ≥ 88 cm female, $n$ (%) | 0 (0) | 17 (23.6) | 119 (39.7) | 0 (0) | <0.0001 | MS vs. LR, $p$ = 0.048; HR vs. LR, $p$ = 0.010; HR vs. NR, $p$ < 0.0001; LR vs. NR, $p$ < 0.0001; MS vs. HR, $p$ = 0.182. |
| WC ≥ 102 cm, male, $n$ (%) | 5 (83.3) | 37 (51.4) | 86 (28.7) | 0 (0) | <0.0001 | MS vs. LR, $p$ = 0.003; MS vs. NR, $p$ < 0.0001; HR vs. LR, $p$ < 0.0001; HR vs. NR, $p$ < 0.0001; LR vs. NR, $p$ < 0.0001; MS vs. HR, $p$ = 0.135; |
| HDL < 40 mg/dL, male, $n$ (%) | 4 (66.6) | 7 (9.7) | 8 (2.7) | 0 (0) | <0.0001 | MS vs. HR, $p$ < 0.0001; MS vs. LR, $p$ < 0.0001; MS vs. NR, $p$ < 0.0001; HR vs. LR, $p$ = 0.006; HR vs. NR, $p$ < 0.0001; LR vs. NR, $p$ = 0.0008. |
| HDL < 50 mg/dL, female, $n$ (%) | 0 (0) | 8 (11.1) | 15 (5) | 0 (0) | <0.0001 | HR vs. NR, $p$ < 0.0001; LR vs. NR, $p$ < 0.0001; MS vs. HR, $p$ = 0.395; MS vs. LR, $p$ = 0.575; HR vs. LR, $p$ = 0.053; |
| SBP ≥ 130 mmHg, $n$ (%) | 4 (66.6) | 33 (45.8) | 28 (9.3) | 0 (0) | <0.0001 | MS vs. LR, $p$ < 0.0001; MS vs. NR, $p$ < 0.0001; HR vs. LR, $p$ < 0.0001; HR vs. NR, $p$ < 0.0001; LR vs. NR, $p$ < 0.0001; MS vs. HR, $p$ = 0.332. |
| DBP ≥ 85 mmHg, $n$ (%) | 0 (0) | 7 (9.7) | 2 (0.7) | 0 (0) | <0.0001 | HR vs. LR, $p$ < 0.0001; HR vs. NR, $p$ < 0.0001; MS vs. HR, $p$ = 0.430; MS vs. LR, $p$ = 0.841; LR vs. NR, $p$ = 0.096. |
| TG ≥ 150 mg/dL, $n$ (%) | 3 (50) | 12 (16.7) | 6 (2) | 0 (0) | <0.0001 | MS vs. HR, $p$ = 0.043; MS vs. LR, $p$ < 0.0001; MS vs. NR, $p$ < 0.0001; HR vs. LR, $p$ < 0.0001; HR vs. NR, $p$ < 0.0001; LR vs. NR, $p$ = 0.003. |
| GI, $n$ (%) | 4 (66.6) | 23 (31.9) | 36 (12) | 0 (0) | <0.0001 | MS vs. LR, $p$ < 0.0001; MS vs. NR, $p$ < 0.0001; HR vs. LR, $p$ < 0.0001; HR vs. NR, $p$ < 0.0001; LR vs. NR, $p$ < 0.0001; MS vs. HR, $p$ = 0.088. |
| Rest HR, bpm | 85 ± 16.6 | 73 ± 13 | 70.3 ± 7.6 | 69.4 ± 13 | 0.009 | MS vs. HR, $p$ = 0.038; MS vs. LR, $p$ = 0.013; MS vs. NR, $p$ = 0.004; HR vs. NR, $p$ = 0.032; HR vs. LR, $p$ = 0.148; LR vs. NR, $p$ = 0.379. |
| Power, $n$ (%) | 3 (50) | 22 (30.5) | 84 (28) | 137 (33) | 0.382 | - |
| Skill, $n$ (%) | 1 (16.7) | 11 (15.3) | 43 (14.3) | 35 (8.4) | 0.059 | LR vs. NR, $p$ = 0.012; MS vs. HR, $p$ = 0.929; MS vs. LR, $p$ = 0.872; MS vs. NR, $p$ = 0.475; HR vs. LR, $p$ = 0.838; HR vs. NR, $p$ = 0.067; |
| Endurance, $n$ (%) | 0 (0) | 4 (5.5) | 32 (10.7) | 81 (19.5) | 0.0006 | HR vs. NR, $p$ = 0.003; LR vs. NR, $p$ = 0.001; MS vs. HR, $p$ = 0.559; MS vs. LR, $p$ = 0.399; MS vs. NR, $p$ = 0.229; HR vs. LR, $p$ = 0.188. |
| Mixed, $n$ (%) | 2 (33.3) | 35 (48.6) | 141 (47) | 162 (39) | 0.123 | - |

Abbreviations: BMI: body mass index; BSA: body surface area; CMI: cardiometabolic index; CVD: cardiovascular diseases; DBP: diastolic blood pressure; GI: glucose intolerance; HDL: high-density lipoprotein; HR: heart rate; LAP: lipid accumulation product; LDL: low-density lipoprotein; MS: metabolic syndrome; SBP: systolic blood pressure; TC: total cholesterol; TG: triglycerides; WC: waist circumference.

In athletes with at least two criteria (HR and MS), a higher prevalence of male athletes was registered (respectively, 100% and 73.6%) compared to athletes with one or no criteria (respectively, 49% and 54.7%, $p = 0.0002$). Significant differences in anthropometric parameters were highlighted in those with HR and MS, with higher body weight ($p < 0.0001$), higher BMI and BSA ($p < 0.0001$), and higher prevalence of overweight athletes ($p < 0.0001$). The lipid profile comparison showed progressively lower concentrations of TC, LDL, and TG and higher HDL-cholesterol values from MS athletes to athletes with no risk for MS (all $p < 0.0001$). The same results were observed also for SBP, DBP, and glycemia (all $p < 0.0001$). The type of sport did not show a relationship with the number of criteria for MS.

In fact, in power and mixed athletes, similar prevalence values were found (respectively, 0.382 and 0.123). In skill athletes, only between NR and LW was a significant difference found ($p = 0.012$). In athletes practicing endurance disciplines, a lower number of criteria were observed ($p = 0.0006$), with a progressive prevalence reduction from 19.5% in those with no criteria to 10.7% in those with one criteria and 5.5% with two criteria. No athletes with MS practiced endurance disciplines.

Finally, we have grouped athletes with MS and those with high risk in "likely MS" ($n = 78$, 9.8%) and athletes with low and no risk in "unlikely MS" ($n = 715$, 90.2%). The usefulness of the LAP and CMI for identifying athletes with likely MS through ROC curves is presented in Table 2. For the LAP, the AUC was 0.80 (95% CI, 0.77–0.83) for all of the participants, 0.81 (95% CI, 0.77–0.84) for male athletes, and 0.77 (95% CI, 0.72–0.81) for female athletes. For the CMI, the AUC was 0.79 (95% CI, 0.76–0.82) for all of the participants, 0.78 (95% CI, 0.74–0.82) for male athletes, and 0.74 (95% CI, 0.69–0.78) for female athletes, thereby indicating good discrimination ability. In addition, the optimal cut-off values for identifying the likely MS group were, respectively, 34.66 for LAP and 0.776 for CMI (general population). Different gender cut-offs were identified with a LAP of 38.79 for men and 14.16 for women and a CMI of 0.881 for men and 0.965 for women. The adjusted OR (95% CI) of the LAP and CMI for the "likely MS" athletes is presented in Table 3. In the overall population, after controlling for age, sex, fat mass, TC, LDL, and BMI, the LAP $\geq$ 34.66 had a hazard ratio of 7.22 [3.75–13.89], $p < 0.0001$, and the CMI $\geq$ 0.776 had a hazard ratio of 5.37 [2.96–9.73], $p < 0.0001$. For males, after adjusting for age, fat mass, TC, LDL, and BMI, the LAP $\geq$ 38.79 had a hazard ratio of 6.22 [2.92–13.24], $p < 0.0001$, and CMI $\geq$ 0.881 had a hazard ratio of 4.80 [2.42–9.50], $p < 0.0001$. On the other hand, for female athletes, LAP $\geq$ 14.16 and CMI $\geq$ 0.965 had, respectively, a hazard ratio of 29.70 [3.50–252.06], $p = 0.002$, and 97.18 [16.00–590.37], $p < 0.0001$.

**Table 2.** Areas under the receiver operating characteristics curve (AUC) for detecting athletes with likely Metabolic Syndrome with LAP and CMI. Abbreviations: AUC: area under the curve; CMI: cardiometabolic index; LAP: lipid accumulation product.

| | AUC (Continuous Variable) | Cut-Off (Youden) | Sensitivity | Specificity | AUC (Cut-Off) | Youden Index |
|---|---|---|---|---|---|---|
| LAP | 0.80 (0.77–0.83) | 34.66 | 67% | 80% | 0.73 | 0.468 |
| CMI | 0.79 (0.76–0.82) | 0.776 | 68% | 79% | 0.74 | 0.474 |
| Males, $n = 433$ | | | | | | |
| LAP | 0.81 (0.77–0.84) | 38.79 | 68% | 82% | 0.75 | 0.499 |
| CMI | 0.78 (0.74–0.82) | 0.881 | 66% | 79% | 0.72 | 0.450 |
| Females, $n = 360$ | | | | | | |
| LAP | 0.77 (0.72–0.81) | 14.16 | 95% | 52% | 0.73 | 0.466 |
| CMI | 0.74 (0.69–0.78) | 0.965 | 53% | 94% | 0.73 | 0.465 |

**Table 3.** OR and 95% CI of cut-offs for the identification of athletes with "likely Metabolic Syndrome" associated with LAP and CMI. Abbreviations: BMI: body mass index; CI: confidence intervals; CMI: cardiometabolic index; H: high risk; L: low risk; LAP: lipid accumulation product; LDL: low-density lipoprotein; MS: metabolic syndrome; No: no risk; OR: odds ratio; TC: total cholesterol.

| | Unadjusted | Adjusted [1] | Unadjusted [2] | | | Adjusted [1,2] | | |
|---|---|---|---|---|---|---|---|---|
| **Cut-Off** | **"Likely MS" (MS + H vs. L + No)** | **"Likely MS" (MS + H vs. L + No)** | **Low** | **High** | **MS** | **Low** | **High** | **MS** |
| All athletes | | | | | | | | |
| LAP ≥ 34.66 | 8.07 [4.87–13.38] $p < 0.001$ | 7.22 [3.75–13.89] $p < 0.001$ | 6.07 [3.86–12.37] $p < 0.001$ | 57.06 [26.32–123.72] $p < 0.001$ | >1000 $p < 0.001$ | 6.73 [2.98–13.99] $p < 0.001$ | 48.60 [21.69–108.89] $p < 0.001$ | >1000 $p < 0.001$ |
| CMI ≥ 0.776 | 8.19 [4.92–13.62] $p < 0.001$ | 5.37 [2.96–9.73] $p < 0.001$ | 6.06 [3.42–10.00] $p < 0.001$ | 8.19 [4.92–13.63] $p < 0.001$ | 15.12 [1.76–130.72] $p = 0.013$ | 4.01 [1.30–8.93] $p < 0.001$ | 6.30 [4.08–9.74] $p < 0.001$ | 4.84 [0.44–0.52] $p = 0.195$ |
| Sex: male | | | | | | | | |
| LAP ≥ 38.79 | 9.64 [5.25–17.69] $p < 0.001$ | 6.22 [2.92–13.24] $p < 0.001$ | 7.64 [3.25–15.69] $p < 0.001$ | 55.74 [19.98–155.49] $p < 0.001$ | >1000 $p < 0.001$ | 4.36 [1.95–11.67] $p < 0.001$ | 38.24 [13.09–111.71] $p < 0.001$ | >1000 $p < 0.001$ |
| CMI ≥ 0.881 | 7.16 [3.96–12.96] $p < 0.001$ | 4.80 [2.42–9.50] $p < 0.001$ | 5.16 [1.96–10.99] $p < 0.001$ | 7.74 [4.64–12.89] $p < 0.001$ | 13.72 [1.58–118.76] $p = 0.017$ | 2.72 [1.38–7.39] $p < 0.001$ | 5.30 [3.07–9.16] $p < 0.001$ | 4.33 [0.37–50.14] $p = 0.240$ |
| Sex: female | | | | | | | | |
| LAP ≥ 14.16 | 19.42 [2.56–147.15] $p = 0.004$ | 29.70 [3.50–252.06] $p = 0.002$ | 7.6 [4.25–13.23] $p < 0.001$ | 19.42 [2.56–147.15] $p = 0.004$ | - | 34.49 [17.18–69.27] $p < 0.001$ | 96.03 [8.87–1039.27] $p < 0.001$ | - |
| CMI ≥ 0.965 | 16.93 [6.21–46.15] $p < 0.001$ | 97.18 [16.00–590.37] $p < 0.001$ | 4.21 [1.71–11.55] $p < 0.001$ | 16.93 [6.21–46.15] $p < 0.001$ | - | 21.75 [3.75–120.24] $p < 0.001$ | 83.01 [14.44–477.06] $p < 0.001$ | - |

[1] Adjusted for age, sex (if not in sub-analysis), fat mass, TC, LDL, and BMI. [2] Reference variable: "no risk".

In Table 4 are presented the proposed gender specific cut-offs for both LAP and CMI for identifying athletes with MS or those that will likely develop MS.

**Table 4.** Sex-specific cut-offs proposed by the study. Abbreviations: CMI: cardiometabolic index; LAP: lipid accumulation product.

| | Male | Female |
|---|---|---|
| LAP | ≥38.79 | ≥14.16 |
| CMI | ≥0.881 | ≥0.965 |

## 4. Discussion

Currently, MS is considered one of the major public health issues [17]. Indeed, MS has been related to a 1.5-fold increase in the risk of all-cause death and a 2-fold increase in the risk of CVD mortality and stroke [4].

A large portion of the population encounters undiagnosed MS, despite the prevalence of MS being significant [8,18,19]. Indeed, accurate diagnosis and treatment of MS are crucial for global- and individual-level prevention efforts, since the disease is becoming more common in all age groups. Moreover, primary prevention is essential for lowering the burden and expense of healthcare-related illnesses in the future [2]. In this setting, regular moderate physical activity (PA) improves blood pressure, body composition, lipid profile, and insulin sensitivity. Conversely, one of the main risk factors for MS and overall mortality is poor levels of physical fitness [20,21]. Research indicates that fulfilling or exceeding PA guidelines has a negative correlation with the likelihood of developing MS and enhances parameters in those who already have MS or are at risk [22]. In addition, patients who no longer fit MS criteria may be reclassified as a result of an exercise program that improves any of the MS markers. About 30.5% of healthy people enrolled in the study by Katzmarzyk et al. were reclassified as no longer having MS due to the combined effect on the improvement of MS indicators following 20 weeks of supervised exercise [23].

Different anthropometric measures like body mass index (BMI), WC, and WHtR have been proposed for predicting MS. However, they present different limits, and new index parameters such as LAP and CMI have recently shown promising results [5–12]. Currently, WC and the concentration of TG at fasting are combined to form LAP, a measure of visceral obesity. Anatomical and biochemical alterations associated with lipid overaccumulation in humans can be described by using anthropometric and biochemical data to compute LAP simultaneously [8,24]. LAP is frequently utilized as a predictor of CVD and as a marker of metabolic disorders. It is a clinical indicator of visceral obesity and has been suggested as an easy, affordable, and reliable way to calculate cardiovascular risk and death because the gold-standard techniques for assessing visceral fat are costly and the measurement of WC cannot differentiate between visceral and subcutaneous fat [25,26]. According to Rotter et al., people with T2DM, obesity, and MS had far greater LAP values than people without these disorders [25]. Additionally, these authors discovered a negative link with HDL-cholesterol and a positive and substantial correlation with insulin, glycemia, and total cholesterol [25]. Moreover, Guo et al. investigated the relationship between LPA and metabolic parameters and discovered that this index is a helpful indicator for MS diagnosis and screening [26]. However, the LAP of men and women cannot easily be compared, since different WC corrections are employed. Compared to WC and BMI, WHtR has been demonstrated to be a more accurate predictor of coronary heart disease and cardiovascular risk factors. Consequently, the product of the TG/HDL-C ratio and WHtR has led to the proposal of a new parameter, the CMI. Furthermore, CMI has been demonstrated to be a key factor in MS and a strong predictor of CVD [7]. With a cut-off of 0.84, the CMI is the most practical and trustworthy index to be used in clinical practice for identifying MS in obese women [27]. However, these indexes have not been studied in a healthy population practicing physical activity, such as athletes.

In our study, we enrolled 794 Olympic athletes, practicing different sports, who were mostly (90.1%) at low or no risk for MS. Remarkably, only a small subset of individuals (9.9%) showed MS or high risk for MS. This confirms that physical activity is associated with lower prevalence of MS [20]. Indeed, regular–moderate PA contributes to improving insulin sensitivity, lipid profile, blood pressure, and body composition [20,21]. However, some athletes may present higher blood pressure values, cholesterol levels, and glycemia levels, being exposed to higher risk for developing MS, as in our cohort. Indeed, athletes are not immune to MS onset and, consequently, to a higher risk for CAD [28]. Thus, individuating patients at risk is crucial to prevent MS development and reduce the risk of adverse outcomes.

From a gender-specific perspective, males are more likely than females to have MS, while females who have MS are more likely to develop CVD. Males are said to be more at risk of T2DM and hypertension among the MS components, whereas females are more likely to have dyslipidemia and abdominal obesity [29]. In our study, sex had also an impact when in comes to MS risk classifying of athletes. Indeed, all of the individuals at HR and more than 70% of those with MS were males. However, the prevalence of MS varies depending on the population examined, the definition employed, and the age, ethnicity, and sex of the affected person. A person's diet, degree of physical activity, genetic background, and degree of over- or under-nutrition all have an impact on how common the condition and its components are. Age-related increases in the prevalence of MS are particularly noticeable during the pre-menopausal to post-menopausal transition [30]. However, in our study, all of the athletes were young. Thus, generalized statements regarding sex differences in prevalence may be misleading due to the potential influence of these numerous confounding factors.

On the other hand, athletes with increased BMI, BSA, or overweight were more frequently individuals satisfying the criteria for HR MS or MS. Thus, preventing measures should be applicated in the early stage or before developing MS. Methods that can effectively reduce body fat include changing diet and modifying energy expenditure through exercise, especially visceral fat.

Moreover, the prevalence of most sporting categories did not significantly change according to the number of criteria. In fact, in power, mixed, and skill athletes, there were no significant differences between those at HR and LW or NR. However, endurance athletes were more frequently individuals with NR or LW than HR (19.5%, 10.7%, and 5.5%, respectively). Indeed, it seems that endurance training has a more favorable effect on glucose and insulin homeostasis and lipid profile than strength training and, consequently, on MS [31].

However, the primary strength of this study is the assessment of LAP and CMI in identifying patients at risk for MS. Indeed, athletes at HR or with MS presented significantly higher values of LAP and CMI than those LR or NR, as illustrated in Table 1. In the sub-analysis, patients were classified into those "likely" to develop MS, if there were at least two criteria, and "unlikely" if there were no or one criteria for MS. Indeed, LAP and CMI confirmed to be good predictors of patients at risk for MS, with good accuracy in both male and female athletes (AUCs of 0.80 and 0.79, respectively). This confirms the good accuracy of both markers in predicting MS already studied in the general population, especially individuals with obesity [32–34].

Individuating athletes at risk would help focus on the frequent monitoring of MS components, the further evaluations of early screenings for MS-related diseases, and mitigating the modifiable underlying risk factors through lifestyle and physical activity changes [35]. For that purpose, we individuated the ideal cut-off, corrected for potential confounders, for identifying athletes likely to develop MS. Indeed, in the general population, LAP $\geq$ 34.66 and CMI $\geq$ 0.776 conferred a 7-fold and 5-fold risk for developing MS, respectively. However, these values had different adjusted cut-offs between males and females. Our study individuated LAP cut-offs as between 38.79 and 14.16 and CMI cut-offs as between 0.881 and 0.965 for male and female athletes, respectively. These cut-offs are slightly different from those described in other studies. Because adipose tissue accumulates around the hips and thighs in women and around the trunk and lower abdominal part in men, physiological variances in height, weight, and body composition between the sexes may be the cause of the disparities in LAP measures between the performance of males and females [36]. According to Haijiang Dai et al. [37], MS prevalence rose in both the male and female groups when LAP levels increased. For men and women, respectively, LAPs $\geq$ 30.5 and 23.0 were shown to be the maximum values for sensitivity and specificity in the diagnosis of MS. On the contrary, the highest sensitivity and specificity were found with LAP cut-off values of 34.2 for the entire sample in a study by Nascimento-Ferreira et al. [5]. Following age stratification, the LAP cut-off values for males and females under 50 were 64.1 and 38, respectively, while for subjects over 50, the values were 36.4 and 34.2 for males and females, respectively. On the other hand, Lazzer et al. individuated 0.84 as a CMI cut-off for individuating women with obesity at risk for developing MS, while male cut-offs for CMI seem to be lower [15,27,38]. As young athletes generally present lower WC and triglyceride levels, this could explain the lower LAP and CMI values in our study compared to those reported in the other studies. Nevertheless, this study highlights the good accuracy of both indexes in predicting MS risk and their usefulness in the early diagnosis of MS among athletes.

LAP and CMI may be routinely calculated for all athletes to identify those at risk for metabolic syndrome. This would allow for the early detection of potential cardiometabolic issues and enable clinicians to place "high risk" athletes under more intensive follow-up and monitoring. By incorporating these indices into regular health assessments, we could ensure that athletes who may be predisposed to metabolic syndrome receive timely interventions, promoting better long-term health outcomes and reducing the risk of developing more severe conditions.

## 5. Limitations

Our study presents several limitations. Firstly, it is a retrospective observational study. Therefore, future prospective studies are needed to verify the suggested instruments and assess their predictive significance for athletes' cardiovascular health on a large scale. The population's demographics, which included a narrow age range (most of them had median age of 25), a sizable sample size, and were restricted to a single center, indicate another limit. Furthermore, this restricts generalizability because this study primarily consists of athletes of Italian nationality and Caucasian ethnicity. Lastly, a variety of factors, including food and prolonged periods of hard training, can affect body composition. Olympic athletes were assessed by our research at all stages throughout the year, including peak training, competitions, and post-training periods like holidays. Furthermore, our indexes' therapeutic efficacy has not yet been established, but they do represent an effort to develop models and scores that will help identify athletes who may be at risk for MS. Large-scale randomized trials are nevertheless required.

## 6. Conclusions

Athletes have lower prevalence of MS compared to the general population. However, they are not immune to developing MS and related issues, including CVD. Therefore, using prediction models, including LAP and CMI, aids in the individuation of athletes at different risks for MS. Indeed, the ROC curve analyses of LAP and CMI showed good diagnostic accuracy as a supplementary screening tool in predicting athletes at high risk for MS, despite the low prevalence of MS in our cohort. The early detection of individuals at risk for MS may contribute to establishing an early prevention strategy, including physical, nutraceutical, or pharmacological management. Randomized prospective studies are necessary to validate their role on a larger scale and their utility in everyday clinical practice. New trials are required to validate the role of LAP and CMI in predicting cardiovascular events and mortality among athletes at risk.

**Author Contributions:** G.D.G. and A.F.: conception and design of the study; F.M.: methodology; G.D.G., A.F., M.C., and E.L.: acquisition of data, review of the literature; R.M., M.C., and M.R.S.: drafting the article and revising it critically for important intellectual content, E.L., M.R.S., and A.P.: final approval of the version that was submitted. All authors have read and agreed to the published version of the manuscript.

**Funding:** This research did not receive any specific grant from funding agencies in the public, commercial, or non-profit sectors.

**Institutional Review Board Statement:** The study design of the present investigation was evaluated and approved by the Review Board of the Institute of Medicine and Sports Science. The research was performed in accordance with The Code of Ethics of the World Medical Association (Declaration of Helsinki).

**Informed Consent Statement:** All of the athletes included in this study were fully informed of the types and nature of the evaluation and signed a consent form, according to the Italian Law and Institute's policy.

**Data Availability Statement:** The original contributions presented in the study are included in the article, further inquiries can be directed to the corresponding author.

**Conflicts of Interest:** The authors declare no financial interests or affiliations with the institutions, organizations, or companies mentioned in the manuscript.

## References


1. Zimmet, P.Z.; Alberti, K.G.; Shaw, J.E. Mainstreaming the metabolic syndrome: A definitive definition. *Med. J. Aust.* **2005**, *183*, 175–176. [CrossRef] [PubMed]
2. Obokata, M.; Negishi, K.; Ohyama, Y.; Okada, H.; Imai, K.; Kurabayashi, M. A Risk Score with Additional Four Independent Factors to Predict the Incidence and Recovery from Metabolic Syndrome: Development and Validation in Large Japanese Cohorts. *PLoS ONE* **2015**, *10*, e0133884. [CrossRef] [PubMed] [PubMed Central]
3. Saklayen, M.G. The Global Epidemic of the Metabolic Syndrome. *Curr. Hypertens. Rep.* **2018**, *20*, 12. [CrossRef] [PubMed] [PubMed Central]
4. Mottillo, S.; Filion, K.B.; Genest, J.; Joseph, L.; Pilote, L.; Poirier, P.; Rinfret, S.; Schiffrin, E.L.; Eisenberg, M.J. The metabolic syndrome and cardiovascular risk a systematic review and meta-analysis. *J. Am. Coll. Cardiol.* **2010**, *56*, 1113–1132. [CrossRef] [PubMed]

5. Nascimento-Ferreira, M.V.; Rendo-Urteaga, T.; Vilanova-Campelo, R.C.; Carvalho, H.B.; da Paz Oliveira, G.; Paes Landim, M.B.; Torres-Leal, F.L. The lipid accumulation product is a powerful tool to predict metabolic syndrome in undiagnosed Brazilian adults. *Clin. Nutr.* **2017**, *36*, 1693–1700. [CrossRef]
6. Ray, L.; Ravichandran, K.; Nanda, S.K. Comparison of Lipid Accumulation Product Index with Body Mass Index and WC as a Predictor of Metabolic Syndrome in Indian Population. *Metab. Syndr. Relat. Disord.* **2018**, *16*, 240–245. [CrossRef]
7. Wakabayashi, I.; Daimon, T. The "cardiometabolic index" as a new marker determined by adiposity and blood lipids for discrimination of diabetes mellitus. *Clin. Chim. Acta* **2015**, *438*, 274–278. [CrossRef] [PubMed]
8. Kahn, H.S. The "lipid accumulation product" performs better than the body mass index for recognizing cardiovascular risk: A population-based comparison. *BMC Cardiovasc. Disord.* **2005**, *5*, 26, Erratum in: *BMC Cardiovasc. Disord.* **2006**, *6*, 5. [CrossRef] [PubMed] [PubMed Central]
9. Chiang, J.K.; Koo, M. Lipid accumulation product: A simple and accurate index for predicting metabolic syndrome in Taiwanese people aged 50 and over. *BMC Cardiovasc. Disord.* **2012**, *12*, 78. [CrossRef] [PubMed] [PubMed Central]
10. Cheng, Y.L.; Wang, Y.J.; Lan, K.H.; Huo, T.I.; Huang, Y.H.; Su, C.W.; Hsieh, W.Y.; Hou, M.C.; Lin, H.C.; Lee, F.Y.; et al. Fatty Liver Index and Lipid Accumulation Product Can Predict Metabolic Syndrome in Subjects without Fatty Liver Disease. *Gastroenterol. Res. Pract.* **2017**, *2017*, 9279836. [CrossRef] [PubMed] [PubMed Central]
11. Li, H.; Zhang, Y.; Luo, H.; Lin, R. The lipid accumulation product is a powerful tool to diagnose metabolic dysfunction-associated fatty liver disease in the United States adults. *Front. Endocrinol.* **2022**, *13*, 977625. [CrossRef] [PubMed] [PubMed Central]
12. Piepoli, M.F.; Hoes, A.W.; Agewall, S.; Albus, C.; Brotons, C.; Catapano, A.L.; Cooney, M.T.; Corrà, U.; Cosyns, B.; Deaton, C.; et al. 2016 European Guidelines on cardiovascular disease prevention in clinical practice: The Sixth Joint Task Force of the European Society of Cardiology and Other Societies on Cardiovascular Disease Prevention in Clinical Practice (constituted by representatives of 10 societies and by invited experts) Developed with the special contribution of the European Association for Cardiovascular Prevention & Rehabilitation (EACPR). *Eur. Heart J.* **2016**, *37*, 2315–2381. [CrossRef] [PubMed] [PubMed Central]
13. Expert Panel on Detection, Evaluation, and Treatment of High Blood Cholesterol in Adults. Executive summary of the third report of The National Cholesterol Education Program (NCEP) expert panel on detection, evaluation, and treatment of high blood cholesterol in adults (Adult Treatment Panel III). *J. Am. Med. Assoc.* **2001**, *285*, 2486–2497. [CrossRef]
14. Khandekar, M.J.; Cohen, P.; Spiegelman, B.M. Molecular mechanisms of cancer development in obesity. *Nat. Rev. Cancer* **2011**, *11*, 886–895. [CrossRef]
15. Kim, M.Y.; An, S.; Shim, Y.S.; Lee, H.S.; Hwang, J.S. Waist-height ratio and body mass index as indicators of obesity and cardiometabolic risk in Korean children and adolescents. *Ann. Pediatr. Endocrinol. Metab.* **2024**, *29*, 182–190. [CrossRef] [PubMed] [PubMed Central]
16. Di Gioia, G.; Crispino, S.P.; Monosilio, S.; Maestrini, V.; Nenna, A.; Segreti, A.; Squeo, M.R.; Lemme, E.; Ussia, G.P.; Grigioni, F.; et al. Cardiovascular and metabolic effects of hyperbilirubinemia in a cohort of Italian Olympic athletes. *Scand. J. Med. Sci. Sports* **2023**, *33*, 2534–2547. [CrossRef] [PubMed]
17. Rochlani, Y.; Pothineni, N.V.; Kovelamudi, S.; Mehta, J.L. Metabolic syndrome: Pathophysiology, management, and modulation by natural compounds. *Ther. Adv. Cardiovasc. Dis.* **2017**, *11*, 215–225. [CrossRef] [PubMed] [PubMed Central]
18. Silveira Rossi, J.L.; Barbalho, S.M.; Reverete de Araujo, R.; Bechara, M.D.; Sloan, K.P.; Sloan, L.A. Metabolic syndrome and cardiovascular diseases: Going beyond traditional risk factors. *Diabetes Metab. Res. Rev.* **2022**, *38*, e3502. [CrossRef] [PubMed]
19. Kassi, E.; Pervanidou, P.; Kaltsas, G.; Chrousos, G. Metabolic syndrome: Definitions and controversies. *BMC Med.* **2011**, *9*, 48. [CrossRef] [PubMed] [PubMed Central]
20. Caro, J.; Navarro, I.; Romero, P.; Lorente, R.I.; Priego, M.A.; Martínez-Hervás, S.; Real, J.T.; Ascaso, J.F. Metabolic effects of regular physical exercise in healthy population. *Endocrinol. Nutr.* **2013**, *60*, 167–172. [CrossRef] [PubMed]
21. Shariful Islam, M.; Fardousi, A.; Sizear, M.I.; Rabbani, M.G.; Islam, R.; Saif-Ur-Rahman, K.M. Effect of leisure-time physical activity on blood pressure in people with hypertension: A systematic review and meta-analysis. *Sci. Rep.* **2023**, *13*, 10639. [CrossRef] [PubMed] [PubMed Central]
22. Joseph, M.S.; Tincopa, M.A.; Walden, P.; Jackson, E.; Conte, M.L.; Rubenfire, M. The Impact Of Structured Exercise Programs On Metabolic Syndrome And Its Components: A Systematic Review. *Diabetes Metab. Syndr. Obes.* **2019**, *12*, 2395–2404. [CrossRef] [PubMed] [PubMed Central]
23. Katzmarzyk, P.T.; Leon, A.S.; Wilmore, J.H.; Skinner, J.S.; Rao, D.C.; Rankinen, T.; Bouchard, C. Targeting the metabolic syndrome with exercise: Evidence from the HERITAGE Family Study. *Med. Sci. Sports Exerc.* **2003**, *35*, 1703–1709. [CrossRef] [PubMed]
24. Kaneva, A.M.; Bojko, E.R. Lipid accumulation product or lap as an up-to-date clinical biochemical marker of human obesity. *Health Risk Anal.* **2019**, *2019*, 164–174. [CrossRef]
25. Rotter, I.; Rył, A.; Szylińska, A.; Pawlukowska, W.; Lubkowska, A.; Laszczyńska, M. Lipid Accumulation Product (LAP) as an Index of Metabolic and Hormonal Disorders in Aging Men. *Exp. Clin. Endocrinol. Diabetes* **2017**, *125*, 176–182. [CrossRef] [PubMed]
26. Guo, S.X.; Zhang, X.H.; Zhang, J.Y.; He, J.; Yan, Y.Z.; Ma, J.L.; Ma, R.L.; Guo, H.; Mu, L.T.; Li, S.G.; et al. Visceral Adiposity and Anthropometric Indicators as Screening Tools of Metabolic Syndrome among Low Income Rural Adults in Xinjiang. *Sci. Rep.* **2016**, *6*, 36091. [CrossRef] [PubMed] [PubMed Central]

27. Lazzer, S.; D'Alleva, M.; Isola, M.; De Martino, M.; Caroli, D.; Bondesan, A.; Marra, A.; Sartorio, A. Cardiometabolic Index (CMI) and Visceral Adiposity Index (VAI) Highlight a Higher Risk of Metabolic Syndrome in Women with Severe Obesity. *J. Clin. Med.* **2023**, *12*, 3055. [CrossRef] [PubMed] [PubMed Central]
28. Celeski, M.; Di Gioia, G.; Nusca, A.; Segreti, A.; Squeo, M.R.; Lemme, E.; Mango, F.; Ferrera, A.; Ussia, G.P.; Grigioni, F. The Spectrum of Coronary Artery Disease in Elite Endurance Athletes-A Long-Standing Debate: State-of-the-Art Review. *J. Clin. Med.* **2024**, *13*, 5144. [CrossRef] [PubMed] [PubMed Central]
29. Alipour, P.; Azizi, Z.; Raparelli, V.; Norris, C.M.; Kautzky-Willer, A.; Kublickiene, K.; Herrero, M.T.; Emam, K.E.; Vollenweider, P.; Preisig, M.; et al. Role of sex and gender-related variables in development of metabolic syndrome: A prospective cohort study. *Eur. J. Intern. Med.* **2024**, *121*, 63–75. [CrossRef] [PubMed]
30. Ziaei, S.; Mohseni, H. Correlation between Hormonal Statuses and Metabolic Syndrome in Postmenopausal Women. *J. Fam. Reprod. Health* **2013**, *7*, 63–66. [PubMed] [PubMed Central]
31. Jamka, M.; Makarewicz-Bukowska, A.; Bokayeva, K.; Śmidowicz, A.; Geltz, J.; Kokot, M.; Kaczmarek, N.; Żok, A.; Kononets, V.; Cielecka-Piontek, J.; et al. Comparison of the Effect of Endurance, Strength and Endurance-Strength Training on Glucose and Insulin Homeostasis and the Lipid Profile of Overweight and Obese Subjects: A Systematic Review and Meta-Analysis. *Int. J. Environ. Res. Public Health* **2022**, *19*, 14928. [CrossRef] [PubMed] [PubMed Central]
32. Tamini, S.; Bondesan, A.; Caroli, D.; Sartorio, A. The Lipid Accumulation Product Index (LAP) and the Cardiometabolic Index (CMI) Are Useful for Predicting the Presence and Severity of Metabolic Syndrome in Adult Patients with Obesity. *J. Clin. Med.* **2024**, *13*, 2843. [CrossRef] [PubMed] [PubMed Central]
33. Radetti, G.; Fanolla, A.; Grugni, G.; Lupi, F.; Sartorio, A. Indexes of adiposity and body composition in the prediction of metabolic syndrome in obese children and adolescents: Which is the best? *Nutr. Metab. Cardiovasc. Dis.* **2019**, *29*, 1189–1196. [CrossRef] [PubMed]
34. Barazzoni, R.; Gortan Cappellari, G.; Semolic, A.; Ius, M.; Zanetti, M.; Gabrielli, A.; Vinci, P.; Guarnieri, G.; Simon, G. Central adiposity markers, plasma lipid profile and cardiometabolic risk prediction in overweight-obese individuals. *Clin. Nutr.* **2019**, *38*, 1171–1179. [CrossRef] [PubMed]
35. American Heart Association; National Heart, Lung, and Blood Institute; Grundy, S.M.; Cleeman, J.I.; Daniels, S.R.; Donato, K.A.; Eckel, R.H.; Franklin, B.A.; Gordon, D.J.; Krauss, R.M.; et al. Diagnosis and management of the metabolic syndrome. An American Heart Association/National Heart, Lung, and Blood Institute Scientific Statement. Executive summary. *Cardiol. Rev.* **2005**, *13*, 322–327. [CrossRef] [PubMed]
36. Bredella, M.A. Sex Differences in Body Composition. *Adv. Exp. Med. Biol.* **2017**, *1043*, 9–27. [CrossRef] [PubMed]
37. Dai, H.; Wang, W.; Chen, R.; Chen, Z.; Lu, Y.; Yuan, H. Lipid accumulation product is a powerful tool to predict non-alcoholic fatty liver disease in Chinese adults. *Nutr. Metab.* **2017**, *14*, 49. [CrossRef] [PubMed] [PubMed Central]
38. Duan, S.; Yang, D.; Xia, H.; Ren, Z.; Chen, J.; Yao, S. Cardiometabolic index: A new predictor for metabolic associated fatty liver disease in Chinese adults. *Front. Endocrinol.* **2022**, *13*, 1004855. [CrossRef] [PubMed] [PubMed Central]


**Disclaimer/Publisher's Note:** The statements, opinions and data contained in all publications are solely those of the individual author(s) and contributor(s) and not of MDPI and/or the editor(s). MDPI and/or the editor(s) disclaim responsibility for any injury to people or property resulting from any ideas, methods, instructions or products referred to in the content.

*life*

MDPI

*Review*

# The Impact of Diet on Lipoprotein(a) Levels

**Michał Stojko [1,*], Aleksandra Spychał [1], Kamil Nikel [1], Rafał Kołodziej [2] and Jolanta Zalejska-Fiolka [3]**

1 Scientific Society of the Department and Chair of Biochemistry, Faculty of Medical Sciences in Zabrze, Medical University of Silesia in Katowice, 40-055 Katowice, Poland; s81359@365.sum.edu.pl (A.S.); s79826@365.sum.edu.pl (K.N.)
2 Students Scientific Association, Department of Immunology, Faculty of Medical Science, University of Rzeszów, 35001 Rzeszów, Poland; rk112690@stud.ur.edu.pl
3 Department and Chair of Biochemistry, Faculty of Medical Sciences in Zabrze, Medical University of Silesia in Katowice, 40-055 Katowice, Poland; jzalejskafiolka@sum.edu.pl
* Correspondence: 83148@365.sum.edu.pl; Tel.: +48-792-477-772

**Abstract:** Background: Lipoprotein(a) [Lp(a)] is recognized as an independent risk factor for cardiovascular diseases; however, the impact of fat-based diets on its levels remains unclear. Objective: This study aims to assess and analyze current evidence on the impact of various types of fat-based diets on Lp(a) levels. Material and Methods: A comprehensive search of the PubMed database was conducted on 9 July 2024, focusing on clinical and randomized trials published since 2000. Out of 697 identified studies, 33 met the inclusion criteria and were selected for analysis. Results: The findings suggest that modifications in fat-based diets, particularly concerning the type and amount of consumed fats and fatty acids, can significantly influence plasma Lp(a) levels. Diets rich in unsaturated fats, including polyunsaturated and monounsaturated fatty acids, were associated with more favorable effects in lowering Lp(a) levels. In contrast, diets high in saturated fats were linked to elevated Lp(a) levels. However, these conclusions were not consistent across all studies considered. Conclusions: This work highlights the importance of a personalized dietary approach, considering both genetic predispositions and dietary habits. While diet alone may not drastically alter Lp(a) levels due to their strong genetic determination, a comprehensive strategy involving a healthy diet rich in unsaturated fats, regular physical activity, and effective weight management is recommended to reduce the risk of cardiovascular diseases. Further research is needed to clarify the mechanisms through which different fats affect Lp(a) and to develop targeted dietary recommendations.

**Keywords:** lipoprotein(a); diet; fats; lipids

## 1. Introduction

Lipoprotein(a) [Lp(a)] is a complex present in blood plasma, consisting of one LDL particle containing apoB-100 and a large, polymorphic glycoprotein apo(a). The LPA gene responsible for the production of Lp(a) is primarily transcribed in the liver [1]. Plasma Lp(a) concentrations exhibit significant individual variability and are inherited. Discovered by Kåre Berg in 1963, Lp(a) has attracted interest due to its association with atherosclerotic diseases, particularly coronary heart disease (CHD), despite its unclear physiological role [2].

One of the challenges in quantifying Lp(a) is the size polymorphism of apo(a). It is hypothesized that differences in apo(a) size may affect test results, depending on the assay used and its antibody specificity [3]. Despite diagnostic challenges, the fact remains that high Lp(a) levels impact cardiovascular risk (CVR). Epidemiological studies suggest that approximately 20% of the European population has high Lp(a) levels, which is also more common in individuals with familial hypercholesterolemia, further increasing CVR. Effective early treatment to reduce Lp(a) levels is crucial in lowering this risk [4].

Lp(a) also inhibits fibrinolysis, linking cholesterol transport with the coagulation system [5]. Studies also indicate the potential of Lp(a) as an acute-phase protein and its ability to carry oxidized phospholipids, which may contribute to atherosclerosis development [6,7]. This includes its mediation in monocyte adhesion and migration through interaction with β2-integrin Mac-1, which is key in the inflammatory process and plaque formation [8].

To date, several therapeutic options exist to lower Lp(a) levels in the blood [9]. Statins lower LDL cholesterol levels, but their effect on Lp(a) is variable. For example, ezetimibe reduces Lp(a) by about 7%, PCSK9 inhibitors by 23–25%, and mipomersen by 26.4% [10,11]. Other methods, such as microsomal triglyceride transfer protein inhibitors and cholesterol ester transfer protein inhibitors, niacin, and thyroid hormone mimetics, can reduce Lp(a) by 20–30% [12–14]. Aspirin may also lower Lp(a), particularly in individuals with high baseline levels [15]. Lipoprotein apheresis is the most effective, reducing Lp(a) by 60–90% [16]. However, therapy choice remains dependent on the individual characteristics of the patient [9].

For this reason, a detailed literature review was conducted to evaluate the impact of the least invasive method of changing plasma Lp(a) levels, namely dietary modification. This work compares how dietary changes may influence Lp(a) levels, which could be crucial in preventing cardiovascular events in individuals with high levels of this lipoprotein.

Dietary interventions can influence Lp(a) levels through several biological pathways. One key pathway is via alterations in hepatic lipid metabolism, as the liver is the primary site of Lp(a) production. Diets rich in unsaturated fats, particularly omega-3 fatty acids, may reduce Lp(a) synthesis by modulating transcription factors involved in lipid homeostasis, such as peroxisome proliferator-activated receptors (PPARs) and sterol regulatory element-binding proteins (SREBPs). Furthermore, diets high in fiber, especially soluble fiber, may improve bile acid excretion, leading to a compensatory increase in hepatic LDL receptor activity, which can lower circulating Lp(a) levels indirectly. Certain dietary patterns, like those rich in polyphenols, have been shown to reduce oxidative stress and inflammation, both of which are associated with increased Lp(a) levels. In contrast, diets high in saturated fats and trans fats can elevate Lp(a) by upregulating inflammatory pathways and LDL particle production, potentially increasing the hepatic secretion of Lp(a). Additionally, certain amino acids, like lysine, have been proposed to interfere with the binding of Lp(a) to fibrinogen, reducing its pro-atherogenic effects. Finally, alcohol consumption in moderate amounts has been shown to lower Lp(a) levels, possibly through enhanced clearance mechanisms, although the exact mechanisms remain under investigation.

## 2. Materials and Methods

Search Methods: The "PubMed" database was searched. As of 9 July 2024, entering the keywords "lipoprotein (a), diet" into the PubMed search engine yielded 697 results, of which 128 remained after narrowing down to research studies. Ultimately, 33 studies were included in the review. The time criteria included studies published from 2000 to the date of the search. There were no restrictions on the publication status regarding entries in the registry.

Objectives: The objective of this study was to analyze and evaluate current evidence on the effects of various fat-based diets on Lp(a) levels.

Selection Criteria: This review included clinical and randomized controlled trials involving humans. Only English-language studies were considered. Studies that ambiguously demonstrated the effect of diet on Lp(a), lacked lipid fractionation, including the separation of Lp(a), or involved changes in pharmacological treatment during the study period were excluded.

Main Results: The review included 33 records of varying quality and sample size. The selected studies are research papers that are statistically significant and directly related to the topic of the impact of diet on Lp(a) levels. An additional 7 studies were included to supplement the review with information provided in the introduction. The results are shown in the PRISMA diagram (Figure 1).

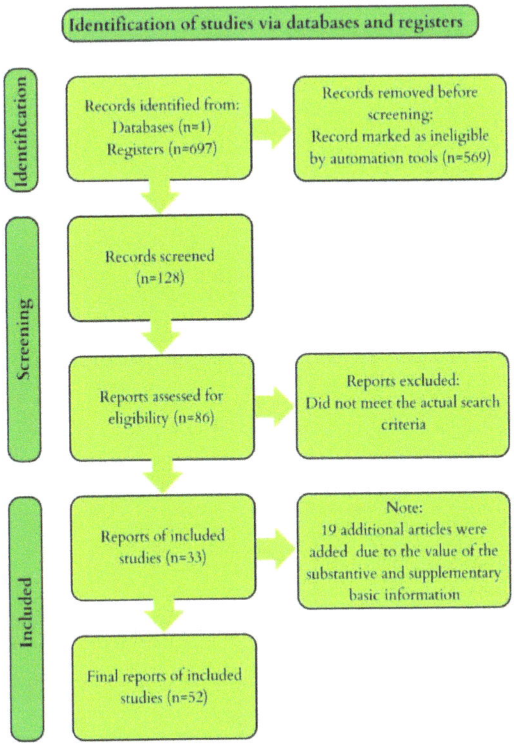


**Figure 1.** The results of our research visualized in the PRISMA diagram.

## 3. Results

The results we collected are presented in the form of a table (Table 1) with detailed descriptions of all studies included in the review.

**Table 1.** Publications Investigating the Impact of Diet on Lp(a) Levels.

| Authors and Year of Publication | Study Population | Dietary Interventions | Conclusions |
|---|---|---|---|
| H.G. Prawo et al., 2023, [17] | A total of 166 African American individuals aged 18–65 years, without comorbidities. | Diet 1—similar to the average American diet, Diet 2—with lower levels of total fat (25% of energy intake) and saturated fats (6% of energy intake). Carbohydrates were mainly derived from fruits and vegetables. Duration: 12 weeks. | Reducing saturated fatty acid intake significantly increased Lp(a) levels while simultaneously decreasing LDL-C. |
| J.M. Delgado-Alarcón et al., 2020, [18] | A total of 66 women at risk of cardiovascular disease. | Participants were randomly assigned to three groups, each consuming the following for breakfast for 30 days: Group A: breakfast rich in polyunsaturated fatty acids (PUFA); Group B: breakfast rich in saturated fatty acids (SFA); Group C: breakfast rich in monounsaturated fatty acids (MUFA) | Breakfast rich in PUFA or MUFA reduced Lp(a) levels. |
| A.M. Tindall et al., 2020, [19] | A total of 34 individuals at risk of cardiovascular disease, including 62% men, average age 44 ± 10 years, with BMI 30.1 ± 4.9 kg/m$^2$. | Participants underwent three different diets in random order, each lasting 6 weeks: nut diet: 57–99 g/d walnuts, 7% SFA, 16% PUFA, 9% MUFA. Fat-adjusted nut diet: 7% SFA, 16% PUFA, 9% MUFA. Oleic acid diet replaces α-linolenic acid diet: 7% SFA, 14% PUFA, 12% MUFA. | Lp(a) did not change with any of the diets. |

**Table 1.** *Cont.*

| Authors and Year of Publication | Study Population | Dietary Interventions | Conclusions |
|---|---|---|---|
| W. Stonehouse et al., 2019, [20] | A total of 38 healthy participants aged 20–40 years. | Participants underwent three different diets in random order, each lasting 4 weeks: palm olein: rich in SFA with unsaturated fatty acids cocoa butter: rich in SFA with unsaturated fatty acids olive oil: unsaturated fatty acids | No significant differences between diets concerning Lp(a). |
| A.A. Hashemzadeh et al., 2017, [21] | A total of 60 patients with overweight, type 2 diabetes, and coronary artery disease. | Participants were randomly assigned to two groups. The study group received 1000 mg of n−3 fatty acids from flaxseed oil, containing 400 mg α-linolenic acid (ALA, 18:3n−3), twice daily for 12 weeks. The control group received a placebo. | Flaxseed oil supplementation significantly reduced Lp(a) gene expression in peripheral blood mononuclear cells compared to the placebo group. |
| C. Bamberger et al., 2017, [22] | A total of 194 healthy individuals, average age 63 ± 7 years, with BMI of 25.1 ± 4.0 kg/m$^2$. | Participants underwent two 8-week dietary periods: (1) diet enriched with 43 g of walnuts daily (saturated fats) and reduced fat and carbohydrate intake; (2) diet without walnuts. | Walnut consumption had no significant impact on Lp(a) levels. |
| D. Iggman et al., 2011, [23] | A total of 20 individuals with hypercholesterolemia. | The study assessed the impact of canola oil, a source of unsaturated fatty acids, on lipid profiles compared to a dairy-based diet rich in saturated fatty acids. Participants followed two different diets for two 3-week periods: saturated fat diet from dairy products (DF); diet with fat based on canola oil (RO). Both diets were isocaloric and differed only in fat composition. | RO diet slightly increased Lp(a) levels by 6% (P = 0.05). |
| S. Gulati et al., 2017, [24] | A total of 50 individuals aged 25–70 with type 2 diabetes, taking stable doses of metformin, with HbA1c < 9% and LDL-c ≥ 100 mg/dl. | Patients underwent a 3-week control diet and exercise period, followed by a 24-week period consuming raw almonds (MUFA and PUFA) making up 20% of daily energy intake, replacing fats and a portion of carbohydrates. | Changes in Lp(a) levels did not reach statistical significance. |
| R. Loganathan et al., 2022, [25] | A total of 40 healthy individuals aged 20–50 years. | Participants were randomly assigned to one of three groups, each receiving baked goods enriched with unsaturated fatty acids (brownies for breakfast and cookies for a snack) prepared with: (1) palm olein, (2) cocoa butter, (3) extra virgin olive oil. | No significant differences in Lp(a) between the different diets. |
| S. Vega-Lopez et al., 2006, [26] | A total of 15 volunteers aged ≥50 years with LDL cholesterol ≥130 mg/dL. | Participants consumed food based on one of four diets for 35 days per phase. The diets differed by type of fat: partially hydrogenated soybean oil, soybean oil, palm oil, or canola oil, with two-thirds of the fat coming from the respective oil, comprising 20% of the diet's energy. | No effect of the studied fats on Lp(a) in plasma. |
| A.H. Lichtenstein et al., 2006, [27] | A total of 30 individuals (16 women and 14 men) over 50 years old with moderate (LDL cholesterol > 130 mg/dl) hypercholesterolemia. | Participants consumed five different diets, each for 35 days in random order. The diets contained the same foods and provided 30% of energy from fat, with two-thirds from one of the following oils: soybean oil (SO), low SFA soybean oil (LoSFA-SO), high oleic soybean oil (HiOleic-SO), low ALA soybean oil (LoALA-SO), partially hydrogenated soybean oil (Hydrog-SO). | Consumption of the studied oils had no significant impact on Lp(a) levels in blood. |
| D. Zambón et al., 2000, [28] | A total of 55 individuals, average age 56 years with polygenic hypercholesterolemia. | Participants followed two different diets for 6 weeks each: Mediterranean diet and a diet with a similar energy and fat content, with walnuts replacing about 35% of energy from monounsaturated fats. | Reduction of Lp(a) by 6.2%, with a significant decrease observed only in men. |
| B. Vessby et al., 2001, [29] | A total of 162 healthy, randomly selected individuals. | The main goal was to check whether a diet rich in MUFA affects insulin sensitivity. Participants were divided into two groups, receiving isocaloric diets rich in saturated fats and monounsaturated fats. Additionally, participants were randomly assigned to subgroups supplementing with fish oil (3.6 g n−3 fatty acids daily) or placebo. | Consumption of a diet rich in MUFA increased Lp(a) by 12%. |

**Table 1.** *Cont.*

| Authors and Year of Publication | Study Population | Dietary Interventions | Conclusions |
|---|---|---|---|
| S. Vega-Lopez et al., 2009, [30] | A total of 30 postmenopausal women aged ≥50 years with LDL cholesterol ≥120 mg/dL. | Participants consumed diets enriched with two different fats for two periods of 35 days each: corn oil (control), partially hydrogenated soybean oil. Each diet included two-thirds of fat from the respective oil. All meals and drinks were provided to maintain stable body weight. | Corn oil diet, compared to partially hydrogenated soybean oil diet, lowered Lp(a) levels. |
| S. Jaranam et al., 2001, [31] | A total of 23 healthy participants, average age 38 years. | In a double-blind, randomized controlled trial, the effect of a diet rich in pecans (unsaturated fats) on lipid profiles was compared. Participants were randomly assigned to a diet containing 28.3% energy from fat or a diet enriched with pecans. Participants replaced 20% of calories from Step I diet with pecans. | A diet enriched with pecans led to a significant decrease in Lp(a) levels. |
| D.J.A. Jenkins et al., 2002 [32] | 27 men and women with hypercholesterolemia | In a randomized crossover trial, the effect of consuming almonds (unsaturated fat) as a snack was compared with low-fat (<5% energy) whole-grain muffins as a control group, participants consumed an isocaloric diet for 1 month | Lp(a) concentration decreased significantly (7.8 ± 3.5%, P = 0.034) |
| J.F. Ruisinger et al., 2015 [33] | 48 people who received a stable dose of a statin for years. | Subjects were randomly assigned to two groups: Almond (unsaturated fat) group (n = 22): addition of 100 g almonds per day to the diet and dietary advice consistent with the Third Assessment Report of the Adult Treatment Panel on Lifestyle Changes.<br>No almond group (n = 26): dietary advice only consistent with the Third Assessment Report of the Adult Treatment Panel on Lifestyle Changes. | No significant differences were observed in Lp(a) |
| J.M. Gaullier et al., 2004 [34] | 180 healthy overweight adults (BMI 25–30 kg/m$^2$) | Participants were randomly assigned to one of three groups for 12 months: linoleic acid (CLA)-free fatty acid (FFA) CLA-triacylglycerol Placebo (olive oil) | A statistically significant increase in Lp(a) was observed in the study groups. |
| J.M. Gaullier et al., 2005 [34] | The study included 134 of 157 participants who completed the initial 12-month study. All participants were healthy overweight adults. | In this study, all participants received 3.4 g of CLA daily as triglycerides for the next 12 months. | Conjugated linoleic acid supplementation for 24 months significantly increased blood Lp(a) concentration |
| T. Tholstrup et al., 2004 [35] | 16 healthy young men | The aim of the study was to investigate the effect of individual fatty acids on postprandial Lp(a) levels and its relationship with lipemia and tissue plasminogen activator (t-PA). Participants consumed meals containing the tested fats (1 g fat/kg body weight) after a 12-h fast. The tested fats were dominated by (approximately 43% g/kg) stearic (S), palmitic (P), oleic, C18:1 trans (T), or linoleic acid. The fats were administered on random days separated by 3-week washout periods. | After consuming meals containing the tested fats, a significant increase in Lp(a) concentration was observed, and the Lp(a) response was different depending on the type of fat.<br>T fat did not change Lp(a) concentration during the study.<br>No relationship was observed between Lp(a) and t-PA concentrations.<br>S and P saturated fats caused an increase in Lp(a), T fat showed a higher response to triacylglycerols (TAG) |
| C. Seidel et al., 2004 [36] | 31 people (15 women and 16 men), nine of whom had hypercholesterolemia | The aim of the study was to compare the effect of dairy products with modified milk fat (ModFat—reduced content of saturated fatty acids) with regular milk fat (RegFat) and soft margarine (Marg) on the concentration of cholesterol, TAG, Lp(a) in the blood of the subjects. The study lasted 13 weeks. | The lowest Lp(a) concentration was shown during the ModFat treatment period compared to other diets. |
| S.S. AbuMweis et al., 2006 [37] | 30 people with mild to moderate hypercholesterolemia | The study aimed to determine the effects of two novel plant sterol formulations on plasma lipids: plant sterols combined with fatty acids from fish oil or esterified to these fatty acids. Participants consumed the following formulations for 29 days as a single dose with a morning meal | None of the plant sterol preparations significantly changed Lp(a) concentration. |

**Table 1.** *Cont.*

| Authors and Year of Publication | Study Population | Dietary Interventions | Conclusions |
|---|---|---|---|
| Y.M. Chan et al., 2007 [38] | 21 moderately overweight individuals with hypercholesterolemia | Patients consumed three different treatment diets, each for 28 days, with 4-week washout periods between diets, in a randomized crossover design:<br>Diet containing olive oil (OO).<br>Diet containing plant sterols esterified to sunflower oil fatty acids (PS-SO).<br>Diet containing plant sterols esterified to olive oil fatty acids (PS-OO).<br>Each diet contained 30% energy from fat, of which 70% came from olive oil. PS-SO and PS-OO provided 1.7 g of plant sterols per day. | No differences in Lp(a) concentrations were observed between diets. However, Lp(a) concentrations increased after OO and PS-SO diets (P = 0.0050 and 0.0421, respectively). |
| A. Garoufi et al., 2014 [39] | 59 children aged 4.5 to 15.9 years, 25 of whom had an initial LDL-C level of 3.4 mmol/l (130 mg/dl) or higher and 34 had lower | Children with hypercholesterolemia received a yogurt drink enriched with 2 g of plant sterols daily for 6–12 months as an addition to their diet. After this period, participants' lipid profiles were reassessed. | Lp(a) concentration remained unchanged |
| M.B. Madsen, 2007 [40] | 6 people with mild hypercholesterolemia, mean age 50.6 ± 9.8 years | In the run-in period and two intervention periods, each lasting 4 weeks. The study products consisted of 20 g low-fat margarine (35% fat) and 250 ml low-fat milk (0.7% fat), providing a total of 2.3 g plant sterols per day. | Consumption of products enriched with plant sterols had no effect on Lp(a) concentration |
| Gebauer S.K. et al., 2015 [41] | 106 healthy adults, mean age: 47 ± 10.8 years,<br>BMI: 28.5 ± 4.0 kg/m$^2$,<br>LDL cholesterol: 3.24 ± 0.63 mmol/l | The study was a 24-day, double-blind, randomized, crossover feeding trial.<br>Control diet (0.1% mixed trans fatty acid (TFA))<br>Diet containing ~3% vaccenic acid (VA)<br>Diet containing ~3% industrially produced trans fatty acids (iTFA)<br>Diet containing 1% cis-9, trans-11 conjugated linoleic acid (c9,t11-CLA)<br>Dietary fat content: 34% energy | VA increased Lp(a) concentration compared to the control diet (2–6% change). The other diets did not significantly affect Lp(a) concentration. |
| S.H. Vermunt et al., 2001 [42] | 88 healthy men from three European countries: France, Scotland and The Netherlands. | In the study, participants were put on a diet with experimental oils purified from trans alpha-linolenic acid for 6 weeks. In the next stage (study period), participants were randomly assigned to a diet with a high content of trans alpha-linolenic acid (1410 mg per day) or a low content of these isomers. | No effect of a diet rich in trans-linolenic acid isomers on Lp(a) concentration was observed in the study group compared to a diet low in trans-linolenic acid isomers. |
| M. Pfeuffer et al., 2011 [43] | 85 overweight men (aged 45–68, BMI 25–35 kg/m$^2$) | 4-week, double-blind study. Participants were randomly assigned to one of four groups: 4.5 g/day of a mixture of conjugated linoleic acid (CLA), 4.5 g/day of safflower oil, 4.5 g/day of heated safflower oil, 4.5 g/day of olive oil (control group). | CLA consumption compared to safflower oil did not change Lp(a) concentration |
| M. Fito et al., 2014, [44] | 930 people at high risk of cardiovascular disease, including 420 men and 510 women | A multicenter, randomized, controlled, parallel-group clinical trial that lasted 6 months. The study patients were randomly assigned to three dietary intervention groups: control group (KT) (changes in current dietary habits), low-fat diet (LD) (reduction of total fat intake to <30% of total calories), and plant-rich diet (PD) (reduction of total fat intake to <30% of total calories and increased consumption of plants and dietary fiber) | Lp(a) concentration was significantly reduced in the PD group (mean decrease of 15%), compared to the KT group (no significant change) and the LD group (no significant change). |
| M.P. St-Onge et al., 2009 [45] | 45 study participants. Adult men and women aged 19–65 years, with LDL concentration in the range of 3.37–4.66 mmol/L | The nutritional study was divided into three phases, each lasting 25 days. Participants consumed three different diets that differed in the type of snacks: Low-fat diet (30.8% energy), Moderate-fat diet with saturated fat (37.9% energy from fat, including 11.4% energy from saturated fat), Moderate-fat diet with polyunsaturated fat (36.3% energy from fat, including 9.7% energy from polyunsaturated fat) | The high polyunsaturated fat diet increased Lp(a) in all groups. The low-fat diet decreased Lp(a) in all groups. Participants with low and intermediate baseline CRP had greater decreases in Lp(a) than those with high baseline CRP with the low-fat diet. |

**Table 1.** *Cont.*

| Authors and Year of Publication | Study Population | Dietary Interventions | Conclusions |
| --- | --- | --- | --- |
| M. Ohman et al., 2008 [46] | 19 healthy volunteers | The study aimed to evaluate the effect of omega-3 enriched eggs on the lipid profile of volunteers. Participants consumed one additional egg per day: a standard egg or an egg enriched with omega-3 fatty acids. Each period lasted 1 month. | No significant changes in Lp(a) concentration were observed |
| U. Hoppu et al., 2013 [47] | 256 mothers in the first trimester of pregnancy. The number of mothers and their children participating in the study decreased in the following years. Finally, 127 mothers and their children participated in the study by the end of the four-year follow-up period. | Dietary counseling was provided to mothers during pregnancy and breastfeeding. The infants were monitored with 3-day dietary records. Participants were randomly assigned to three groups: diet/probiotics, diet/placebo, and control/placebo. The probiotics included Lactobacillus rhamnosus GG and Bifidobacterium lactis. The study lasted 4 years. Dietary counseling focused on reducing the intake of saturated fatty acids (SFA) and increasing monounsaturated (MUFA) and polyunsaturated (PUFA) | Lp(a) levels increased from baseline to year 4, with mean values increasing from 22.6 mg/dL to 28.6 mg/dL |
| P.T. Voon et al., 2011 [48] | 45 healthy Malaysian adults (9 men, 36 women) | The study examined the effects of a Malaysian high-protein diet prepared with 3 different fats on CVD risk markers in the blood. in 3 dietary periods, each lasting 5 weeks. Participants consumed three different diets in which fats accounted for two-thirds of the 30% of calories from fat: a diet containing palm olein (PO) rich in palmitate (palmitic acid, 16:0), a diet containing coconut oil (CO) rich in lauric acid (12:0) and myristic acid (14:0), and a diet containing olive oil (OO) rich in oleic acid (18:1). | The CO diet reduced postprandial Lp(a) concentration (postprandial concentration in the CO diet 1.31 +/− 6 1.11 mmol/L vs 1.42 in PO and 1.41 in OO) in contrast to the PO and OO diets. |

## 4. Discussion

Research on the impact of different types of diets on Lp(a) levels has shown effects dependent on the type of fat. In the context of dietary interventions that may affect Lp(a) levels, it is crucial to consider both the amount and type of fats consumed. Literature examples indicate varying effects of different types of fats. For instance, H.G. Prawo et al., using a diet with reduced total fat and SFA for 12 weeks, observed an increase in Lp(a) levels while simultaneously reducing LDL-C. Similarly, in the study by M.P. St-Onge et al., involving 45 participants over three phases lasting 25 days each, a diet rich in PUFA led to an increase in Lp(a), while a low-fat diet decreased Lp(a) levels. On the other hand, U. Hoppu et al. observed a gradual increase in Lp(a) from the beginning of the study to the fourth year in 127 mothers and their children with reduced SFA intake and increased MUFA and PUFA intake. It is possible that the increase in Lp(a) in this research may be related to other long-term changes in the body that are not directly linked to diet [17,45,47].

Delgado-Alarcón et al. compared the impact of three different breakfasts on Lp(a) levels over a month, finding that meals rich in PUFA and MUFA led to significant reductions of Lp(a). In contrast, the 6-week study by A.M. Tindall et al., with similar diets, did not show changes in Lp(a) levels, although the sample size was about half as large (34 people). Similarly, W. Stonehouse et al. found no change in Lp(a) in a study with a similar number of participants and diets. Likewise, S. Gulati et al., in a 24-week period enriched with MUFA and PUFA, did not achieve statistically significant changes in Lp(a). The studies by R. Loganathan et al., S. Vega-Lopez et al., and A.H. Lichtenstein et al. also did not observe significant differences in Lp(a) between different diets enriched with unsaturated fatty acids [18–20,24–27].

The study by S. Vega-Lopez et al. with 30 participants tested a diet enriched with partially hydrogenated soybean oil, which led to a decrease in Lp(a). Soybean oil is primarily a source of PUFA but also contains MUFA and saturated fats [49]. In a larger group (124 people), C. Bamberger et al.'s 8-week study found no significant impact of walnut-enriched diets on Lp(a) levels. Walnuts are rich in various types of fats, including

MUFA and PUFA and a small amount of saturated fats [50], making them a focus of interest as a dietary addition. Similarly, pecans, which have a higher MUFA content compared to PUFA, were included in the diet in the study by S. Jaranam et al. and led to a decrease in Lp(a). A decrease in Lp(a) was also observed in the study by D.J.A. Jenkins et al. with almond supplementation, which is mainly a source of monounsaturated fats, while the same dietary addition in J.F. Ruisinger et al.'s study did not result in significant differences in Lp(a) [21,31–33].

A small group of 20 participants in D. Iggman's study examined the effect of canola oil, a source of unsaturated fatty acids, on lipid profiles compared to a dairy-based diet rich in saturated fatty acids. The canola oil diet increased Lp(a) levels. In a study with 162 participants, B. Vessby et al. found that consuming a diet rich in MUFA increased Lp(a) by 12%, although trans fats were at the same level across all tested diets. Conversely, D. Zambón et al. demonstrated a reduction of Lp(a) with a diet supplemented with monounsaturated fats over 6 weeks, with significant decreases observed only in men. Supplementation with flaxseed oil significantly reduced Lp(a) gene expression in peripheral blood mononuclear cells compared to the placebo group in the study by A.A. Hashemzadeh et al. Flaxseed oil is a rich source of fats, particularly PUFA [21,23,28,29].

J.M. Gaullier et al. studied the impact of linoleic acid, free fatty acids, and triglycerides at different concentrations in diets with 180 overweight adults, observing a significant increase in Lp(a). The following year, the same authors published a study where 134 participants from the first study received 3.4 g of linoleic acid daily for another year, which significantly increased Lp(a) after 24 months [34].

In the study by Gebauer S.K. et al. with 106 healthy adults over 24 days, diets with vascenic acid, industrially produced trans fatty acids, and conjugated linoleic acid cis-9, trans-11 (c9,t11-CLA) showed a change only with vascenic acid (increasing Lp(a)). In the study by S.H. Vermunt et al., neither a diet high in trans isomers of alpha-linolenic acid nor a low one showed changes in Lp(a). Similarly, in M. Pfeuffer et al.'s study, including safflower oil, showed no changes. The study by M. Ohman et al. on omega-3 fatty acid supplementation also showed no changes in Lp(a). Participants in P.T. Voon et al.'s study consumed three different diets over 5 weeks, where fats constituted two-thirds of 30% of calories from fat, and only the diet containing coconut oil reduced postprandial Lp(a). This is because long-chain SFA increases postprandial Lp(a), but coconut oil contains shorter-chain fatty acids that lower postprandial Lp(a) [41–43,46,48].

The study by T. Tholstrup et al. with 16 healthy men consuming meals with 1 g of fat (mainly saturated) per kg of body weight after a 12 h fast, including stearic and palmitic acids, led to elevated Lp(a) levels. In contrast, the study by C. Seidel et al. with 15 women and 16 men showed that a diet with reduced saturated fatty acids over 13 weeks resulted in the lowest Lp(a) levels compared to standard diets.

It is also worth noting the variability in the results obtained by researchers. When analyzing the available data, it should be emphasized that some studies were based on smaller sample sizes or were of variable quality, which could have affected the reliability and clarity of the results [35,36].

Some studies focused on phytosterols, natural compounds present in various plant parts. The average person consumes 100–400 mg of phytosterols daily, mainly from vegetable oils, bread, cereals, nuts, and vegetables. Due to their cholesterol-like structure, they compete with cholesterol in the intestine, reducing its absorption and lowering LDL-C levels in plasma [51,52]. However, studies by S.S. AbuMweis et al., Y.M. Chan et al., A. Garoufi et al., and M.B. Madsen did not show an impact on Lp(a) levels with phytosterol-enriched diets. In contrast, J.M.M. Fito et al. found a significant reduction of Lp(a) after 6 months of a plant-rich diet among 930 individuals with high CVD risk [37–39,44].

Research has demonstrated that the type of fat in the diet can influence Lp(a) levels. Diets high in SFA generally increase Lp(a) levels, whereas reducing SFA in the diet sometimes leads to an increase in Lp(a) levels but more commonly results in a reduction of LDL-C without affecting Lp(a). Diets rich in MUFA and PUFA can have varying effects. Increasing

MUFA in the diet may either increase or decrease Lp(a) levels, depending on whether it is the sole dietary supplement and the percentage of fats in the diet as well as the duration of the intervention. Similarly, PUFA can affect Lp(a) in different ways. Some studies show an increase in Lp(a) with PUFA-rich diets, while others show a decrease. Reducing SFA intake and increasing MUFA and PUFA can have a beneficial impact on the overall lipid profile, though the effect on Lp(a) may vary. The diversity in the effects of SFA, MUFA, and PUFA on Lp(a) levels results from genetics, metabolism, diet composition, and the specific characteristics of each fat. Each of these variables can influence study outcomes and the body's response. Lifestyle and physical activity can also significantly influence Lp(a) levels. Regular physical activity contributes to improving the lipid profile, which can lead to a reduction of Lp(a) levels by decreasing inflammation and enhancing lipid metabolism. Conversely, lifestyle factors such as smoking, excessive alcohol consumption, and obesity can raise Lp(a) levels and increase the risk of cardiovascular diseases. This phenomenon is associated with hormonal and metabolic changes, as well as the development of chronic inflammation, which can stimulate Lp(a) production and lead to disturbances in lipid metabolism. An important topic to address is the adaptation of the diet to demographic and genetic profiles. Dietary interventions must be tailored to genetic and demographic profiles, as responses to dietary changes vary between individuals. For example, people with familial hypercholesterolemia or certain ethnic groups may metabolize fats differently, requiring a more targeted approach. Personalized nutrition, which takes into account genotype and ethnic background, allows for better control of Lp(a) levels and other lipids, potentially reducing the risk of cardiovascular diseases more effectively.

Coconut oil: containing short-chain fatty acids, coconut oil may lower postprandial Lp(a). Nuts and seeds: dietary supplementation with nuts, such as almonds, pecans, or walnuts, may contribute to lowering Lp(a) levels. Flaxseed oil: flaxseed oil has been shown to reduce Lp(a) gene expression, which could be beneficial for individuals with high levels of this lipoprotein. Limiting trans fats: trans fats, such as vascenic acid, increase Lp(a) levels, so their elimination from the diet is beneficial. The impact of dietary fats on lipid levels is variable. Generally, increasing dietary cholesterol raises LDL-C levels, but individual responses can differ. Current dietary guidelines recommend consuming a high amount of vegetables, fruits, legumes, nuts, whole grains, and fish, replacing SFA with MUFA and PUFA, reducing cholesterol intake, avoiding processed meats, refined carbohydrates, and sugary drinks, and eliminating trans fats.

## 5. Summary

Elevated Lp(a) levels are a genetically regulated, independent CVD risk factor. However, variability in Lp(a) levels among individuals and population groups also suggests a role for non-genetic factors. Diets with lower saturated fat content have a moderate impact on Lp(a) levels, usually increasing them, in contrast to LDL cholesterol, which decreases. Diets rich in MUFA and PUFA can either decrease or increase Lp(a) depending on the diet duration, fat content percentage, and supplements used.

Research shows that the effect of diet on Lp(a) levels is variable; however, a common trend is the claim that adopting a diet rich in vegetables, fruits, legumes, nuts, whole grains, and fish, replacing SFA with MUFA and PUFA, reducing cholesterol intake, and avoiding trans fats may benefit the overall lipid profile and cardiovascular health. Nevertheless, this subject requires further study to draw firm conclusions and establish recommendations for controlling Lp(a) levels.

**Author Contributions:** Conceptualization, M.S. and A.S.; methodology, K.N.; software, R.K.; validation, M.S., A.S. and J.Z.-F.; formal analysis, J.Z.-F.; investigation, R.K.; resources, M.S.; data curation, M.S.; writing—original draft preparation, K.N.; writing—review and editing, R.K.; visualization, K.N.; supervision, J.Z.-F.; project administration, M.S.; funding acquisition, A.S. All authors have read and agreed to the published version of the manuscript.

**Funding:** This research received no external funding.

Conflicts of Interest: The authors declare no conflicts of interest.

## References


1. Jawi, M.M.; Frohlich, J.; Chan, S.Y. Lipoprotein(a) the Insurgent: A New Insight into the Structure, Function, Metabolism, Pathogenicity, and Medications Affecting Lipoprotein(a) Molecule. *J. Lipids* **2020**, *2020*, e3491764. [CrossRef] [PubMed]
2. Sandholzer, C.; Hallman, D.M.; Saha, N.; Sigurdsson, G.; Lackner, C.; Császár, A.; Boerwinkle, E.; Utermann, G. Effects of the apolipoprotein(a) size polymorphism on the lipoprotein(a) concentration in 7 ethnic groups. *Hum. Genet.* **1991**, *86*, 607–614. [CrossRef] [PubMed]
3. Vinci, P.; Di Girolamo, F.G.; Panizon, E.; Tosoni, L.M.; Cerrato, C.; Pellicori, F.; Altamura, N.; Pirulli, A.; Zaccari, M.; Biasinutto, C.; et al. Lipoprotein(a) as a Risk Factor for Cardiovascular Diseases: Pathophysiology and Treatment Perspectives. *Int. J. Environ. Res. Public Health* **2023**, *20*, 6721. [CrossRef] [PubMed]
4. Kronenberg, F.; Mora, S.; Stroes, E.S.G. Consensus and guidelines on lipoprotein(a)—Seeing the forest through the trees. *Curr. Opin. Infect. Dis.* **2022**, *33*, 342–352. [CrossRef]
5. Nordestgaard, B.G.; Chapman, M.J.; Ray, K.; Borén, J.; Andreotti, F.; Watts, G.F.; Ginsberg, H.; Amarenco, P.; Catapano, A.; Descamps, O.S.; et al. Lipoprotein(a) as a cardiovascular risk factor: Current status. *Eur. Heart J.* **2010**, *31*, 2844–2853. [CrossRef]
6. Schmidt, K.; Noureen, A.; Kronenberg, F.; Utermann, G. Structure, function, and genetics of lipoprotein (a). *J. Lipid Res.* **2016**, *57*, 1339–1359. [CrossRef]
7. McCormick, S.P.A. Lipoprotein(a): Biology and Clinical Importance. *Clin. Biochem. Rev.* **2004**, *25*, 69–80.
8. Sotiriou, S.N.; Orlova, V.V.; Al-Fakhri, N.; Ihanus, E.; Economopoulou, M.; Isermann, B.; Bdeir, K.; Nawroth, P.P.; Preissner, K.T.; Gahmberg, C.G.; et al. Lipoprotein(a) in atherosclerotic plaques recruits inflammatory cells through interaction with Mac-1 integrin. *FASEB J.* **2006**, *20*, 559–561. [CrossRef]
9. Paragh, G.; Zilahi, P.; Kolozsvári, L.R.; Lőrincz, H.; Fülöp, P.; Harangi, M. Novel Therapeutic Approaches for the Management of Elevated Lipoprotein(a): From Traditional Agents to Future Treatment Options. *Life* **2024**, *14*, 374. [CrossRef]
10. Awad, K.; Mikhailidis, D.P.; Katsiki, N.; Muntner, P.; Banach, M. Effect of Ezetimibe Monotherapy on Plasma Lipoprotein(a) Concentrations in Patients with Primary Hypercholesterolemia: A Systematic Review and Meta-Analysis of Randomized Controlled Trials. *Drugs* **2018**, *78*, 453–462. [CrossRef]
11. Santos, R.D.; Raal, F.J.; Catapano, A.L.; Witztum, J.L.; Steinhagen-Thiessen, E.; Tsimikas, S. Mipomersen, an Antisense Oligonucleotide to Apolipoprotein B-100, Reduces Lipoprotein(a) in Various Populations with Hypercholesterolemia. *Arterioscler. Thromb. Vasc. Biol.* **2015**, *35*, 689–699. [CrossRef] [PubMed]
12. Sahebkar, A.; Reiner, Ž.; Simental-Mendía, L.E.; Ferretti, G.; Cicero, A.F.G. Effect of extended-release niacin on plasma lipoprotein(a) levels: A systematic review and meta-analysis of randomized placebo-controlled trials. *Metabolism* **2016**, *65*, 1664–1678. [CrossRef] [PubMed]
13. Samaha, F.F.; McKenney, J.M.; Bloedon, L.T.; Sasiela, W.J.; Rader, D.J. Inhibition of microsomal triglyceride transfer protein alone or with ezetimibe in patients with moderate hypercholesterolemia. *Nat. Clin. Pract. Cardiovasc. Med.* **2008**, *5*, 497–505. [CrossRef] [PubMed]
14. Grover, G.J.; Egan, D.M.; Sleph, P.G.; Beehler, B.C.; Chiellini, G.; Nguyen, N.-H.; Baxter, J.D.; Scanlan, T.S. Effects of the Thyroid Hormone Receptor Agonist GC-1 on Metabolic Rate and Cholesterol in Rats and Primates: Selective Actions Relative to 3,5,3′-Triiodo-l-Thyronine. *Endocrinology* **2004**, *145*, 1656–1661. [CrossRef] [PubMed]
15. Akaike, M.; Azuma, H.; Kagawa, A.; Matsumoto, K.; Hayashi, I.; Tamura, K.; Nishiuchi, T.; Iuchi, T.; Takamori, N.; Aihara, K.-I.; et al. Effect of Aspirin Treatment on Serum Concentrations of Lipoprotein(a) in Patients with Atherosclerotic Diseases. *Clin. Chem.* **2002**, *48*, 1454–1459. [CrossRef]
16. Korneva, V.A.; Kuznetsova, T.Y.; Julius, U. Modern Approaches to Lower Lipoprotein(a) Concentrations and Consequences for Cardiovascular Diseases. *Biomedicines* **2021**, *9*, 1271. [CrossRef]
17. Law, H.G.; Khan, M.A.; Zhang, W.; Bang, H.; Rood, J.; Most, M.; Lefevre, M.; Berglund, L.; Enkhmaa, B. Reducing saturated fat intake lowers LDL-C but increases Lp(a) levels in African Americans: The GET-READI feeding trial. *J. Lipid Res.* **2023**, *64*, 100420. [CrossRef]
18. Delgado-Alarcón, J.M.; Hernández Morante, J.J.; Aviles, F.V.; Albaladejo-Otón, M.D.; Morillas-Ruíz, J.M. Effect of the Fat Eaten at Breakfast on Lipid Metabolism: A Crossover Trial in Women with Cardiovascular Risk. *Nutrients* **2020**, *12*, 1695. [CrossRef]
19. Tindall, A.M.; Kris-Etherton, P.M.; Petersen, K.S. Replacing Saturated Fats with Unsaturated Fats from Walnuts or Vegetable Oils Lowers Atherogenic Lipoprotein Classes Without Increasing Lipoprotein(a). *J. Nutr.* **2020**, *150*, 818–825. [CrossRef]
20. Stonehouse, W.; Benassi-Evans, B.; James-Martin, G.; Abeywardena, M. Fatty acid regio-specificity of triacylglycerol molecules may affect plasma lipid responses to dietary fats—A randomised controlled cross-over trial. *Eur. J. Clin. Nutr.* **2019**, *74*, 268–277. [CrossRef]
21. Hashemzadeh, A.A.; Nasoohi, N.; Raygan, F.; Aghadavod, E.; Akbari, E.; Taghizadeh, M.; Memarzadeh, M.R.; Asemi, Z. Flaxseed Oil Supplementation Improve Gene Expression Levels of PPAR-$\gamma$, LP(a), IL-1 and TNF-$\alpha$ in Type 2 Diabetic Patients with Coronary Heart Disease. *Lipids* **2017**, *52*, 907–915. [CrossRef] [PubMed]
22. Bamberger, C.; Rossmeier, A.; Lechner, K.; Wu, L.; Waldmann, E.; Stark, R.G.; Altenhofer, J.; Henze, K.; Parhofer, K.G. A Walnut-Enriched Diet Reduces Lipids in Healthy Caucasian Subjects, Independent of Recommended Macronutrient Replacement and Time Point of Consumption: A Prospective, Randomized, Controlled Trial. *Nutrients* **2017**, *9*, 1097. [CrossRef] [PubMed]

23. Iggman, D.; Gustafsson, I.B.; Berglund, L.; Vessby, B.; Marckmann, P.; Risérus, U. Replacing dairy fat with rapeseed oil causes rapid improvement of hyperlipidaemia: A randomized controlled study. *J. Intern. Med.* **2011**, *270*, 356–364. [CrossRef] [PubMed]
24. Gulati, S.; Misra, A.; Pandey, R.M. Effect of Almond Supplementation on Glycemia and Cardiovascular Risk Factors in Asian Indians in North India with Type 2 Diabetes Mellitus: A 24-Week Study. *Metab. Syndr. Relat. Disord.* **2017**, *15*, 98–105. [CrossRef] [PubMed]
25. Loganathan, R.; Nagapan, G.; Teng, K.T.; Voon, P.T.; Yap, S.Y.; Ng, Y.T.; Ng, T.K.; Choo, Y.M.; Ong, A.S.; Ong, S.H.; et al. Diets enriched with palm olein, cocoa butter and extra virgin olive oil exhibited similar lipid response: A randomized controlled study in young healthy adults. *Nutr. Res.* **2022**, *105*, 113–125. [CrossRef]
26. Vega-López, S.; Ausman, L.M.; Jalbert, S.M.; Erkkilä, A.T.; Lichtenstein, A.H. Palm and partially hydrogenated soybean oils adversely alter lipoprotein profiles compared with soybean and canola oils in moderately hyperlipidemic subjects. *Am. J. Clin. Nutr.* **2006**, *84*, 54–62. [CrossRef]
27. Lichtenstein, A.H.; Matthan, N.R.; Jalbert, S.M.; Resteghini, N.A.; Schaefer, E.J.; Ausman, L.M. Novel soybean oils with different fatty acid profiles alter cardiovascular disease risk factors in moderately hyperlipidemic subjects. *Am. J. Clin. Nutr.* **2006**, *84*, 497–504. [CrossRef]
28. Zambón, D.; Sabaté, J.; Munoz, S.; Campero, B.; Casals, E.; Merlos, M.; Laguna, J.C.; Ros, E. Substituting Walnuts for Monounsaturated Fat Improves the Serum Lipid Profile of Hypercholesterolemic Men and Women. *Ann. Intern. Med.* **2000**, *132*, 538. [CrossRef]
29. Vessby, B.; Uusitupa, M.; Hermansen, K.; Riccardi, G.; Rivellese, A.A.; Tapsell, L.C.; Nälsén, C.; Berglund, L.; Louheranta, A.; Rasmussen, B.M.; et al. Substituting Dietary Saturated for Monounsaturated Fat Impairs Insulin Sensitivity in Healthy Men and Women: The KANWU Study. *Diabetologia* **2001**, *44*, 312–319. [CrossRef]
30. Vega-López, S.; Matthan, N.R.; Ausman, L.M.; Ai, M.; Otokozawa, S.; Schaefer, E.J.; Lichtenstein, A.H. Substitution of vegetable oil for a partially-hydrogenated fat favorably alters cardiovascular disease risk factors in moderately hypercholesterolemic postmenopausal women. *Atherosclerosis* **2009**, *207*, 208–212. [CrossRef]
31. Rajaram, S.; Burke, K.; Connell, B.; Myint, T.; Sabaté, J. A Monounsaturated Fatty Acid–Rich Pecan-Enriched Diet Favorably Alters the Serum Lipid Profile of Healthy Men and Women. *J. Nutr.* **2001**, *131*, 2275–2279. [CrossRef] [PubMed]
32. Jenkins, D.J.; Kendall, C.W.; Marchie, A.; Parker, T.L.; Connelly, P.W.; Qian, W.; Haight, J.S.; Faulkner, D.; Vidgen, E.; Lapsley, K.G.; et al. Dose Response of Almonds on Coronary Heart Disease Risk Factors: Blood Lipids, Oxidized Low-Density Lipoproteins, Lipoprotein(a), Homocysteine, and Pulmonary Nitric Oxide. *Circulation* **2002**, *106*, 1327–1332. [CrossRef] [PubMed]
33. Ruisinger, J.F.; Gibson, C.A.; Backes, J.M.; Smith, B.K.; Sullivan, D.K.; Moriarty, P.M.; Kris-Etherton, P. Statins and almonds to lower lipoproteins (the STALL Study). *J. Clin. Lipidol.* **2015**, *9*, 58–64. [CrossRef] [PubMed]
34. Gaullier, J.-M.; Halse, J.; Høye, K.; Kristiansen, K.; Fagertun, H.; Vik, H.; Gudmundsen, O. Conjugated linoleic acid supplementation for 1 y reduces body fat mass in healthy overweight humans. *Am. J. Clin. Nutr.* **2004**, *79*, 1118–1125. [CrossRef] [PubMed]
35. Tholstrup, T.; Samman, S. Postprandial Lipoprotein(a) Is Affected Differently by Specific Individual Dietary Fatty Acids in Healthy Young Men. *J. Nutr.* **2004**, *134*, 2550–2555. [CrossRef]
36. Seidel, C.; Deufel, T.; Jahreis, G. Effects of Fat-Modified Dairy Products on Blood Lipids in Humans in Comparison with Other Fats. *Ann. Nutr. Metab.* **2005**, *49*, 42–48. [CrossRef]
37. AbuMweis, S.S.; A Vanstone, C.; Ebine, N.; Kassis, A.; Ausman, L.M.; Jones, P.J.H.; Lichtenstein, A.H. Intake of a Single Morning Dose of Standard and Novel Plant Sterol Preparations for 4 Weeks Does Not Dramatically Affect Plasma Lipid Concentrations in Humans. *J. Nutr.* **2006**, *136*, 1012–1016. [CrossRef]
38. Chan, Y.M.; Demonty, I.; Pelled, D.; Jones, P.J.H. Olive oil containing olive oil fatty acid esters of plant sterols and dietary diacylglycerol reduces low-density lipoprotein cholesterol and decreases the tendency for peroxidation in hypercholesterolaemic subjects. *Br. J. Nutr.* **2007**, *98*, 563–570. [CrossRef]
39. Garoufi, A.; Vorre, S.; Soldatou, A.; Tsentidis, C.; Kossiva, L.; Drakatos, A.; Marmarinos, A.; Gourgiotis, D. Plant sterols–enriched diet decreases small, dense LDL-cholesterol levels in children with hypercholesterolemia: A prospective study. *Ital. J. Pediatr.* **2014**, *40*, 42. [CrossRef]
40. Madsen, M.B.; Jensen, A.M.; Schmidt, E.B. The effect of a combination of plant sterol-enriched foods in mildly hypercholesterolemic subjects. *Clin. Nutr.* **2007**, *26*, 792–798. [CrossRef]
41. Gebauer, S.K.; Destaillats, F.; Dionisi, F.; Krauss, R.M.; Baer, D.J. Vaccenic acid and trans fatty acid isomers from partially hydrogenated oil both adversely affect LDL cholesterol: A double-blind, randomized controlled trial. *Am. J. Clin. Nutr.* **2015**, *102*, 1339–1346. [CrossRef] [PubMed]
42. Vermunt, S.H.F.; Beaufrère, B.; Riemersma, R.A.; Sébédio, J.L.; Chardigny, J.M.; Mensink, R.P. Dietarytransα-linolenic acid from deodorised rapeseed oil and plasma lipids and lipoproteins in healthy men: The TransLinE Study. *Br. J. Nutr.* **2001**, *85*, 387–392. [CrossRef] [PubMed]
43. Pfeuffer, M.; Fielitz, K.; Laue, C.; Winkler, P.; Rubin, D.; Helwig, U.; Giller, K.; Kammann, J.; Schwedhelm, E.; Böger, R.H.; et al. CLA does not impair endothelial function and decreases body weight as compared with safflower oil in overweight and obese male subjects. *J. Am. Coll. Nutr.* **2011**, *30*, 19–28. [CrossRef] [PubMed]

44. Fitó, M.; Estruch, R.; Salas-Salvadó, J.; Martínez-Gonzalez, M.A.; Arós, F.; Vila, J.; Corella, D.; Díaz, O.; Sáez, G.; de la Torre, R.; et al. Effect of the Mediterranean diet on heart failure biomarkers: A randomized sample from the PREDIMED trial. *Eur. J. Heart Fail.* **2014**, *16*, 543–550. [CrossRef] [PubMed]
45. St-Onge, M.P.; Zhang, S.; Darnell, B.; Allison, D.B. Baseline Serum C-Reactive Protein Is Associated with Lipid Responses to Low-Fat and High-Polyunsaturated Fat Diets. *J. Nutr.* **2009**, *139*, 680–683. [CrossRef]
46. Öhman, M.; Åkerfeldt, T.; Nilsson, I.; Rosen, C.; Hansson, L.-O.; Carlsson, M.; Larsson, A. Biochemical effects of consumption of eggs containing omega-3 polyunsaturated fatty acids. *Upsala J. Med. Sci.* **2008**, *113*, 315–324. [CrossRef]
47. Hoppu, U.; Isolauri, E.; Koskinen, P.; Laitinen, K. Diet and blood lipids in 1–4 year-old children. *Nutr. Metab. Cardiovasc. Dis.* **2013**, *23*, 980–986. [CrossRef]
48. Voon, P.T.; Ng, T.K.W.; Lee, V.K.M.; Nesaretnam, K. Diets high in palmitic acid (16:0), lauric and myristic acids (12:0 + 14:0), or oleic acid (18:1) do not alter postprandial or fasting plasma homocysteine and inflammatory markers in healthy Malaysian adults. *Am. J. Clin. Nutr.* **2011**, *94*, 1451–1457. [CrossRef]
49. Yang, Z.-H.; Nill, K.; Takechi-Haraya, Y.; Playford, M.P.; Nguyen, D.; Yu, Z.-X.; Pryor, M.; Tang, J.; Rojulpote, K.V.; Mehta, N.N.; et al. Differential Effect of Dietary Supplementation with a Soybean Oil Enriched in Oleic Acid versus Linoleic Acid on Plasma Lipids and Atherosclerosis in LDLR-Deficient Mice. *Int. J. Mol. Sci.* **2022**, *23*, 8385. [CrossRef]
50. Petrović-Oggiano, G.; Debeljak-Martačić, J.; Ranković, S.; Pokimica, B.; Mirić, A.; Glibetić, M.; Popović, T. The Effect of Walnut Consumption on n-3 Fatty Acid Profile of Healthy People Living in a Non-Mediterranean West Balkan Country, a Small Scale Randomized Study. *Nutrients* **2020**, *12*, 192. [CrossRef]
51. Li, X.; Xin, Y.; Mo, Y.; Marozik, P.; He, T.; Guo, H. The Bioavailability and Biological Activities of Phytosterols as Modulators of Cholesterol Metabolism. *Molecules* **2022**, *27*, 523. [CrossRef] [PubMed]
52. Tasdighi, E.; Adhikari, R.; Almaadawy, O.; Leucker, T.M.; Blaha, M.J. LP(a): Structure, Genetics, Associated Cardiovascular Risk, and Emerging Therapeutics. *Annu. Rev. Pharmacol. Toxicol.* **2023**, *64*, 135–157. [CrossRef] [PubMed]


**Disclaimer/Publisher's Note:** The statements, opinions and data contained in all publications are solely those of the individual author(s) and contributor(s) and not of MDPI and/or the editor(s). MDPI and/or the editor(s) disclaim responsibility for any injury to people or property resulting from any ideas, methods, instructions or products referred to in the content.

life

*Article*

# Lymphocyte to White Blood Cell Count Ratio an Independent Risk Factor for Heart Failure

**Lior Charach [1,*], Avishay Spitzer [2], Lior Zusmanovitch [3] and Gideon Charach [4]**

1 Division of Gastroenterology, Laniado Medical Center, Netanya 4244916, Israel
2 Oncology Institute, Tel Aviv Sourasky Medical Center, Tel Aviv University, Tel Aviv 6423906, Israel
3 Meuhedet Health Service, Tel-Aviv 6473813, Israel
4 Holon Institute of Technology Israel, Holon 5810201, Israel
* Correspondence: drliorcharach@gmail.com

**Abstract:** Objective: Heart failure affects 1–2% of the population in developed countries. Hemogram biomarkers are cheap, rapid, readily accessible and are known to have prognostic benefit in cardiovascular, infectious and oncologic diseases. Methods: The aim of the current study is to evaluate lymphocyte-to-white-blood-cell ratio (LWR) as a prognostic predictor in patients with heart failure. Patients with heart failure were recruited between January 2000 and July 2001. Exclusion criteria included metastatic malignancy, exposure to chemotherapy, radiotherapy or medications known to affect complete blood count. Results: 338 patients were enrolled, 33 were excluded. Mean age was 70.1 ± 10.8, 225 patients were male (73%) and 80 were female (27%). All patients were divided into three groups according to LWR. Group 1 < 0.2, group 2—0.2 < LWR < 0.35 and group 3 > 0.35. Patients with LWR ratio < 0.2 had the poorest survival while patients in the highest LWR (ratio > 0.35) had the best long-term survival. Conclusions: Patients with congestive heart failure and LWR < 0.2 showed significant increased mortality. LWR was shown as independent prognostic predictor for HF patients compared to other main outcome parameters, including CRP, NYHA, EF and LDL.

**Keywords:** lymphocyte to white blood cell ratio; heart failure; biomarkers

## 1. Introduction

Inflammation plays a crucial role in the atherogenic process and can lead to cardiovascular sequela including ischemic heart disease and heart failure (HF) [1,2]. Non-ischemic cardiomyopathy (NICM) may lead to heart failure and known etiologies of NICM include genetic, infiltrative, medications, radiation, viruses, parasites, post-partum and valvular diseases [3].

Heart failure affects approximately 65 million people worldwide, with a prevalence of 1–2% among the general adult population in developed countries [4]. Heart failure classification had several modifications during the past 25 years [5]. Previously, HF was classified as either systolic or diastolic dysfunction and the current study used this classification because it started at 2000. Since 2005, the American College of Cardiology/American Heart Association guidelines adopted a new classification based on ejection fraction, which is also known as heart failure with reduced ejection fraction (HFrEF) and heart failure with preserved ejection fraction (HFpEF). During 2020, the Heart Failure society of America together with the Heart Failure Association of the European Society of Cardiology and the Japanese Heart Failure Society suggested four different classes according to left ventricular ejection fraction (LVEF): HF with reduced ejection fraction (LVEF $\leq$ 40%), HF with mildly reduced ejection fraction (LVEF 41–49%), HF with preserved ejection fraction (LVEF $\geq$ 50%) and a new classification, HF with improved ejection fraction, which is defined as symptomatic HF with LVEF $\leq$ 40%, a $\geq$10-point increase from baseline LVEF, and a second measurement of LVEF >40% [5,6].

Cheap, rapid and easily accessible biomarkers are needed to prognosticate heart failure. Hemogram biomarkers raise great interest due to their characteristics which reflect an organism's health condition. Several studies tested biomarkers as prognostic factors in cardiovascular diseases, including monocytes, lymphocytes and neutrophils. Neutrophil-to-lymphocyte ratio (NLR) has been extensively studied among patients with heart failure, and high NLR was shown to be associated with worse outcomes [7–10]. Furthermore, platelet-to-lymphocyte ratio (PLR), monocyte-to-lymphocyte ratio (MLR) and lymphocyte-to-monocyte ratio (LMR) were studied in patients with heart failure and are used as prognostic biomarkers [11–14].

Lymphocytes play a role in systemic inflammatory response and thus contribute to atherosclerosis development [15,16]. Low lymphocyte count is considered as a predictive biomarker of unfavorable outcomes in patients with heart failure, chronic ischemic heart disease and acute coronary syndromes [17–19]. Possible etiologies for this finding may be associated with the sympathetic nervous system and renin–angiotensin–aldosterone hormones, which show that elevated angiotensin, cortisol and adrenaline are associated with oxidative stress, proapoptotic effect on lymphocytes and increase in WBC [20–22].

Lymphocyte-to-white-blood-cell ratio has been shown to be a prognostic biomarker in infectious diseases such as endocarditis, hepatitis B and COVID-19 as well as in oncological diseases [23–25].

The aim of this study is to evaluate the prognostic role of lymphocyte-to-white-blood-cell ratio in patients with congestive heart failure.

## 2. Methods

All patients in this prospective study were successfully recruited from an out-patient heart failure clinic in Tel Aviv Medical Center. The study was approved by the institutional ethics committee (No-0554-17-TLV) and each subject provided informed consent to participate. Patients included were between age 18–95 years with symptoms of congestive heart failure and history of ischemic heart disease who were followed between January 2000 and July 2001. Baseline blood samples were collected, including complete blood count with differential counts, lipid profile and kidney function test. On the first visit, all participants were examined by a physician, medical history was obtained, blood pressure, heart rate and weight were measured, New York Heart Association (NYHA) was determined and trans-thoracic echocardiography was performed. Systolic heart failure was defined as left ventricular ejection fraction less than 40% and diastolic dysfunction was defined as ejection fraction above 40%. Ischemic heart disease was defined according to confirmed myocardial infarction per electrocardiography, cardiac biomarkers including creatine phosphorkinase MB, troponin or both, pathological stress test (thallium or technetium), pathological coronary angiography or coronary artery bypass grafting. Follow-up was at least every quartile.

Exclusion criteria included patients with metastatic malignancy, exposure to chemotherapy, radiotherapy or medications that are known to affect the complete blood count; acute and severe renal failure; active liver disease; severe pulmonary disease; active infectious disease; recent acute myocardial infarction, which was defined as less than 3 months and heart surgery diseases that have an impact on lymphocyte and total leucocyte count.

## 3. Statistical Analyses

All statistical analyses were performed with R version 4.0.3. Survival analysis was performed using the R survival and survminer packages. All reported tests were 2-sided, and $p < 0.05$ was considered significant.

All continuous variables are displayed as mean (SD). Categorical variables are displayed as numbers (percentages) of participants within each group. Continuous normally distributed variables were compared with a *t*-test, continuous non-normally distributed variable with the Kruskal–Wallis test and categorical variables with the $\chi 2$ test. Participants with missing data were excluded from all analyses.

## 4. Patient Assignment to Groups

Patients were classified into three groups based on the ratio of lymphocytes count to WBC ($\frac{Lymphocytes}{WBC}$). This ratio was calculated for each patient, and the distribution of these ratios was then divided into three groups based on the 25th and 75th percentiles of the distribution. Patients with $\frac{Lymphocytes}{WBC}$ ratio falling below the 25th percentile were assigned to the *Low* group, those between the 25th and 75th percentiles to the Medium group, and those above the 75th percentile to the High group. The Medium group was set as the baseline level of the categorical variable. Similarly, the patients were divided into three groups for other measured variables—left ventricular ejection fraction, New York Heart Association creatinine, hemoglobin, total cholesterol, low-density lipoprotein (LDL), high-density lipoprotein (HDL), triglyceride, C-reactive protein (CRP), polymorphonuclear (PMN) to lymphocyte ratio, monocyte to lymphocyte ratio, platelet to lymphocyte ratio, absolute monocyte count, absolute lymphocyte count and N-terminal pro b-type natriuretic peptide (NT-pro-BNP).

## 5. Cox Regression Analysis

Participants were censored on event occurrence (i.e., death) or at the end of the study period. All measured variables and the age and gender covariates were tested with Schoenfeld tests to evaluate the assumption of hazard proportionality, revealing that age was a non-proportional hazard. Then, the effect associated with each measured variable was estimated by generating an age-stratified Cox regression model including the measured variable and gender as a covariate. Finally, the results of all Cox models were pulled into a single table.

Survival curves were estimated with the Kaplan–Meier method for each measured variable independently.

## 6. Results

A total of 338 patients were enrolled in this study, 33 patients were excluded due to lack of follow up, noncompliance or technical reasons. The mean age of the patients that were included in this study was 70.1 ± 10.8 years. The mean follow up was 11.3 years and 78% of the patients necessitated hospitalization during follow-up. A total of 60% of the patients had systolic dysfunction and 40% had diastolic dysfunction.

Table 1 describes general characteristics, clinical and laboratory parameters divided into three lymphocyte/white blood cell groups (group 1 ratio < 0.2, group 2 ratio 0.2–0.35, group 3 ratio > 0.35). Patients in group 1 (<0.2) were older, (mean 74.8 ± 10.6), had higher NYHA classification, higher NT-proBNP levels and lower LDL levels ($p < 0.001$) compared to group 3 (LWR > 0.35). Patients in group 3 (LWR > 0.35) were younger (mean 67.4 ± 9.4), had higher monocyte count, creatinine clearance, LDL count ($p < 0.001$) and lower NT-pro-BNP levels ($p < 0.001$).

Kaplan–Meier survival curves divided into three groups of LWR is shown in Figure 1. Patients in group 1 had the poorest survival, 10% for 16 years (192 months), while patients in group 3 demonstrated the best long term survival, 84%. We examined main HF clinical characteristics, such as LVEF and NYHA class according to LWR, and their impact on survival. Figures 2 and 3 present the Kaplan–Meier curve according to LVEF and NYHA class, showing that patients with LVEF above 40% and high LWR had substantial better survival compared to patients with low ratio, 89% vs. 10% respectively ($p < 0.0001$). Patients with LVEF < 40% showed significant difference in survival, patients with high ratio (LWR > 0.35) had 89% ($p < 0.0001$) compared to 9% in the low ratio group. Table 2 shows the hazard ratio (HR) in comparison to group 2 (25th and 75th percentiles). HR was lower in the highest LWR ($p < 0.05$). Patients in group 3 (LWR > 0.35) with NYHA class 1–2 showed better survival compared to group 1, 85% versus 17%, respectively. In NYHA class 3–4 patients in group 3 (LWR > 0.35) showed better survival as well, 84%, versus 5% in group 1 ($p < 0.0001$). These findings demonstrate high predictive value of LWR. Similar results of better outcome and prolonged survival were seen in Kaplan–Meier analysis between LWR, CRP, LDL, creatinine and hemoglobin. The highest HR was seen in LWR $\leq$ 0.2; moreover, patients with poor cardiac function manifested by NT-pro BNP above 4336 pg/mL, LVEF $\leq$ 25% and NYHA 3 had high HR as well. Polymorphonuclear (PMN) to lymphocyte ratio $\geq$ 3.2 also exhibited high HR and can partially be explained by the high neutrophil fraction in white blood cell count (WBC). Further clinical and demographic parameters including hypertension, hemoglobin, HDL and LDL did not show statistical significance. Pearson's correlation index analysis did not show any correlation between LWR and mentioned variables. Chi Square analysis assessed the dependency of the categorical variables and LWR was shown to be independent prognostic parameter when compared with CRP, NYHA, EF and LDL.

**Table 1.** Baseline demographic, clinical and laboratory characteristics according to lymphocyte to WBC groups.

| | Group1 LWR < 0.2 | Group2 0.2 < LWR < 0.35 | Group3 LWR > 0.35 | *p*-Value |
|---|---|---|---|---|
| N | 76 | 158 | 71 | |
| Age (mean (SD)) | 74.82 (10.62) | 69.12 (10.96) | 67.42 (9.46) | <0.001 |
| Male (%) | 61 (80.3) | 112 (70.9) | 52 (73.2) | 0.31 |
| LVEF (%) (mean (SD)) | 34.63 (15.67) | 37.94 (14.3) | 37.73 (13.29) | 0.37 |
| DM (%) | 32 (42.1) | 67 (42.4) | 23 (32.4) | 0.328 |
| Smoking (%) | 31 (40.8) | 40 (25.3) | 23 (32.4) | 0.053 |
| Hyperlipidemia (%) | 44 (57.9) | 100 (63.3) | 44 (62.0) | 0.727 |
| Hypertension (%) | 46 (60.5) | 89 (56.7) | 48 (67.6) | 0.296 |
| Ischemic heart disease (%) | 58 (76.3) | 120 (75.9) | 52 (73.2) | 0.887 |
| Valve disease (%) | 17 (22.4) | 30 (19.0) | 10 (14.1) | 0.432 |
| Weight (kg) (mean (SD)) | 74.40 (17.44) | 77.89 (16.18) | 79.62 (14.66) | 0.137 |
| LVEF group > 40 (%) | 26 (34.2) | 68 (43.0) | 28 (39.4) | 0.432 |
| NYHA (mean (SD)) | 3.04 (0.64) | 2.66 (0.56) | 2.69 (0.63) | <0.001 |
| NYHA 1–2 | 12 (15.8) | 44 (27.8) | 22 (31.0) | |
| NYHA > 3 | 32 (42.1) | 17 (10.8) | 14 (19.7) | |
| Follow up time years (mean (SD)) | 2.29 (3.83) | 9.78 (5.49) | 12.79 (2.92) | <0.001 |
| Hospitalizations (%) | 46 (60.5) | 81 (51.3) | 49 (69.0) | 0.036 |
| Mortality (%) | 69 (90.8) | 47 (29.7) | 8 (11.3) | <0.001 |
| Hemoglobin (g%) (mean (SD)) | 14.74 (1.41) | 12.94 (1.73) | 12.61 (1.48) | 0.182 |
| Platelets ($10^9$/L) (mean (SD)) | 235.60 (97.16) | 227.22 (74.20) | 190.78 (74.91) | 0.005 |
| White blood cell ($10^9$/L) (mean (SD)) | 10.49 (4.91) | 7.45 (1.76) | 5.02 (1.18) | <0.001 |
| Lymphocytes (K/µL) (mean (SD)) | 16.81 (6.06) | 29.65 (6.84) | 33.95 (6.84) | <0.001 |
| Polymorphonuclear (K/µL) (mean (SD)) | 70.34 (24.27) | 63.69 (16.97) | 59.26 (9.71) | 0.003 |
| Monocytes (K/µL) (mean (SD)) | 5.95 (3.82) | 10.84 (5.03) | 13.96 (5.40) | <0.001 |
| GPT (IU/L) (mean (SD)) | 23.14 (21.56) | 23.28 (15.60) | 20.49 (11.75) | 0.493 |
| Alkaline phosphate (IU/L) (mean (SD)) | 73.29 (54.16) | 64.32 (39.40) | 64.58 (42.38) | 0.322 |
| Creatinine (mg/dL) (mean (SD)) | 2.28 (1.48) | 1.74 (1.21) | 1.53 (0.60) | <0.001 |
| Cholesterol (mg/dL) (mean (SD)) | 186.28 (53.73) | 185.64 (37.60) | 186.08 (44.56) | 0.994 |
| LDL (mg/dL) (mean (SD)) | 121.07 (46.07) | 125.10 (33.45) | 139.92 (43.21) | 0.008 |
| HDL (mg/dL) (mean (SD)) | 44.71 (11.70) | 44.79 (11.51) | 44.19 (11.35) | 0.933 |
| Triglyceride (mg/dL) (mean (SD)) | 171.33 (116.18) | 160.31 (91.70) | 141.13 (63.67) | 0.152 |
| CRP mg/dL (mean (SD)) | 10.43 (15.83) | 8.42 (14.91) | 5.18 (7.62) | 0.074 |
| NT-proBNP (pg/mL) (mean (SD)) | 5670.62 (7493.15) | 3422.98 (5522.27) | 2526.21 (3990.99) | 0.003 |
| Albumin (g/L) (mean (SD)) | 39.72 (9.05) | 39.29 (9.36) | 39.62 (7.40) | 0.931 |

LVEF—Left ventricular ejection fraction; DM—Diabetes mellitus; NYHA—New-York Heart Association; CRP—C-reactive protein; NT-proBNP-N-terminal pro b-type natriuretic peptide; LDL—low density lipoprotein; HDL—high density lipoprotein; GPT—glutamate pyruvate alanine aminotransferase.

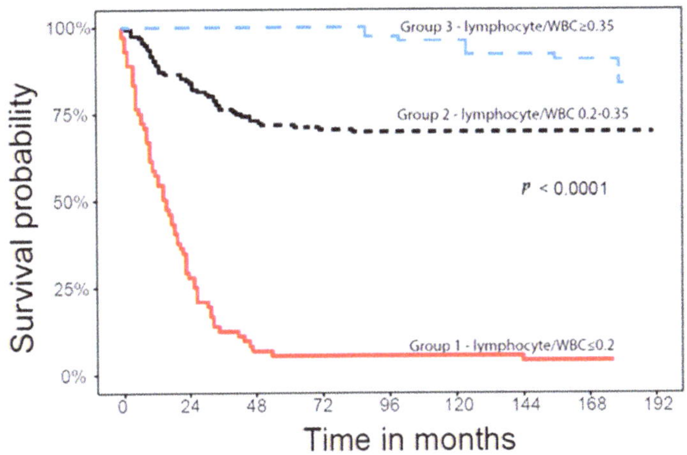


**Figure 1.** Kaplan–Meier survival curves divided into three groups according to lymphocytes to WBC ratio.

**Table 2.** Mortality Hazard ratio of main clinical and laboratory parameters related to heart failure according to variables groups.

| Variable Group | HR | *p* Value | conf.low | conf.high |
|---|---|---|---|---|
| Lymphocytes to WBC ratio $\leq$ 0.2 | 5.74 | <0.001 | 3.81 | 8.66 |
| Lymphocytes to WBC ratio $\geq$ 0.35 | 0.26 | <0.001 | 0.12 | 0.57 |
| LVEF $\leq$ 25% | 1.91 | <0.01 | 1.26 | 2.91 |
| LVEF $\geq$ 50% | 1.07 | 0.74 | 0.68 | 1.69 |
| NYHA 1–2 | 0.6 | 0.05 | 0.35 | 1.02 |
| NYHA > 3 | 1.82 | <0.01 | 1.23 | 2.7 |
| Creatinine (mg/dL) $\leq$ 1.2 | 0.58 | 0.06 | 0.32 | 1.03 |
| Creatinine (mg/dL) $\geq$ 1.5 | 1.81 | <0.01 | 1.23 | 2.66 |
| Hemoglobin $\leq$ 12 g% | 1.15 | 0.48 | 0.76 | 1.74 |
| Hemoglobin $\geq$ 14 g% | 0.76 | 0.29 | 0.47 | 1.25 |
| Total Cholesterol $\leq$ 162 (mg/dL) | 1.43 | 0.08 | 0.95 | 2.16 |
| Total Cholesterol $\geq$ 203 (mg/dL) | 1.1 | 0.65 | 0.7 | 1.75 |
| LDL Cholesterol $\leq$ 102 (mg/dL) | 1.36 | 0.13 | 0.9 | 2.05 |
| LDL Cholesterol $\geq$ 147 (mg/dL) | 0.83 | 0.44 | 0.52 | 1.32 |
| HDL Cholesterol $\leq$ 36 (mg/dL) | 0.79 | 0.31 | 0.5 | 1.24 |
| HDL Cholesterol $\geq$ 52 (mg/dL) | 0.97 | 0.92 | 0.64 | 1.49 |
| Triglycerides $\leq$ 95 (mg/dL) | 1.26 | 0.27 | 0.83 | 1.91 |
| Triglycerides $\geq$ 195 (mg/dL) | 1.33 | 0.2 | 0.85 | 2.08 |
| CRP (mg/dL) $\leq$ 1.52 | 0.71 | 0.17 | 0.44 | 1.15 |
| CRP (mg/dL) $\geq$ 8.67 | 1.72 | <0.01 | 1.15 | 2.57 |
| PMN to lymphocytes ratio $\leq$ 1.75 | 0.21 | <0.001 | 0.09 | 0.5 |
| PMN to lymphocytes ratio $\geq$ 3.2 | 3.34 | <0.001 | 2.27 | 4.92 |
| Monocytes to lymphocytes ratio $\leq$ 0.27 | 2.01 | <0.001 | 1.36 | 2.97 |
| Monocytes to lymphocytes ratio $\geq$ 0.47 | 0.56 | 0.02 | 0.33 | 0.94 |
| Platelets to lymphocytes ratio $\leq$ 80 | 0.32 | <0.001 | 0.17 | 0.6 |
| Platelets to lymphocytes ratio $\geq$ 154 | 2.07 | <0.001 | 1.41 | 3.04 |
| NT-proBNP $\leq$ 653 (pg/mL) | 0.55 | 0.04 | 0.3 | 0.99 |
| NT-proBNP $\geq$ 4336 (pg/mL) | 2.29 | <0.001 | 1.56 | 3.35 |

LVEF—Left ventricular ejection fraction; NYHA—New-York Heart Association Functional Class; PMN—polymorphonuclear; CRP-C–reactive protein; NT-proBNP—N-terminal pro b-type natriuretic peptide.

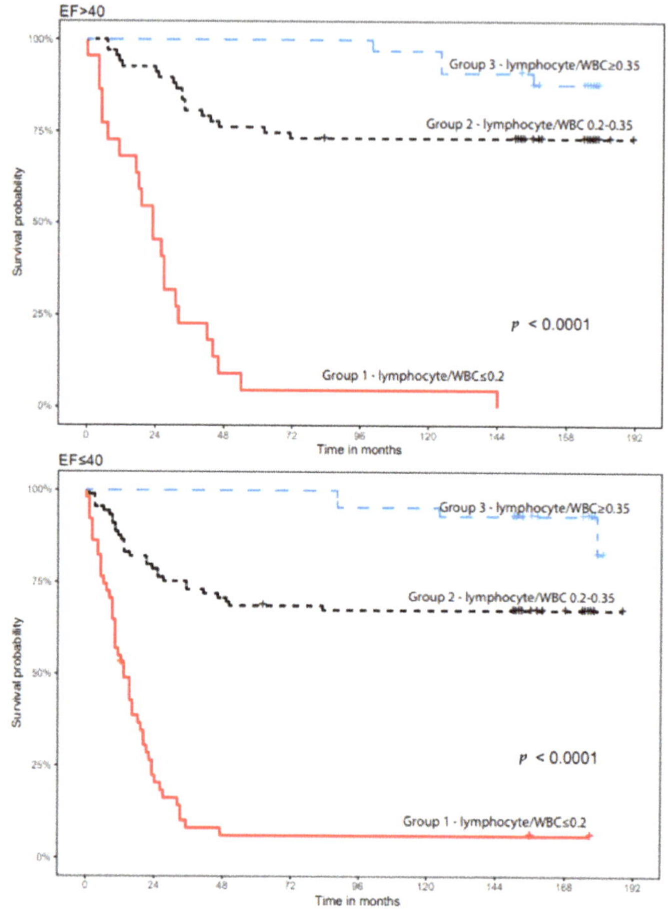


**Figure 2.** Kaplan–Meier curve according to left ventricular ejection fraction.

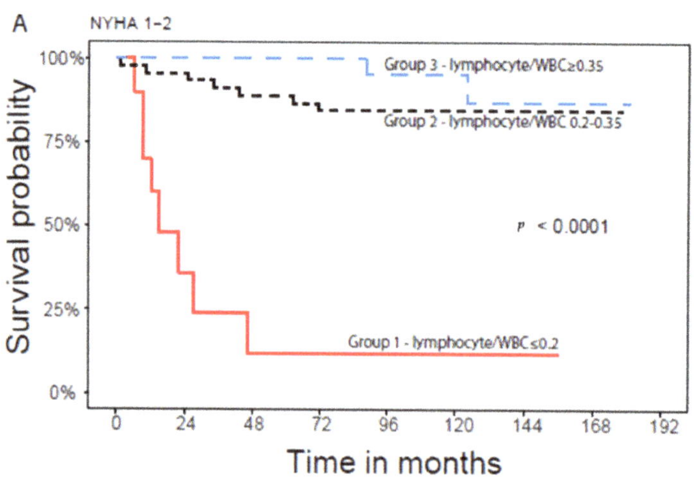


**Figure 3.** *Cont.*

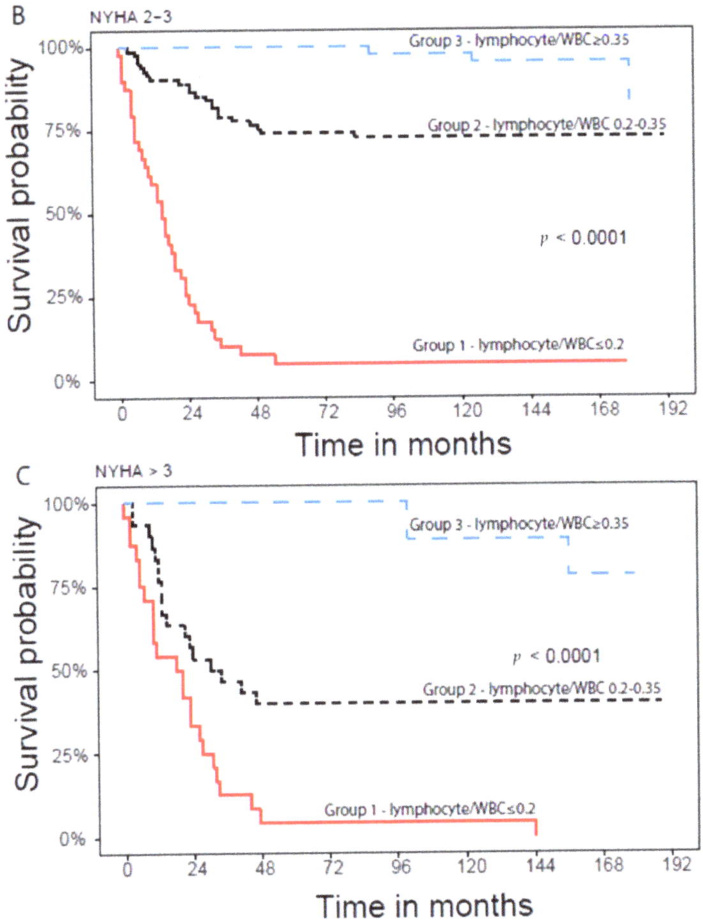


**Figure 3.** Kaplan–Meier curve according to NYHA class. Figure (**A**) shows survival probability among patients with NYHA classes 1–2; figure (**B**) shows survival probability among patients with NYHA classes 2–3; figure (**C**) shows survival probability among patients with NYHA class above 3.

## 7. Discussion

Lymphocytes are a valuable component in the inflammatory process and low levels are associated with increased risk of atherosclerosis and its sequela, such as heart failure and ischemic heart disease [15–19]. Previous studies evaluated different hemogram components and ratios in relation to atherosclerosis and heart failure. High neutrophil counts and neutrophil-to-lymphocyte ratio were associated with increased atherosclerotic cardiovascular risk and mortality among patients with heart failure [26–29]. Low lymphocytes count was shown to be associated with increased mortality in patients with acute decompensated heart failure [30]. Monocytes count was considered as a useful predictive biomarker and indicator of unfavorable outcomes among patients with acute coronary syndrome, post-infarction, heart failure, coronary artery disease and atherosclerosis [7,8]. Previous studies showed a relationship between total WBC, including eosinophil, neutrophil, and monocyte counts separately. Total WBC counts were related to the severity of coronary artery disease, and higher WBC counts increased the risk of cardiovascular diseases [31,32].

One pathophysiological explanation for these observations can be the activation of the renin-angiotensin system and adrenergic nervous system, which leads to elevated stress hormones and to programmed cell death in lymphocytes. These hormonal changes lead to an increase in neutrophil count and to relative lymphocytopenia [20–22]. Moreover, oxidative stress was shown to be associated with the activation of inflammatory cells, which leads to myocardial damage and thus contributes to heart failure progression [33].

LWR has been studied in association with infectious diseases, including infective endocarditis, COVID-19, acute on chronic liver failure secondary to hepatitis B virus and in patients with cancer [23–25,34]. Zhang Y. et al. [23] stated that in patients with acute on chronic liver failure secondary to hepatitis B virus, LWR can be used as an independent risk factor for poor outcomes after 28 days with a cutoff of 0.11 [23]. Zhang M. et al. [24] evaluated the prognostic value of LWR in patients with endocarditis and showed higher mortality among patients with low LWR, with cutoff of 0.1. Zhao et al. [25] showed that, in patients with advanced malignancy receiving palliative care, low LWR is associated with increased hazard ratio for mortality compared to high LWR. Formiga et al. [35] assessed LWR among elderly with first acute HF hospitalization and showed that patients with low LWR had higher mortality rates.

The current study divided patients with heart failure into three groups according to LWR. Patients with lowest LWR, which was set below 0.2, showed significant increased mortality compared to patients with higher LWR. The highest HR, 5.74, was in group 1, with LWR < 0.2 ($p < 0.001$) and the lowest HR, 0.26, was in the group 3, LWR > 0.35. It makes possible to consider that LWR is a simple, low cost and important predictor of outcome in patients with HF. Moreover, LWR can be considered as an independent prognostic predictor when compared to other main outcome parameters, including CRP, NYHA, EF and LDL.

NYHA class was higher in group 1, although LDL was lower ($p < 0.001$). One possible explanation for this finding is cardiac cachexia phenomena, which is seen in advanced heart failure, where high catabolic state is associated with low cholesterol levels and implies poor prognosis [22,36].

Other biomarkers were evaluated as well in this study. CRP was reported to bind to oxidized low-density lipoprotein (OxLDL) as part of the innate immune response to oxidized phosphorylcholine-bearing phospholipids in this modified lipoprotein [18]. In the current study, the HR for CRP above 8.67 showed statistical significance; however, lower values were not statistically significant. This may suggest that, while CRP may be related to myocardial injury, it is not a good predictor for long-time outcomes of HF. This finding is in concordance with previous reports [18,37].

Natriuretic peptides improve discrimination for HF prognosis above conventional risk factors and improve risk classification for heart failure [38]. Previous studies compared CRP to NT-pro BNP or other biomarkers like OxLDL. CRP has prognostic value based on mechanism of inflammation and oxidative stress which occurs in atherosclerosis; however, other biomarkers like NT-proBNP or OxLDL were more sensitive and are associated with better prediction [18]. In this study, total lymphocyte count showed the best correlation and was the best predictor of survival, including NT-pro BNP [18]. Previously, we evaluated the prognostic value of NT-proBNP in a 3.7-year follow-up study in patients with chronic HF [18]. NT-proBNP emerged as potential biomarker of clinical interest in HF management. NT-proBNP is related to HF severity and to clinical status. NT-proBNP was strongly associated with prognosis across the entire spectrum of HF. However, NT-proBNP can be low or normal in balanced HF [29,39].

Vitamin D binding (VDB) protein levels have been shown to correlate with cardiovascular disease, including myocardial infarction and HF. VDB protein was not available at the time of recruitment and there was not enough data about the prognostic effect of VDB protein and HF, thus it was not measured at HF units [40,41].

There were limitations to this study, which included relatively small sample size and enrollment being limited to a single center. We did not evaluate biomarkers such as vascular cell adhesion protein 1, CD34+ cells, endothelial progenitor cells, vascular endothelial growth factor receptor-2, tumor necrosis factor alpha and its receptor and stromal derived factor-1, which are known to increase in HF. Procalcitonin, which also shown prognostic value, and its levels correlate with adverse clinical outcomes and severity was not evaluated, because the information was not available at the study onset. Further prospective, multicenter studies with larger cohort will be needed to establish the conception of LWR as good prognostic predictor in patients with HF.

## 8. Conclusions

This study assesses LWR biomarker in relation to patients with congestive heart failure. LWR is an easily accessible, inexpensive and reliable prognostic biomarker and may help clinicians assessing high-risk patients as early as possible. Patients with congestive heart failure and LWR < 0.2 showed significant increased mortality while patients with LWR > 0.35 expressed better survival. LWR is independent prognostic predictor for HF patients when compared to main outcome parameters including CRP, NYHA, EF and LDL.

**Author Contributions:** Conceptualization, L.C. and G.C.; methodology, G.C.; formal analysis, A.S.; investigation, L.C.; data curation, L.Z.; writing—original draft preparation, L.C. and L.Z; writing—review and editing, L.C. and L.Z.; supervision, G.C.; All authors have read and agreed to the published version of the manuscript.

**Funding:** This research received no external funding.

**Institutional Review Board Statement:** The study was conducted in accordance with the Declaration of Helsinki, and approved by the Institutional Review Board Committee of Tel-Aviv Medical Center (0554-17-TLV).

**Informed Consent Statement:** Informed consent was obtained from all subjects involved in the study.

**Data Availability Statement:** Available data can be made public, in accordance with the journal's policy.

**Conflicts of Interest:** The authors declare no conflict of interest.

## References


1. Frąk, W.; Wojtasińska, A.; Lisińska, W. Pathophysiology of cardiovascular diseases: New insights into molecular mechanisms of atherosclerosis, arterial hypertension, and coronary artery disease. *Biomedicines* **2022**, *10*, 1938. [CrossRef] [PubMed]
2. Björkegren, J.L.; Lusis, A.J. Atherosclerosis: Recent developments. *Cell* **2022**, *185*, 1630–1645. [CrossRef] [PubMed]
3. Fayol, A.; Wack, M.; Livrozet, M. Aetiological classification and prognosis in patients with heart failure with preserved ejection fraction. *ESC Heart Fail.* **2022**, *9*, 519–530. [CrossRef] [PubMed]
4. Groenewegen, A.; Rutten, F.H.; Mosterd, A. Epidemiology of heart failure. *Eur. J. Heart Fail.* **2020**, *22*, 1342–1356. [CrossRef]
5. Lam, C.S.; Yancy, C. Universal definition and classification of heart failure: Is it universal? Does it define heart failure? *J. Card. Fail.* **2021**, *27*, 509–511. [CrossRef]
6. Fonarow, G.C. Refining classification of heart failure based on ejection fraction. *JACC Heart Fail.* **2017**, *5*, 808–809. [CrossRef]
7. Curran, F.M.; Bhalraam, U.; Mohan, M. Neutrophil-to-lymphocyte ratio and outcomes in patients with new-onset or worsening heart failure with reduced and preserved ejection fraction. *ESC Heart Fail.* **2021**, *8*, 3168–3179. [CrossRef]
8. Benites-Zapata, V.A.; Hernandez, A.V.; Nagarajan, V. Usefulness of neutrophil-to-lymphocyte ratio in risk stratification of patients with advanced heart failure. *Am. J. Cardiol.* **2015**, *115*, 57–61. [CrossRef]
9. Bhat, T.; Teli, S.; Rijal, J. Neutrophil to lymphocyte ratio and cardiovascular diseases: A review. *Expert Rev. Cardiovasc. Ther.* **2013**, *11*, 55–59. [CrossRef]
10. Durmus, E.; Kivrak, T.; Gerin, F. Neutrophil-to-lymphocyte ratio and platelet-to-lymphocyte ratio are predictors of heart failure. *Arq. Bras. Cardiol.* **2015**, *105*, 606–613. [CrossRef]
11. Naylor, S. Biomarkers: Current perspectives and future prospects. *Expert Rev. Mol. Diagn.* **2003**, *3*, 525–529. [CrossRef] [PubMed]
12. Shahid, F.; Lip, G.Y.; Shantsila, E. Role of monocytes in heart failure and atrial fibrillation. *J. Am. Heart Assoc.* **2018**, *7*, e007849. [CrossRef] [PubMed]
13. Wong, K.L.; Yeap, W.H.; Tai, J.J.Y. The three human monocyte subsets: Implications for health and disease. *Immunol. Res.* **2012**, *53*, 41–57. [CrossRef] [PubMed]

14. Vakhshoori, M.; Nemati, S.; Sabouhi, S. Selection of monocyte-to-lymphocyte ratio (MLR) or lymphocyte-to-monocyte ratio (LMR) as best prognostic tool in heart failure: A systematic review. *SN Compr. Clin. Med.* **2023**, *5*, 227. [CrossRef]
15. Frostegård, J. Immunity, atherosclerosis and cardiovascular disease. *BMC Med.* **2013**, *11*, 117. [CrossRef]
16. Hedrick, C.C. Lymphocytes in atherosclerosis. *Arterioscler. Thromb. Vasc. Biol.* **2015**, *35*, 253–257. [CrossRef]
17. Núñez, J.; Miñana, G.; Bodí, V. Low lymphocyte count and cardiovascular diseases. *Curr. Med. Chem.* **2011**, *18*, 3226–3233. [CrossRef]
18. Charach, G.; Grosskopf, I.; Roth, A. Usefulness of total lymphocyte count as predictor of outcome in patients with chronic heart failure. *Am. J. Cardiol.* **2011**, *107*, 1353–1356. [CrossRef]
19. Acanfora, D.; Gheorghiade, M.; Trojano, L.; CHF Italian Study Investigators. Relative lymphocyte count: A prognostic indicator of mortality in elderly patients with congestive heart failure. *Am. Heart J.* **2001**, *142*, 167–173. [CrossRef]
20. Marra, S.; Hoffman-Goetz, L. β-adrenergic receptor blockade during exercise decreases intestinal lymphocyte apoptosis but not cell loss in mice. *Can. J. Physiol. Pharmacol.* **2004**, *82*, 465–473. [CrossRef]
21. Abrams, M.T.; Robertson, N.M.; Yoon, K. Inhibition of glucocorticoid-induced apoptosis by targeting the major splice variants of BIM mRNA with small interfering RNA and short hairpin RNA. *J. Biol. Chem.* **2004**, *279*, 55809–55817. [CrossRef]
22. Anker, S.D.; Chua, T.P.; Ponikowski, P. Hormonal changes and catabolic/anabolic imbalance in chronic heart failure and their importance for cardiac cachexia. *Circulation* **1997**, *96*, 526–534. [CrossRef] [PubMed]
23. Zhang, Y.; Chen, P.; Zhu, X. Lymphocyte-to-white blood cell ratio is associated with outcome in patients with hepatitis B virus-related acute-on-chronic liver failure. *World J. Gastroenterol.* **2023**, *29*, 3678–3687. [CrossRef]
24. Zhang, M.; Ge, Q.; Qiao, T. Prognostic Value of Lymphocyte-to-White Blood Cell Ratio for In-Hospital Mortality in Infective Endocarditis Patients. *Int. J. Clin. Pract.* **2022**, *2022*, 8667054. [CrossRef] [PubMed]
25. Zhao, W.; Wang, P.; Jia, H. Lymphocyte count or percentage: Which can better predict the prognosis of advanced cancer patients following palliative care? *BMC Cancer* **2017**, *17*, 514. [CrossRef] [PubMed]
26. Luo, J.; Thomassen, J.Q.; Nordestgaard, B.G. Neutrophil counts and cardiovascular disease. *Eur. Heart J.* **2023**, *44*, 4953–4964. [CrossRef] [PubMed]
27. Vakhshoori, M.; Nemati, S.; Sabouhi, S. Neutrophil to lymphocyte ratio (NLR) prognostic effects on heart failure; a systematic review and meta-analysis. *BMC Cardiovasc. Disord.* **2023**, *23*, 555. [CrossRef]
28. Charach, G.; Rogowski, O.; Karniel, E. Monocytes may be favorable biomarker and predictor of long-term outcome in patients with chronic heart failure: A cohort study. *Medicine* **2019**, *98*, e17108. [CrossRef]
29. Silva, N.; Bettencourt, P.; Guimarães, J.T. The lymphocyte-to-monocyte ratio: An added value for death prediction in heart failure. *Nutr. Metab. Cardiovasc. Dis.* **2015**, *25*, 1033–1040. [CrossRef]
30. Uthamalingam, S.; Patvardhan, E.A.; Subramanian, S. Utility of the neutrophil to lymphocyte ratio in predicting long-term outcomes in acute decompensated heart failure. *Am. J. Cardiol.* **2011**, *107*, 433–438. [CrossRef]
31. Kim, J.H.; Lim, S.; Park, K.S. Total and differential WBC counts are related with coronary artery atherosclerosis and increase the risk for cardiovascular disease in Koreans. *PLoS ONE* **2017**, *12*, e0180332. [CrossRef] [PubMed]
32. Kounis, N.G.; Soufras, G.D.; Tsigkas, G. White blood cell counts, leukocyte ratios, and eosinophils as inflammatory markers in patients with coronary artery disease. *Clin. Appl. Thromb./Hemost.* **2015**, *21*, 139–143. [CrossRef] [PubMed]
33. Aimo, A.; Castiglione, V.; Borrelli, C. Oxidative stress and inflammation in the evolution of heart failure: From pathophysiology to therapeutic strategies. *Eur. J. Prev. Cardiol.* **2020**, *27*, 494–510. [CrossRef] [PubMed]
34. Pitre, T.; Jones, A.; Su, J. Inflammatory biomarkers as independent prognosticators of 28-day mortality for COVID-19 patients admitted to general medicine or ICU wards: A retrospective cohort study. *Intern. Emerg. Med.* **2021**, *16*, 1573–1582. [CrossRef] [PubMed]
35. Formiga, F.; Chivite, D.; Salvatori, M. Lymphocyte-to-white blood cells ratio in older patients experiencing a first acute heart failure hospitalization. *Eur Geriatr Med.* **2018**, *9*, 365–370. [CrossRef]
36. Von Haehling, S.; Schefold, J.C.; Springer, J. The cholesterol paradox revisited: Heart failure, systemic inflammation, and beyond. *Heart Fail. Clin.* **2008**, *4*, 141–151. [CrossRef]
37. George, J.; Wexler, D.; Roth, A. Usefulness of anti-oxidized LDL antibody determination for assessment of clinical control in patients with heart failure. *Eur. J. Heart Fail.* **2006**, *8*, 58–62. [CrossRef]
38. Smith, J.G.; Newton-Cheh, C.; Almgren, P. Assessment of conventional cardiovascular risk factors and multiple biomarkers for the prediction of incident heart failure and atrial fibrillation. *J. Am. Coll. Cardiol.* **2010**, *56*, 1712–1719. [CrossRef]
39. Anand, I.S.; Latini, R.; Florea, V.G. C-reactive protein in heart failure: Prognostic value and the effect of valsartan. *Circulation* **2005**, *112*, 1428–1434. [CrossRef]
40. Gasparri, C.; Curcio, A.; Torella, D. Proteomics reveals high levels of vitamin D binding protein in myocardial infarction. *Front Biosci Elite Ed* **2010**, *2*, 796–804.
41. Petrone, A.B.; Weir, N.L.; Steffen, B.T. Plasma vitamin D-binding protein and risk of heart failure in male physicians. *Am. J. Cardiol.* **2013**, *112*, 827–830. [CrossRef]

**Disclaimer/Publisher's Note:** The statements, opinions and data contained in all publications are solely those of the individual author(s) and contributor(s) and not of MDPI and/or the editor(s). MDPI and/or the editor(s) disclaim responsibility for any injury to people or property resulting from any ideas, methods, instructions or products referred to in the content.

*life*

MDPI

*Review*

# Unveiling the Potential: Remote Monitoring and Telemedicine in Shaping the Future of Heart Failure Management

**Ju-Chi Liu [1,2,†], Chun-Yao Cheng [3], Tzu-Hurng Cheng [4,†], Chen-Ning Liu [5], Jin-Jer Chen [6,7] and Wen-Rui Hao [1,2,*]**

1 Division of Cardiology, Department of Internal Medicine, Shuang Ho Hospital, Ministry of Health and Welfare, Taipei Medical University, New Taipei City 23561, Taiwan; liumdcv@s.tmu.edu.tw
2 Division of Cardiology, Department of Internal Medicine, School of Medicine, College of Medicine, Taipei Medical University, Taipei City 11002, Taiwan
3 Department of Medical Education, National Taiwan University Hospital, Taipei 100225, Taiwan; b05401143@ntu.edu.tw
4 Department of Biochemistry, School of Medicine, College of Medicine, China Medical University, Taichung City 404333, Taiwan; thcheng@mail.cmu.edu.tw
5 Center of Integrated, Shuang Ho Hospital, Ministry of Health and Welfare, Taipei Medical University, New Taipei City 23561, Taiwan; 12585@s.tmu.edu.tw
6 Division of Cardiology, Department of Internal Medicine and Graduate Institute of Clinical Medical Science, China Medical University, Taichung 115201, Taiwan; jc8510@yahoo.com
7 Institute of Biomedical Sciences, Academia Sinica, Taipei 11529, Taiwan
* Correspondence: b8501043@tmu.edu.tw
† The author contributed as the first co-authors.

**Abstract:** Heart failure (HF) remains a significant burden on global healthcare systems, necessitating innovative approaches for its management. This manuscript critically evaluates the role of remote monitoring and telemedicine in revolutionizing HF care delivery. Drawing upon a synthesis of current literature and clinical practices, it delineates the pivotal benefits, challenges, and personalized strategies associated with these technologies in HF management. The analysis highlights the potential of remote monitoring and telemedicine in facilitating timely interventions, enhancing patient engagement, and optimizing treatment adherence, thereby ameliorating clinical outcomes. However, technical intricacies, regulatory frameworks, and socioeconomic factors pose formidable hurdles to widespread adoption. The manuscript emphasizes the imperative of tailored interventions, leveraging advancements in artificial intelligence and machine learning, to address individual patient needs effectively. Looking forward, sustained innovation, interdisciplinary collaboration, and strategic investment are advocated to realize the transformative potential of remote monitoring and telemedicine in HF management, thereby advancing patient-centric care paradigms and optimizing healthcare resource allocation.

**Keywords:** heart failure (HF); remote monitoring; telemedicine; cardiovascular care; personalized medicine; patient engagement; treatment adherence; healthcare innovation; artificial intelligence (AI); machine learning; healthcare resource optimization

## 1. Introduction

Heart failure (HF) presents a significant global public health challenge characterized by inefficient blood pumping by the heart, resulting in debilitating symptoms and heightened mortality rates. The escalating burden of HF, driven by an aging populace and an upsurge in cardiovascular risk factors, underscores the necessity for innovative management strategies [1,2]. Remote monitoring and telemedicine have emerged as promising strategies to revolutionize HF care delivery, overcoming constraints in traditional healthcare frameworks. By harnessing telecommunications technology and digital health platforms, remote monitoring allows continuous surveillance of HF patients' clinical parameters beyond conventional healthcare settings. Telemedicine facilitates real-time communication between patients and healthcare providers, enabling prompt intervention and personalized management [3].

This manuscript aims to elucidate the pivotal role of remote monitoring and telemedicine in reshaping HF management. By integrating current evidence and insights from clinical practice, it delineates the benefits, challenges, and personalized approaches associated with these innovative technologies, exploring their potential to enhance access to care, improve early detection of clinical deterioration, promote patient engagement, and optimize treatment outcomes among HF patients.

Moreover, recent advancements in machine learning (ML) have revolutionized healthcare, offering opportunities for personalized medicine and predictive analytics. Studies by Kao et al. (2023) [4] and Hsiu et al. (2022) [5] demonstrate ML applications in predicting atrial fibrillation risk and discriminating vascular aging, respectively, using electronic medical records and arterial pulse spectrum analysis. Similarly, research by Chen et al. (2022) [6] explores ML's potential in understanding physiological responses to interventions, such as the side effects of COVID-19 vaccination. Furthermore, ML techniques have been crucial in hypertension management and cardiovascular risk assessment, as evidenced by studies like Liu et al. (2021) [7] and Lee et al. (2016) [8]. These investigations underscore ML's utility in extracting meaningful insights from complex physiological data, aiding in early detection and personalized intervention strategies, particularly pertinent in HF management.

In the context of HF management, ML integration holds promise for enhancing risk stratification, optimizing treatment algorithms, and predicting clinical outcomes. Leveraging ML algorithms on remote monitoring data can enable early identification of subtle physiological changes indicative of HF exacerbations, empowering timely interventions and preemptive measures to prevent adverse events. Additionally, the manuscript scrutinizes the technical, regulatory, and socioeconomic hurdles impeding the widespread adoption of remote monitoring, telemedicine, and ML in HF care. It emphasizes tailored interventions and advanced technology integration to adeptly cater to individual patient exigencies. Ultimately, this manuscript aims to enrich the burgeoning literature on remote monitoring, telemedicine, and ML in HF management, advocating for sustained innovation, interdisciplinary collaboration, and strategic investment to unlock their transformative potential in advancing patient-centric care paradigms and optimizing healthcare resource allocation.

## 2. Evolution of Remote Monitoring and Telemedicine in Heart Failure

Historically, remote monitoring dates back to the early 20th century with telegraph and telephone-based consultations between physicians and patients. Breakthroughs in the latter half of the century, including portable medical devices and the internet, laid the groundwork for modern remote monitoring and telemedicine solutions, enabling real-time transmission of patient data and consultations [9,10].

In HF management, early remote monitoring efforts focused on transmitting electrocardiographic signals and ambulatory vital signs monitoring to detect arrhythmias and hemodynamic fluctuations. Over time, the integration of wireless technology, wearable sensors, and mobile applications expanded remote monitoring capabilities, enabling continuous monitoring of various physiological parameters, including fluid status, activity levels, and medication adherence [11]. Recent advancements in ML have further propelled the evolution of remote monitoring and telemedicine in HF management. Studies such as those by Kao et al. (2023) [4] and Hsiu et al. (2022) [5] demonstrate ML's application in predicting atrial fibrillation risk and discriminating vascular aging, respectively, utilizing electronic medical records and arterial pulse spectrum analysis. Additionally, research by Chen et al. (2022) [6] highlights ML's potential in understanding physiological responses to interventions, such as the side effects of COVID-19 vaccination. Furthermore, ML techniques have played a pivotal role in enhancing remote monitoring capabilities for hypertensive patients, as evidenced by studies like Liu et al. (2021) [7] and Lee et al. (2016) [8]. These investigations underscore ML's utility in extracting meaningful insights from complex physiological data, aiding in early detection and personalized intervention strategies, particularly pertinent in HF management.

The adoption of remote monitoring and telemedicine in HF management has steadily grown, driven by the recognition of HF as a chronic condition requiring ongoing surveillance, advancements in healthcare informatics facilitating data integration, and the COVID-19 pandemic accelerating telemedicine adoption [12]. However, challenges persist, including technical issues, regulatory barriers, and disparities in access and digital literacy [13]. In summary, the evolution of remote monitoring and telemedicine, coupled with advancements in ML, has revolutionized HF management, offering opportunities for personalized, proactive care delivery. Addressing the remaining challenges is crucial to ensuring equitable access and maximizing benefits for all HF patients.

## 3. Benefits of Remote Monitoring and Telemedicine in Heart Failure Management

Remote monitoring and telemedicine have emerged as invaluable tools in HF management, offering benefits that enhance patient outcomes and optimize healthcare resource utilization (Table 1). Integrating recent literature enriches our understanding of these advantages and their implications for HF management. One significant advantage is the enhanced access to care they provide for HF patients. Enabling real-time monitoring of physiological parameters and symptoms from patients' homes, remote monitoring reduces the need for frequent clinic visits, empowering patients to actively engage in their care [4]. This alleviates travel burdens and ensures timely intervention in cases of clinical deterioration. Studies show that remote monitoring interventions lead to earlier detection of worsening HF symptoms, enabling prompt adjustments to treatment regimens and reducing hospitalization risks [9,14].

Furthermore, remote monitoring and telemedicine foster patient engagement and self-management, which are pivotal to successful HF management. Through these platforms, patients proactively participate in self-care activities such as monitoring fluid intake, adhering to medication regimens, and adopting lifestyle modifications [15]. Recent advances in ML offer opportunities to enhance patient engagement by providing personalized insights and interventions based on real-time data analysis [6]. Moreover, the impact extends beyond individual patient outcomes to optimize broader healthcare resource utilization. By facilitating proactive HF management through early detection of clinical deterioration, remote monitoring reduces hospitalization frequency and duration, alleviating strain on healthcare systems and cutting costs [16]. Additionally, remote monitoring data guides more efficient resource allocation by identifying high-risk patients who may benefit from targeted interventions, maximizing healthcare resources' value [17]. Insights from recent studies on ML applications in healthcare resource utilization underscore the potential for data-driven approaches to further optimize resource allocation and enhance healthcare efficiency [18,19]. In summary, remote monitoring and telemedicine offer benefits for HF management, including improved access to care, enhanced patient engagement and self-management, and optimized healthcare resource utilization. Enabling proactive, personalized care delivery, these technologies have the potential to transform HF management, improving outcomes for patients while relieving strain on healthcare systems. Continued investment in infrastructure, alongside efforts to address barriers, will be crucial to realizing their full potential in enhancing HF care delivery.

**Table 1.** Key benefits and challenges of remote monitoring and telemedicine in heart failure management.

| Aspect | Description |
|---|---|
| **Benefits** | |
| Improved Patient Outcomes | Remote monitoring allows for continuous tracking of patient health, leading to timely interventions and better management of heart failure. |
| Enhanced Patient Engagement | Telemedicine provides patients with easy access to healthcare providers, encouraging active participation in their own care. |
| Reduced Hospital Readmissions | Early detection of symptoms and prompt management via telemedicine can prevent hospital readmissions, which are common in heart failure patients. |
| Cost-Effectiveness | By reducing the need for in-person visits and hospital stays, remote monitoring and telemedicine can lower healthcare costs. |
| Increased Accessibility | Telemedicine bridges the gap for patients in remote or underserved areas, ensuring they receive necessary care. |
| **Challenges** | |
| Technical Issues | Dependence on reliable internet and technology can be a barrier, especially in rural areas with poor connectivity. |
| Data Privacy and Security | Handling sensitive patient data requires robust security measures to prevent breaches and ensure confidentiality. |
| Patient Compliance | Successful remote monitoring relies on patients' adherence to using the technology and following medical advice. |
| Health Literacy | Some patients, particularly the elderly, may struggle with the technology required for remote monitoring and telemedicine. |
| Integration with Existing Systems | Seamless integration of telemedicine platforms with existing electronic health record systems can be complex and resource-intensive. |

This table provides a concise overview of both the advantages and the potential obstacles associated with the use of remote monitoring and telemedicine in managing heart failure.

## 4. Challenges and Considerations

Despite the promising benefits of remote monitoring and telemedicine in HF management, several challenges and considerations must be addressed to realize their full potential and ensure equitable access and utilization (Table 1). Remote monitoring and telemedicine in the management of heart failure present a range of significant benefits and notable challenges. The primary benefits encompass improved patient outcomes through continuous health monitoring, which enables timely interventions and optimal management of the condition. Furthermore, telemedicine enhances patient engagement by providing convenient access to healthcare providers, thereby encouraging active participation in their own care. This approach also contributes to a reduction in hospital readmissions by allowing for early detection of symptoms and prompt management. Additionally, the cost-effectiveness of telemedicine is evident, as it reduces the need for in-person visits and hospital stays, ultimately lowering healthcare costs. Increased accessibility is another critical advantage, as telemedicine bridges the gap for patients residing in remote or underserved areas, ensuring they receive the necessary care.

Despite these benefits, several challenges persist. Technical issues such as the dependence on reliable internet connectivity and advanced technology can be significant barriers, particularly in rural areas with poor connectivity. Data privacy and security concerns are paramount, as handling sensitive patient information requires robust security measures to prevent breaches and maintain confidentiality. Patient compliance with the technology and adhering to medical advice are essential for successful remote monitoring. Health literacy poses another challenge, especially among the elderly, who may struggle with the technology required for telemedicine. Finally, the integration of telemedicine platforms with existing electronic health record systems can be complex and resource-intensive, posing an additional hurdle to widespread adoption.

One significant challenge is the array of technical issues that can impede the seamless operation of remote monitoring and telemedicine systems. Connectivity issues, such as unreliable internet connections or poor cellular coverage in rural areas, can disrupt data transmission and compromise the effectiveness of remote monitoring interventions [4]. Machine learning-based prediction and analysis offer opportunities for innovation in overcoming these barriers. Interoperability—the ability of different devices and systems to exchange and interpret data—remains a challenge, as many remote monitoring platforms operate in silos, leading to fragmented data and inefficiencies in care delivery. Additionally, ensuring robust data security measures to protect sensitive patient information from unauthorized access or cyberattacks is paramount to maintaining patient trust and compliance with privacy regulations [4,8].

Regulatory and reimbursement barriers pose significant problems for the widespread adoption of remote monitoring and telemedicine in HF management. While the COVID-19 pandemic prompted temporary regulatory changes and expanded reimbursement policies to facilitate telehealth services, many of these provisions are subject to revision or expiration [18]. Clarifying regulatory guidelines and establishing sustainable reimbursement models for remote monitoring and telemedicine services are critical to incentivizing healthcare organizations and providers to invest in these technologies and integrate them into routine clinical practice [18,20].

Addressing disparities in access to technology and digital literacy is another pressing concern. Socioeconomic factors, such as income level, education, and geographic location, can influence individuals' ability to access and utilize remote monitoring and telemedicine services effectively. Vulnerable populations, including older adults, low-income individuals, and those residing in rural or underserved areas, may face barriers related to access to broadband internet, affordability of devices, and proficiency in using digital health tools [19]. Efforts to bridge the digital divide and promote digital literacy among diverse patient populations are essential to ensure equitable access to remote monitoring and telemedicine services and mitigate disparities in HF care outcomes [19,21].

Furthermore, patient and provider acceptance and adherence to remote monitoring protocols are critical determinants of success. While some patients may embrace the convenience and flexibility of remote monitoring, others may express concerns about privacy, data security, or the perceived loss of personal connection with their healthcare providers. Similarly, healthcare providers may encounter resistance or skepticism regarding the reliability and accuracy of remote monitoring data or the feasibility of integrating telemedicine into their workflow [8,22,23]. Addressing these concerns through education, training, and ongoing support is essential to foster acceptance and engagement among both patients and providers and promote sustained adherence to remote monitoring protocols [8,15,23].

To conclude, while remote monitoring and telemedicine hold significant promise for improving HF management, several challenges and considerations must be addressed to maximize their impact and ensure equitable access and utilization. By addressing technical, regulatory, socioeconomic, and behavioral barriers, stakeholders can work together to overcome these challenges and harness the full potential of remote monitoring and telemedicine to enhance HF care delivery and outcomes [4,18,19,22].

## 5. Personalized Approaches in Remote Monitoring and Telemedicine

Personalization is emerging as a key principle in remote monitoring and telemedicine for HF management, offering the potential to optimize care delivery and enhance patient outcomes (Table 2). Integrating insights from recent literature further enriches our understanding of these personalized approaches and their implications for HF management. Tailoring remote monitoring protocols based on individual patient characteristics and preferences is fundamental to personalized care. Considering factors such as age, comorbidities, disease severity, and technological proficiency, healthcare providers can design remote monitoring programs that meet the unique needs and preferences of each patient [24]. Insights from studies by Chen et al. (2022) [6] and Kao et al. (2023) [4] on machine learning-based prediction and analysis enable the customization of monitoring parameters and interventions tailored to individual patient profiles.

**Table 2.** Types of remote monitoring technologies and their applications in heart failure management.

| Technology | Description | Applications |
|---|---|---|
| Wearable Devices | Devices such as smartwatches and fitness trackers that monitor vital signs like heart rate, activity levels, and sleep patterns. | Continuous monitoring of heart rate, physical activity, and sleep quality to detect early signs of heart failure exacerbation. |
| Implantable Devices | Devices like cardiac resynchronization therapy (CRT) and implantable cardioverter defibrillators (ICD) that provide real-time monitoring and therapeutic intervention. | Monitoring of cardiac function and automatic delivery of therapy to manage arrhythmias and other cardiac events. |
| Remote Monitoring Platforms | Comprehensive systems that collect and analyze data from various sources, including wearables and implantable devices. | Integration and analysis of patient data to provide holistic insights and enable proactive management of heart failure. |
| Mobile Health Apps | Smartphone applications designed to track symptoms, medication adherence, and lifestyle factors such as diet and exercise. | Facilitating patient self-management, education, and communication with healthcare providers. |
| Telemedicine Platforms | Online systems that enable virtual consultations, remote check-ins, and real-time communication between patients and healthcare providers. | Providing accessible healthcare services, routine check-ups, and emergency consultations without the need for in-person visits. |
| Home-Based Diagnostic Tools | Devices such as digital blood pressure monitors, weight scales, and ECG monitors that patients use at home to track their health metrics. | Daily monitoring of vital signs and early detection of health changes, allowing for timely medical intervention. |
| Artificial Intelligence and Analytics | Advanced software that uses machine learning algorithms to predict patient outcomes and personalize treatment plans based on collected data. | Enhancing decision-making processes for healthcare providers by predicting disease progression and optimizing treatment strategies. |

This table outlines various remote monitoring technologies, their descriptions, and specific applications in the context of heart failure management, providing a clear overview of the tools available and their practical uses.

Furthermore, the integration of AI and ML algorithms holds promise for personalized risk stratification in HF management. AI-driven models can analyze large datasets encompassing clinical, physiological, and behavioral variables to predict individual patient trajectories and proactively intervene to mitigate adverse outcomes [25]. Leveraging insights from Hsiu et al. (2022) [5] on discriminating vascular aging using machine learning analysis, AI-powered decision support tools can assist healthcare providers in interpreting remote monitoring data and making informed clinical decisions tailored to each patient's unique circumstances.

Customizing telemedicine interventions to meet the needs of diverse patient populations is another critical aspect of personalized care in HF management. Telemedicine platforms offer a range of modalities for remote communication, including video consultations, secure messaging, and remote monitoring applications [26]. By offering flexibility in communication channels and adapting communication styles to suit individual preferences and cultural backgrounds, healthcare providers can enhance patient engagement and satisfaction with telemedicine services. Insights from previous studies [19] can guide the customization of telemedicine interventions to accommodate patients with specific needs or limitations, ensuring equitable delivery of telemedicine services to all patients.

Overall, personalized approaches to remote monitoring and telemedicine are essential for optimizing HF management and delivering patient-centered care. By tailoring remote monitoring protocols, integrating AI-driven risk stratification models, and customizing telemedicine interventions to meet the diverse needs of patients, healthcare providers can enhance engagement, improve outcomes, and promote equity in access to care. Continued research, innovation, and collaboration are needed to further develop and implement personalized approaches in remote monitoring and telemedicine, ultimately advancing the field of HF management and improving the lives of patients affected by this chronic condition.

## 6. Future Directions and Implications

The future of remote monitoring and telemedicine in HF management holds significant promise, with ongoing innovations poised to transform healthcare delivery models, enhance patient outcomes, and optimize resource utilization. Integrating insights from recent literature further enriches our understanding of potential future directions and implications of remote monitoring and telemedicine in HF management.

Innovations in remote monitoring technology and telemedicine platforms are expected to drive significant advancements in HF management. The integration of wearable sensors, implantable devices, and Internet of Things (IoT) technologies enables continuous monitoring of physiological parameters relevant to HF progression, such as biomarkers, fluid status, and physical activity levels [27]. These advancements offer opportunities for comprehensive monitoring, facilitating earlier detection of HF exacerbations and timely interventions.

Furthermore, advancements in remote monitoring platforms, such as cloud-based data analytics, AI, and ML, facilitate real-time analysis of patient data and predictive modeling. AI-driven models predict individual patient trajectories and enable personalized interventions tailored to unique circumstances [28]. Leveraging insights from machine learning analyses [5,6], these platforms optimize treatment strategies and enhance patient outcomes through proactive and personalized care delivery.

The potential impact of remote monitoring and telemedicine on healthcare delivery models, patient outcomes, and resource utilization is significant. By enabling remote access to healthcare services and reducing the need for in-person visits, these technologies improve access to care, enhance patient engagement, and optimize treatment outcomes for HF patients [29]. Moreover, by empowering patients to participate in their care and providing healthcare providers with real-time data and decision-support tools, these technologies facilitate more efficient and effective care delivery, ultimately reducing healthcare costs and maximizing resource value [30].

Opportunities for research, collaboration, and overcoming barriers to implementation are essential for realizing the full potential of remote monitoring and telemedicine in HF management. Continued investment in research and development is required to refine and validate remote monitoring technologies, evaluate their impact on patient outcomes, and identify strategies for integrating them into routine clinical practice [31]. Collaboration among stakeholders, including healthcare providers, technology developers, policymakers, and patient advocacy groups, is critical for addressing regulatory, reimbursement, and interoperability challenges, fostering innovation, and driving widespread adoption of these solutions [32].

Efforts to promote digital literacy, address healthcare disparities, and ensure equitable access to remote monitoring and telemedicine services are essential for realizing the promise of these technologies in improving HF care delivery and outcomes for all patients [33]. By addressing these challenges and harnessing the full potential of remote monitoring and telemedicine, stakeholders can advance the field of HF management and improve the lives of patients affected by this chronic condition.

There are some limitations. Given that this is not a systematic review, it inherently possesses certain weaknesses and selection biases that are challenging to mitigate. Additionally, remote monitoring and telemedicine prove to be less practical for patients with hearing or visual impairments or those with lower cultural or intellectual levels. These limitations underscore the need for tailored approaches to ensure equitable access and effectiveness in digital health interventions.

## 7. Conclusions

In conclusion, remote monitoring and telemedicine have emerged as indispensable tools in the management of HF, offering benefits including improved access to care, enhanced patient engagement, and optimized resource utilization (Table 3). Despite challenges, the potential impact of remote monitoring and telemedicine on healthcare delivery models and patient outcomes is profound.

**Table 3.** Comparison of traditional in-person heart failure management and remote monitoring/telemedicine approaches.

| Aspect | Traditional In-Person Management | Remote Monitoring/Telemedicine |
|---|---|---|
| Accessibility | Limited to geographic location and availability of healthcare providers. | Accessible from anywhere with internet connectivity, bridging gaps for remote or underserved areas. |
| Frequency of Monitoring | Periodic check-ups, typically scheduled weeks or months apart. | Continuous or frequent monitoring, allowing for real-time data collection and timely interventions. |
| Patient Engagement | Patient engagement often limited to scheduled visits; may be passive between appointments. | Encourages active patient participation through regular updates, use of apps, and constant feedback loops. |
| Response Time | Potential delays in response to symptoms or health changes, depending on appointment availability. | Rapid response to changes in patient condition, enabling prompt medical attention and adjustments in treatment. |
| Cost | Costs include travel, time off work, and potential hospital admissions for exacerbations. | Reduces overall costs by minimizing travel, preventing hospital readmissions, and facilitating efficient care. |
| Data Collection | Limited data collected during in-person visits, often relying on patient recall and periodic testing. | Comprehensive data collection from multiple sources (wearables, apps, devices) providing a more complete health picture. |
| Care Coordination | Coordination can be fragmented, with different providers handling various aspects of care. | Integrated platforms can streamline communication and coordination among healthcare providers. |
| Health Outcomes | Dependent on the frequency of visits and patient's ability to seek timely care. | Potentially improved outcomes through early detection, continuous monitoring, and personalized interventions. |
| Patient Convenience | Involves travel, waiting times, and possible disruptions to daily routines. | Offers convenience with virtual consultations and home-based monitoring, reducing the need for frequent clinic visits. |
| Technology Dependence | Minimal technology required; primary reliance on face-to-face interactions and physical examinations. | Relies heavily on technology, requiring patients to use devices, apps, and ensure internet connectivity. |

This table provides a side-by-side comparison of traditional in-person heart failure management versus remote monitoring and telemedicine, highlighting the differences in accessibility, frequency of monitoring, patient engagement, response time, cost, data collection, care coordination, health outcomes, patient convenience, and technology dependence.

Continued investment, innovation, and collaboration are essential to harnessing the full potential of remote monitoring and telemedicine in HF management. Insights from recent literature, such as machine learning-based prediction models [4] and analyses revealing distinct arterial pulse variability [5,6], highlight the importance of leveraging technological advancements to improve HF care delivery.

Efforts to promote digital literacy, address healthcare disparities, and ensure equitable access to remote monitoring and telemedicine services are critical for realizing the promise of these technologies in improving HF care delivery and outcomes for all patients. Collaborative initiatives, informed by population-based studies [19], can drive policy changes and resource allocation strategies to address these challenges.

In summary, remote monitoring and telemedicine represent transformative opportunities to advance the field of HF management and improve the lives of patients affected by this chronic condition. By embracing innovation, collaboration, and patient-centered approaches, we can push the boundaries of HF care delivery and achieve better outcomes for patients worldwide. Insights from studies on healthcare resource utilization [19] and the impact of sleep quality on quality of life in HF patients [22] underscore the multidimensional nature of HF management and the importance of holistic approaches in optimizing patient care.

Through ongoing research, interdisciplinary collaboration, and a commitment to addressing healthcare disparities, we can realize the full potential of remote monitoring and telemedicine in HF management, paving the way for more effective, accessible, and patient-centered care delivery.

**Author Contributions:** J.-C.L., C.-Y.C. and T.-H.C. wrote the initial paper. T.-H.C., C.-N.L. and J.-J.C. designed the tables. W.-R.H. revised the paper. All authors have read and agreed to the published version of the manuscript.

**Funding:** This research received no external funding.

**Conflicts of Interest:** The authors declare no conflict of interest.

## References

1. Saito, H.; Maeda, D.; Kagiyama, N.; Sunayama, T.; Dotare, T.; Fujimoto, Y.; Jujo, K.; Saito, K.; Uchida, S.; Hamazaki, N.; et al. Prognostic Value of Objective Social Isolation and Loneliness in Older Patients With Heart Failure: Subanalysis of FRAGILE-HF and Kitasato Cohort. *J. Am. Heart Assoc.* **2024**, *13*, e032716. [CrossRef]
2. Garanin, A.; Rubanenko, A.; Trusov, Y.; Rubanenko, O.; Kolsanov, A. Comparative Effectiveness of Complex Telemedicine Support in Prevention of Hospitalizations and Mortality in Patients with Heart Failure: A Systematic Review and Meta-Analysis. *Life* **2024**, *14*, 507. [CrossRef]
3. Ahmed, F.Z.; Sammut-Powell, C.; Martin, G.P.; Callan, P.; Cunnington, C.; Kahn, M.; Kale, M.; Weldon, T.; Harwood, R.; Fullwood, C.; et al. Association of a device-based remote management heart failure pathway with outcomes: TriageHF Plus real-world evaluation. *ESC Heart Fail.* **2024**. [CrossRef]
4. Kao, Y.T.; Huang, C.Y.; Fang, Y.A.; Liu, J.C.; Chang, T.H. Machine Learning-Based Prediction of Atrial Fibrillation Risk Using Electronic Medical Records in Older Aged Patients. *Am. J. Cardiol.* **2023**, *198*, 56–63. [CrossRef]
5. Hsiu, H.; Liu, J.C.; Yang, C.J.; Chen, H.S.; Wu, M.S.; Hao, W.R.; Lee, K.Y.; Hu, C.J.; Wang, Y.H.; Fang, Y.A. Discrimination of vascular aging using the arterial pulse spectrum and machine-learning analysis. *Microvasc. Res.* **2022**, *139*, 104240. [CrossRef]
6. Chen, C.C.; Chang, C.K.; Chiu, C.C.; Yang, T.Y.; Hao, W.R.; Lin, C.H.; Fang, Y.A.; Jian, W.; Hsu, M.H.; Yang, T.L.; et al. Machine Learning Analyses Revealed Distinct Arterial Pulse Variability According to Side Effects of Pfizer-BioNTech COVID-19 Vaccine (BNT162b2). *J. Clin. Med.* **2022**, *11*, 6119. [CrossRef]
7. Liu, J.C.; Hsu, Y.P.; Zhu, J.C.; Hao, W.R.; Yang, T.Y.; Sung, L.C.; Kao, P.F.; Hwang, J.; Hsiu, H. Beat-to-beat and spectral analyses of the noninvasive radial pulse and laser-Doppler signals in patients with hypertension. *Clin. Hemorheol. Microcirc.* **2021**, *79*, 365–379. [CrossRef]
8. Lee, P.; Liu, J.C.; Hsieh, M.H.; Hao, W.R.; Tseng, Y.T.; Liu, S.H.; Lin, Y.K.; Sung, L.C.; Huang, J.H.; Yang, H.Y.; et al. Cloud-based BP system integrated with CPOE improves self-management of the hypertensive patients: A randomized controlled trial. *Comput. Methods Programs Biomed.* **2016**, *132*, 105–113. [CrossRef]
9. Ploux, S.; Strik, M.; Ramirez, F.D.; Buliard, S.; Chauvel, R.; Dos Santos, P.; Haissaguerre, M.; Jobbe-Duval, A.; Picard, F.; Riocreux, C.; et al. Remote management of worsening heart failure to avoid hospitalization in a real-world setting. *ESC Heart Fail.* **2023**, *10*, 3637–3645. [CrossRef]
10. Zahradka, N.; Pugmire, J.; Lever Taylor, J.; Wolfberg, A.; Wilkes, M. Deployment of an End-to-End Remote, Digitalized Clinical Study Protocol in COVID-19: Process Evaluation. *JMIR Form. Res.* **2022**, *6*, e37832. [CrossRef]
11. Ziacchi, M.; Molon, G.; Giudici, V.; Botto, G.L.; Viscusi, M.; Brasca, F.; Santoro, A.; Curcio, A.; Manzo, M.; Mauro, E.; et al. Integration of a Smartphone HF-Dedicated App in the Remote Monitoring of Heart Failure Patients with Cardiac Implantable Electronic Devices: Patient Access, Acceptance, and Adherence to Use. *J. Clin. Med.* **2023**, *12*, 5528. [CrossRef] [PubMed]

12. Pages, N.; Picard, F.; Barritault, F.; Amara, W.; Lafitte, S.; Maribas, P.; Abassade, P.; Labarre, J.P.; Boulestreau, R.; Chaouky, H.; et al. Remote patient monitoring for chronic heart failure in France: When an innovative funding program (ETAPES) meets an innovative solution (Satelia(R) Cardio). *Digit Health* **2022**, *8*, 20552076221116774. [CrossRef] [PubMed]
13. Auener, S.L.; van Dulmen, S.A.; van Kimmenade, R.; Westert, G.P.; Jeurissen, P.P. Sustainable adoption of noninvasive telemonitoring for chronic heart failure: A qualitative study in the Netherlands. *Digit Health* **2023**, *9*, 20552076231196998. [CrossRef] [PubMed]
14. Ghilencea, L.N.; Chiru, M.R.; Stolcova, M.; Spiridon, G.; Manea, L.M.; Stanescu, A.A.; Bokhari, A.; Kilic, I.D.; Secco, G.G.; Foin, N.; et al. Telemedicine: Benefits for Cardiovascular Patients in the COVID-19 Era. *Front. Cardiovasc. Med.* **2022**, *9*, 868635. [CrossRef] [PubMed]
15. Singhal, A.; Riley, J.P.; Cowie, M.R. Benefits and challenges of telemedicine for heart failure consultations: A qualitative study. *BMC Health Serv. Res.* **2023**, *23*, 847. [CrossRef] [PubMed]
16. Kuan, P.X.; Chan, W.K.; Fern Ying, D.K.; Rahman, M.A.A.; Peariasamy, K.M.; Lai, N.M.; Mills, N.L.; Anand, A. Efficacy of telemedicine for the management of cardiovascular disease: A systematic review and meta-analysis. *Lancet Digit Health* **2022**, *4*, e676–e691. [CrossRef] [PubMed]
17. Zakiyah, N.; Marulin, D.; Alfaqeeh, M.; Puspitasari, I.M.; Lestari, K.; Lim, K.K.; Fox-Rushby, J. Economic Evaluations of Digital Health Interventions for Patients With Heart Failure: Systematic Review. *J. Med. Internet Res.* **2024**, *26*, e53500. [CrossRef] [PubMed]
18. Islam, M.M.; Poly, T.N.; Alsinglawi, B.; Lin, L.F.; Chien, S.C.; Liu, J.C.; Jian, W.S. Application of Artificial Intelligence in COVID-19 Pandemic: Bibliometric Analysis. *Healthcare* **2021**, *9*, 441. [CrossRef] [PubMed]
19. Chen, S.C.; Xirasagar, S.; Liu, J.C.; Kao, Y.W.; Shia, B.C.; Yang, T.H.; Lin, H.C. A Population-Based Study of Healthcare Resource Utilization in Patients with Mitral Valve Prolapse. *Int. J. Environ. Res. Public. Health* **2020**, *17*, 1622. [CrossRef]
20. Storm, M.; Morken, I.M.; Austin, R.C.; Nordfonn, O.; Wathne, H.B.; Urstad, K.H.; Karlsen, B.; Dalen, I.; Gjeilo, K.H.; Richardson, A.; et al. Evaluation of the nurse-assisted eHealth intervention 'eHealth@Hospital-2-Home' on self-care by patients with heart failure and colorectal cancer post-hospital discharge: Protocol for a randomised controlled trial. *BMC Health Serv. Res.* **2024**, *24*, 18. [CrossRef]
21. Zaman, S.B.; Khan, R.K.; Evans, R.G.; Thrift, A.G.; Maddison, R.; Islam, S.M.S. Exploring Barriers to and Enablers of the Adoption of Information and Communication Technology for the Care of Older Adults With Chronic Diseases: Scoping Review. *JMIR Aging* **2022**, *5*, e25251. [CrossRef]
22. Liu, J.C.; Hung, H.L.; Shyu, Y.K.; Tsai, P.S. The impact of sleep quality and daytime sleepiness on global quality of life in community-dwelling patients with heart failure. *J. Cardiovasc. Nurs.* **2011**, *26*, 99–105. [CrossRef]
23. Wang, M.Y.; Chang, N.C.; Hsieh, M.H.; Su, C.T.; Liu, J.C.; Shyu, Y.K.; Tsai, P.S. Effect of Feedback Signal on Blood Pressure Self-regulation Capability in Individuals With Prehypertension or Stage I Hypertension: A Randomized Controlled Study. *J. Cardiovasc. Nurs.* **2016**, *31*, 166–172. [CrossRef]
24. Lee, K.C.; Breznen, B.; Ukhova, A.; Martin, S.S.; Koehler, F. Virtual healthcare solutions in heart failure: A literature review. *Front. Cardiovasc. Med.* **2023**, *10*, 1231000. [CrossRef] [PubMed]
25. Shara, N.; Bjarnadottir, M.V.; Falah, N.; Chou, J.; Alqutri, H.S.; Asch, F.M.; Anderson, K.M.; Bennett, S.S.; Kuhn, A.; Montalvo, B.; et al. Voice activated remote monitoring technology for heart failure patients: Study design, feasibility and observations from a pilot randomized control trial. *PLoS ONE* **2022**, *17*, e0267794. [CrossRef] [PubMed]
26. Abraham, C.; Jensen, C.; Rossiter, L.; Dittman Hale, D. Telenursing and Remote Patient Monitoring in Cardiovascular Health. *Telemed. J. E Health* **2024**, *30*, 771–779. [CrossRef] [PubMed]
27. Ciotola, F.; Pyxaras, S.; Rittger, H.; Buia, V. MEMS Technology in Cardiology: Advancements and Applications in Heart Failure Management Focusing on the CardioMEMS Device. *Sensors* **2024**, *24*, 2922. [CrossRef] [PubMed]
28. Senarath, S.; Fernie, G.; Roshan Fekr, A. Influential Factors in Remote Monitoring of Heart Failure Patients: A Review of the Literature and Direction for Future Research. *Sensors* **2021**, *21*, 3575. [CrossRef]
29. Dickinson, M.G.; Allen, L.A.; Albert, N.A.; DiSalvo, T.; Ewald, G.A.; Vest, A.R.; Whellan, D.J.; Zile, M.R.; Givertz, M.M. Remote Monitoring of Patients With Heart Failure: A White Paper From the Heart Failure Society of America Scientific Statements Committee. *J. Card. Fail.* **2018**, *24*, 682–694. [CrossRef]
30. Di Lenarda, A.; Casolo, G.; Gulizia, M.M.; Aspromonte, N.; Scalvini, S.; Mortara, A.; Alunni, G.; Ricci, R.P.; Mantovan, R.; Russo, G.; et al. The future of telemedicine for the management of heart failure patients: A Consensus Document of the Italian Association of Hospital Cardiologists (A.N.M.C.O), the Italian Society of Cardiology (S.I.C.) and the Italian Society for Telemedicine and eHealth (Digital S.I.T.). *Eur. Heart J. Suppl.* **2017**, *19* (Suppl. D), D113–D129.
31. Clark, D.L.; Desai, N.R.; Owens, G.M.; Stemple, C.A. Rethinking heart failure: Patient classification and treatment. *Am. J. Manag. Care* **2022**, *28* (Suppl. 14), S255–S267. [PubMed]
32. Pina, I.L.; Gibson, G.T.; Zieroth, S.; Kataria, R. Reflecting on the advancements of HFrEF therapies over the last two decades and predicting what is yet to come. *Eur. Heart J. Suppl.* **2022**, *24* (Suppl. L), L2–L9. [CrossRef] [PubMed]
33. Villani, G.Q.; Villani, A.; Zanni, A.; Sticozzi, C.; Maceda, D.P.; Rossi, L.; Pisati, M.S.; Piepoli, M.F. Mobile health and implantable cardiac devices: Patients' expectations. *Eur. J. Prev. Cardiol.* **2019**, *26*, 920–927. [CrossRef] [PubMed]


**Disclaimer/Publisher's Note:** The statements, opinions and data contained in all publications are solely those of the individual author(s) and contributor(s) and not of MDPI and/or the editor(s). MDPI and/or the editor(s) disclaim responsibility for any injury to people or property resulting from any ideas, methods, instructions or products referred to in the content.

MDPI AG
Grosspeteranlage 5
4052 Basel
Switzerland
Tel.: +41 61 683 77 34

*Life* Editorial Office
E-mail: life@mdpi.com
www.mdpi.com/journal/life

Disclaimer/Publisher's Note: The title and front matter of this reprint are at the discretion of the Guest Editors. The publisher is not responsible for their content or any associated concerns. The statements, opinions and data contained in all individual articles are solely those of the individual Editors and contributors and not of MDPI. MDPI disclaims responsibility for any injury to people or property resulting from any ideas, methods, instructions or products referred to in the content.

www.ingramcontent.com/pod-product-compliance
Lightning Source LLC
Chambersburg PA
CBHW061550210926
51850CB00009B/2057
*9783725864881*